ADOLESCENT DEPRESSION

A Johns Hopkins Press Health Book

Francis Mark
MONDIMORE, MD
Patrick
KELLY, MD

ADOLESCENT DEPRESSION
2nd
Edition

A Guide for Parents

Johns Hopkins University Press
Baltimore

Note to the reader: This book is not meant to substitute for medical care of people with depression or other mental disorders, and treatment should not be based solely on its contents. Instead, treatment must be developed in a dialogue between the individual and his or her physician. Our book has been written to help with that dialogue.

Drug dosage: The author and publisher have made reasonable efforts to determine that the selection of drugs discussed in this text conform to the practices of the general medical community. The medications described do not necessarily have specific approval by the U.S. Food and Drug Administration for use in the diseases for which they are recommended. In view of ongoing research, changes in governmental regulation, and the constant flow of information relating to drug therapy and drug reactions, the reader is urged to check the package insert of each drug for any change in indications and dosage and for warnings and precautions. This is particularly important when the recommended agent is a new and/or infrequently used drug.

© 2002 Francis Mark Mondimore
© 2015 Johns Hopkins University Press
All rights reserved. Published 2015
Printed in the United States of America on acid-free paper
9 8 7 6 5 4 3 2 1

Johns Hopkins University Press
2715 North Charles Street
Baltimore, Maryland 21218-4363
www.press.jhu.edu

Library of Congress Cataloging-in-Publication Data
Mondimore, Francis Mark, 1953–
    Adolescent depression : a guide for parents / Francis Mark Mondimore, MD, and Patrick Kelly, MD. — Second edition.
        pages cm. — (A Johns Hopkins press health book)
    Includes bibliographical references and index.
    ISBN 978-1-4214-1789-9 (hardcover : alk. paper) — ISBN 978-1-4214-1790-5 (pbk. : alk. paper) — ISBN 978-1-4214-1791-2 (electronic) — ISBN 1-4214-1789-8 (hardcover : alk. paper) — ISBN 1-4214-1790-1 (pbk. : alk. paper) — ISBN 1-4214-1791-X (electronic) 1. Depression in adolescence—Popular works. I. Kelly, Patrick, 1978– II. Title.
    RJ506.D4M66 2015
    616.85′2700835—dc23   2015002501

A catalog record for this book is available from the British Library.

Figures 3-1, 3-2, 3-3, 5-1, 5-2, 5-3, 7-1, 8-1, and 15-1 by Jacqueline Schaffer.

Special discounts are available for bulk purchases of this book. For more information, please contact Special Sales at 410-516-6936 or specialsales@press.jhu.edu.

Johns Hopkins University Press uses environmentally friendly book materials, including recycled text paper that is composed of at least 30 percent post-consumer waste, whenever possible.

The authors dedicate this book to their parents,

Frank and Winifred Mondimore,

and Pat Kelly, Sr., and Vicki Kelly

CONTENTS

PREFACE

Francis Mondimore's essential publication of the first edition of *Adolescent Depression* fundamentally changed the conversation among adolescents, parents, and providers when it comes to this condition. He brought to light a different (and correct) view of depression as a biological illness that needs to be taken as seriously as diabetes or any other medical condition, altering forever the way in which parents see their children.

But, as with all things, work in the study and treatment of adolescent depression has progressed, and we thought that you, the reader, could benefit from being brought up to date on the latest information. In the thirteen years that have elapsed since the book's initial publication, many changes, large and small, have affected the field of psychiatry. Every chapter in this new edition has been updated to reflect the most current evidence base in terms of diagnosis, treatment, and advice for both parents and children. We cover and explain new treatments, both medication and psychotherapy. In an extensive discussion of bipolar affective disorder in young persons, we attempt to examine rationally how and why this diagnosis, once perceived as extremely rare, has suddenly become so common. We also introduce discussions of new topics, such as the interface between autism and depression. One of the biggest changes in the field of psychiatry, a new version of our basic system of diagnosing patients, has recently rocked the psychiatric field and is an essential change for parents and adolescents to understand so they can have an educated discussion with their physician.

We go through the changes relative to young persons and how this new way of looking at psychiatric conditions may change your child's treatment, diagnosis—or both.

Nonetheless, the central message of this text remains the same. For a long time, mental health professionals thought that serious depression was an illness only adults were likely to develop. The general belief among psychologists and psychiatrists was that children might get a little sad or upset about some disappointment or frustration, but that they weren't emotionally mature enough to experience true depression. Gloominess and "angst" were thought to be almost universal among adolescents, but only temporary —just a developmental stage that they would emerge from unscathed.

Research done in the 1990s demolished these myths. We now realize that young people do indeed get seriously depressed. In fact, as is becoming clear, depressive illnesses and bipolar disorders that start in adolescence may be more serious and more difficult to treat than adult-onset mood disorders. A 2013 study sponsored by the Centers for Disease Control and Prevention estimated that 4 percent of young people between the ages of 3 and 17 years had been diagnosed with a depressive illness, with adolescents more likely than their younger counterparts to be diagnosed (up to 13 percent).[1] It's been estimated that nearly one in five persons will go through a period of serious depression during their lifetime, and research increasingly indicates that many of these people will have had their first encounter with depression as teenagers.

Some parents still struggle with the idea of their child being treated for a psychiatric illness, seeing a therapist, or taking medication for a problem that they may think—and hope—might be "just a phase." We hope to persuade you in this book that serious depression in adolescents is an illness— an illness that can be effectively treated.

Clinical studies have shown that depression is underdiagnosed in young people and undertreated as well. A study in 2000 found that only 20 percent of seriously depressed adolescents in a community sample received any treatment for their problem. The same study found high rates of relapse in these young people, and even more disturbing was the finding that, by their twenty-fourth birthday, many of them had developed other psychiatric problems in addition to depression, most commonly alcoholism and drug abuse.[2]

We now know that depression comes in many forms and is often the symptom of a collection of emotional illnesses that psychiatrists call mood disorders. Some adolescents with a mood disorder are troubled by "down" and sad feelings—the feelings people usually think of when they hear the word *depression*. But other adolescents with a mood disorder have predominantly irritable moods with angry outbursts, temper tantrums, and destructive rages, problems that seem to bear little relationship to what most people think of as depression. Can the same illness really look so different from one young person to the next? Why? These are some of the questions we hope to answer in this book.

This is not a "how to talk to your teenager" book. Adolescent mood disorders are complex, poorly understood, and potentially dangerous illnesses, and parents want the facts about these illnesses. What are the danger signals of serious depression in teenagers? How are mood disorders diagnosed? What are the implications of the different diagnoses? How does depression relate to other problems, like drug abuse, attention-deficit/hyperactivity disorder (ADHD), and eating disorders? What are the available treatments? How can parents of an adolescent with a mood disorder help their child get the best treatment possible? What else can parents do? You'll find answers to all these questions in this book.

We have organized the book by dividing it into four parts. Part I, Symptoms, Syndromes, and Diagnosis, focuses on recognizing serious depression in adolescents and on understanding why mood disorders are real illnesses. It reviews some of the unique issues of emotional development during adolescence that may explain why mood disorders express themselves differently in young people than in adults. We also try to explain something about the diagnostic process in psychiatry and the classification of mood disorders.

Part II, Treatment, reviews the different medications and other medical treatments used to treat depression, as well as the types of psychotherapy and counseling that have been shown to be useful, how these very different treatments relate to each other, and why a combination of both medication and therapy is the most useful approach to treating depression.

Part III, Variations, Causes, and Connections, discusses other problems that often complicate the picture in depressed adolescents, such as ADHD and eating disorders and the dangerous and frightening issues of suicidal behavior and "cutting." A chapter on the inheritance of mood disorders and evidence for the genetic basis of these illnesses rounds out this part of the book.

Part IV, Getting Better and Staying Well, contains the real-world, practical information you need to maximize the effectiveness of treatment and minimize the chances of relapse and complications. Finding a good treatment team, dealing with insurance issues, and handling such emergencies as dangerous behaviors and hospitalization are some of the issues covered here. We specifically seek to open the "black box" of mental health treatment and diagnosis in chapter 16, wherein we describe the various, seemingly innumerable types of mental health professionals and what their particular roles in your child's treatment should be. We also expose our own means of reaching a diagnosis, and give general guidelines (and warnings) to parents about what to look for when seeing a psychiatrist.

WE HOPE THAT AFTER READING THIS BOOK YOU WILL better understand the symptoms, the treatments, the complications, and what we know about the causes of mood disorders in adolescents. More important, we hope you will feel better equipped and more confident about helping your depressed adolescent get the most out of treatment, on the road to recovery, and on the path to becoming a happy and healthy adult.

ACKNOWLEDGMENTS

Patrick Kelly

My first and most gracious acknowledgment goes to Francis Mondimore, without whom this book would not have been possible. This is both for the obvious reason, but also, and more important, for his mentorship. He taught me how to write, how to think, and how to be a good psychiatrist (or at least try, by modeling myself after such a great one).

I'd also like to thank our editor, Jacqueline Wehmueller, whose encouragement and advocacy are critical to any success that this book might have.

And thanks to Michael Lindsay, without whose unwavering support this book would be an unrealized dream.

Above all, I'd like to thank you, the readers of this book. Psychiatrists get to close up their office and go home at night. Any person or family member who has struggled with depression knows that it is a twenty-four-hour-a-day, seven-day-a-week struggle against the darkness, and that continued striving toward success, such as by educating yourself through this work, is sometimes the bravest and most difficult thing you can do. Thank you.

Francis Mark Mondimore

I'd like to thank those who have helped me in the writing of this book. First, many, many thanks to Sallie Mink, RN, of DRADA (Depression and Related Affective Disorders Association) at Johns Hopkins, who suggested the project to me in the first place and who was a constant source of support and encouragement.

Thanks to all my colleagues in the Affective Disorders Section of the Department of Psychiatry and Behavioral Sciences at Johns Hopkins, especially Anthony Drobnick, MD, for feedback, encouragement, and support.

Thanks to Jacqueline Schaffer for her handsome illustrations, and special thanks to all the wonderful staff of Johns Hopkins University Press, most especially my editor, Jacqueline Wehmueller. I have been fortunate indeed to work with such a dedicated and talented group of people.

And thanks, once again, to Jay Allen Rubin, my biggest fan and frankest critic, for always being there.

ADOLESCENT DEPRESSION

Introduction

For many years, psychiatrists and psychologists proposed that serious depression was rare, even impossible, in children and adolescents. We now know this is not true. In fact, you'll see the words *adolescent depression* in magazine articles and newspaper stories practically every day.

Often the term appears in a context that is frightening for parents worried that their child may be depressed: a story about adolescent drug abuse or suicide. Parents can become so frightened at the thought of these destructive and violent problems affecting their family that they can't decide what to do next. Sometimes the thought "my child would *never* do something like *that*" tempts parents to minimize the severity of the symptoms of this treatable illness, perhaps allowing them to talk themselves out of seeking psychiatric evaluation for their teenager. On the other hand, it's possible to panic, perhaps rushing off to an emergency room in the middle of the night after finding some gloomy poetry that a teenager has left lying around. What should parents do if they think their adolescent might have a problem with serious depression? If an adolescent has been diagnosed with serious depression, what are the implications? How best to help?

We would be lying to you if we said that adolescent depression was something psychiatrists understand completely. But there is a lot we *do* know about depression in young people. Admittedly, quite a lot was initially based on what we knew about adults. Using this knowledge as a springboard, psychiatry found some significant differences in the form the depressive illness can take in younger persons who are still undergoing phenomenal amounts of biological growth and development, not to mention the psychological tasks of defining themselves.

That word *illness* is key. What is unequivocally clear is that serious depression is the symptom of an illness—actually a group of illnesses, called *mood disorders*. The symptoms of depression should be approached in the same way we would approach *any* symptoms that might indicate a serious illness: taking the potential problem seriously, getting the adolescent to an evaluation by the proper professional expert as soon as possible, and participating in treatment by monitoring symptoms and treatment response, being supportive and encouraging, and following through on any other recommendations from the treatment team.

The horror stories you read in newspapers are often the result of *not* following this approach—a serious depression that has gone unrecognized or, worse, that was suspected but not treated, for a variety of reasons: fear of a "mental illness" diagnosis, misinformation about psychiatric medications based on rumors and inaccuracies, or the erroneous idea that mood disorders are not "real" diseases. Parents of a child with diabetes don't generally worry over "what the neighbors will think" about their child's diagnosis and treatment. Parents of a child with leukemia don't usually blame themselves for their child's illness or wonder "what did we do wrong?" Serious depression *is* a serious medical illness and should be approached no differently from any other illness.

When physicians see an adolescent who may be suffering from depression (we'll discuss later why a physician, preferably a psychiatrist trained in the treatment of children and adolescents, needs to be one of the first professionals involved), their approach will be the usual medical approach to symptoms and illnesses: getting all the facts about the symptoms, performing an examination of the patient, perhaps doing some lab tests, and making a diagnosis. That symptoms are mostly emotional rather than physical—sadness, loss of interest in things, rather than abdominal pains or fever—doesn't change anything about needing a medical approach to what may turn out to be a medical problem. The examination involves talking and listening to the patient rather than using a stethoscope or blood pressure cuff, but psychiatrists have years of training that enable them, by just this method, to draw out mental experiences from patients and pick up subtle changes in psychological functioning that are the signs of illness.

Like physical illnesses, mood disorders have characteristic patterns of symptoms and a characteristic "natural history," that is, a predictable way in which the illness usually runs its course. To make predictions about a medical problem, a diagnosis must first be made. The most important prediction a diagnosis allows is a prediction of what treatment will be effective at restoring the patient to health.

In psychiatric illnesses, as in no other group of medical problems, people get distracted by "why" questions and forget to focus on "what" questions. For the surgeon treating a person with a broken leg, *why* the patient's leg is broken (a car accident? skiing mishap?) is of relatively little interest. The *what* question (What's wrong with this patient? His leg is broken *here* and *here*) is the focus of attention. The answers to these kinds of questions determine the treatment plan. Psychiatry is not that much different: treatment is determined by answering the question "What kind of depression does this person suffer from?" Major depressive disorder? The depression of bipolar disorder? The minor, temporary depression we call an adjustment disorder? The answer must be determined before other questions become relevant: Is he depressed because he broke up with his girlfriend? Because he didn't get into the college that was his first choice? These kinds of questions are related to the search for diagnosis, but they usually become really relevant only *after* a diagnosis has been made.

This way of thinking about people and their emotions doesn't come naturally to us. We have all experienced being sad after a loss or apprehensive in the face of uncertainty, so we expect that all bad emotional feelings come about in this way. We have become accustomed to expecting to find reasons for unpleasant emotions in a person's life and experience. But this kind of analysis can lead us dangerously astray in the case of serious depression: looking for "reasons" can distract from the diagnosis, and thus delay the treatment, of a serious illness.

A more familiar example will illustrate. Perhaps your child, like many children, went through a period of having "tummy aches" on school mornings if she was nervous about school or simply didn't want to go. But the question that popped into your mind that first morning was probably not

"Why doesn't my child want to go to school?" but rather "What's wrong with my child? What illness might explain these pains?" It's probably a safe bet that you took your child's temperature, put her to bed and watched her closely, and perhaps called or even took her to the pediatrician to make sure it wasn't an illness, such as food poisoning or appendicitis, that needed medical attention. You would wonder about the judgment of any parent who didn't take these steps, wouldn't you? Even a visit to the emergency room wouldn't be an overreaction if the child seemed to be in extreme distress. Only after medical problems had been ruled out, when it was clear that the child wasn't ill, would it have been appropriate to start looking for psychological explanations: reasons that the child might not want to go to school.

The book begins, then, by describing the symptoms of these illnesses: mood disorders. Understanding how psychiatrists approach a problem with adolescent depression, make a diagnosis, and decide on a treatment plan is an important first step for the parent who wants to know how to help.

Since the first version of this work was published in 2002, the field of psychiatry, particularly that branch focusing on younger patients, has experienced many changes. These changes have affected every aspect of this book—including even the meaning of the title. "Adolescent" is now a more ambiguous term and encompasses a larger group. The new generation of millennials, as opposed to Generation X-ers, are experiencing something of a prolonged adolescence. Traditionally, the field of "child" psychiatry focused on patients until they turned 18, at which point they were considered adults. Although this is still true in many legal situations (including some relating to their care, which we deal with later in the book), an entirely new focus on "transitional aged youth," those between approximately 16 and 24, has emerged. These young persons are in many ways more similar to their younger neighbors in age than to their older ones—many are still in school, still struggling to define their individual identity, unmarried and without children, sometimes still depending on (or even living with) their parents. They differ from the prior generation in other ways as well, including an increased suspiciousness of psychiatry and psychiatric treatment, yet an increased willingness to share all aspects of their lives (including psychiatric diagnoses), sometimes with negative social ramifications. Later on in the book, we discuss how adolescents can sometimes misuse social media to spread messages that inadvertently harm themselves or others, including bullying and sharing dark, sometimes graphic, stories of their own struggles. The face of adolescence has shifted, providing an increased challenge to these young persons and to their parents.

The term in the other half of the title, "Depression," has also experienced some changes in what it encompasses and signifies. Since 2002, depression has been increasingly recognized (in many cases, thanks to this book) in younger and younger children. This has been a boon to patients because their symptoms are getting treated, and the stigma surrounding the condition is lessening. Other trends have cropped up, however, that may have been less helpful. Primary pediatricians began to get increasingly involved in psychiatric treatment, and up to around 2005, there was a large increase in antidepressant prescriptions. There seemed to be such a swing of the pendulum that providers saw a particular type of these medications—SSRIs, or selective serotonin reuptake inhibitors—as a sort of cure-all for any low mood, with little to no attention paid to the psychological overlays of real-world problems that were either the causes of or the result of the depression.

In 2005, the situation changed, when the FDA put a black box warning (the most severe warning possible) on these medications based on the results of a study (later debunked) that seemed to indicate that these medications may double the rates of suicide in adolescents. As we now know, the factor most likely to predispose an adolescent to suicide is untreated depression, but the pendulum had swung again. Now no pediatricians would prescribe these critical medications; even general psychiatrists were fearful. Even today, many providers feel uncomfortable prescribing medications to address depression, leaving many people untreated. This is why it is crucial for patients and parents to acquire an in-depth understanding of these medications—including when the medications should and, sometimes more important, should not be used—and to have an educated and enlightened discussion with their psychiatrist before beginning on any path of treatment.

Although we focus in this book on the changes in the psychiatric field, the foundations of our science are still rooted in the same guiding principles. We urge readers not to do that which is most tempting—to skip ahead to the "treatment" section of this text. Treatment must be guided by diagnosis. Medicating a low mood that is not the result of the illness of depression is like trying to treat seasonal allergies with an antibiotic (a drug useful only for addressing bacterial infections)—no effect at all. Similarly, ignoring a serious depression through the misunderstanding that the "blues" will go away on their own can have the same result as withholding antibiotics from a serious bacterial infection—dire consequences indeed. Before jumping ahead to pick your child's medication, first spend some time learning what exactly may be behind her symptoms and which symptoms are important to pay attention to. We want to take you down the same path we as psychiatrists would take in diagnosing a patient and developing a treatment plan. This book is organized to do exactly that. Many complain that psychiatry and psychiatric treatment is at best a mystery, at worst a guessing game. We hope to open this subject up and show you precisely how a good psychiatrist will come to a conclusion about what has been afflicting you or your child and how to best help in recovery.

Part I

SYMPTOMS, SYNDROMES & DIAGNOSIS

WHAT IS DEPRESSION? Doesn't everybody feel down now and then, especially teenagers? How can we tell when depression is serious? These are some of the questions we answer in this first part of the book.

We begin with a chapter on what depression is, how to recognize it, and more important, how it differs from the normal "downs" everyone experiences. This chapter also has an introduction to some of the theories of what causes depression, including a discussion of how we have learned that biological changes in the brain are at the root of serious depressive illness.

In chapter 2, we take a closer look at the psychology of adolescence and explain why depression often takes different forms in adolescents than in adults—so different that it may be hard to recognize.

Chapter 3 gets into the nitty-gritty of the diagnostic process in psychiatry, with an introduction to how psychiatrists think about depression and mood disorders, then an outline and description of the different types of depression that are seen in adolescents.

The part ends with a more detailed look at the diagnostic scheme for mood disorders that is currently used by the American Psychiatric Association: the *Diagnostic and Statistical Manual of Mental Disorders* (the *DSM*). As of this writing, the *DSM* has recently undergone its first revision in over a decade, one that changes the fundamental way it views patients. We discuss how adolescents are seen in both versions. Most important, we explain why it's critical not to view the *DSM* as the "bible of psychiatry," as it has often been called, but rather to see it as an imperfect work in progress that is a helpful guide to, but not the ultimate authority on, understanding treating actual patients in the real world.

Depression

Some Definitions

The word *depression* comes from Latin roots that mean "pressed down." Many of the common words we use to describe the feelings of depression describe, in one way or another, a downward direction or position. People talk about feeling "down in the dumps" or "low" or simply "down." The many synonyms for depression that begin with the same two letters, like "*de*spondent" and "*de*jected," share the Latin-derived prefix *de-*, which signifies a downward direction (as in "*de*scend").

Other words for depression cast it as the *opposite* of something: we say we are "unhappy" or "discontented," emphasizing the opposite of the good feelings of happiness or contentment. Still other words for depression conjure up the *absence* of something: the depressed are said to be "gloomy," a word that denotes an absence of light; or "dispirited," an absence of that vital spark of life we call spirit; or "desolate," the absence of just about everything. All these words capture something of the feeling of depression.

But if you listen to people who have suffered from serious depressive illnesses talk about their experiences (more on why we psychiatrists see this as an illness in a bit), you soon learn that depression is not a moving down or away from something and not really a lack of something; rather, it is a something that comes over its sufferers and imposes itself on them. William James, the great nineteenth-century American psychologist-turned-philosopher, who suffered from depression, said that, far from an absence of something, depression is "positive and active anguish...wholly unknown to healthy life."[1] William Styron, the Pulitzer Prize–winning author of the novel *Sophie's Choice*, wrote in his memoir of severe depressive illness, *Darkness Visible*, of feeling "a poisonous fogbank roll in upon my mind."[2] The prolific author J. K. Rowling introduced us to the Dementors in her Harry Potter novel series. "Dementors are among the foulest creatures that walk this earth...they drain peace, hope, and happiness out of the air around them. Get too near a Dementor and every good feeling, every happy memory will be sucked out of you...You'll be left with nothing but the worst experiences of your life."[3] They were one of the most feared specters in Harry's world and perfectly personified the effects of a depressive episode—which the author is public about having experienced in her life. In a separate interview, she described her bout with depression as the "absence of being able to envisage that you will ever be cheerful again. The absence of hope. That very deadened feeling, which is so very different from feeling sad."[4]

From the ancient Greeks comes the word *melancholy*, derived from their words for "black bile," the bodily fluid whose excess they believed caused the state of misery we now call depression. They conceptualized depression as caused by a disturbance of bodily functioning, an out-of-balance state of the four vital bodily fluids called "humors" (the other three were water, blood, and yellow bile). After several thousand years of attempts at other explanations, this idea should strike us today as an astonishingly modern one, an idea that some have now returned to with such phrases as "chemical imbalance" to describe where depression comes from.

But to define depression accurately, we need to define another word, *mood*, because any definition of depression must include the idea of *low mood*. Our mood includes our happiness or sadness, our state of optimism or pessimism, our feelings of contentedness or dissatisfaction with our situation, even physical feelings such as how fatigued or robust we feel. Mood is like our emotional temperature, a set of feelings that expresses our sense of emotional comfort or discomfort.

When people are in a good mood, they are confident and optimistic, relaxed and friendly, patient, interested, content. The word *happy* captures part of it, but good mood includes a lot more. The mental picture most people have of the boisterous adolescent is a good illustration of what *good mood* means. Many teenagers feel confident and energetic and have a sense of physical well-being; they sleep soundly and eat heartily. It's easy for them to be sociable and affectionate; the future looks bright, and the moment is ripe for starting new projects.

In a low mood, an opposite set of feelings takes over. People tend to turn inward and may seem preoccupied or distracted by their thoughts. The word *sad* captures some of the experience, but low mood is a bit more complicated. There may be a sense of emptiness and loss. People with low mood find it difficult to think about the future and, when they do, find it hard not to be pessimistic or even intimidated by it. Teenagers may be impatient and irritable, losing their temper more easily and then feeling guilty about having done so. They have difficulty being affectionate or sociable, so they avoid others and prefer to be alone. Energy is low, motivation ebbs away, and interest is dulled. Self-doubt takes over; they become preoccupied, worrying even more than usual about how other people see them. As you will see later in this part of the book, depression is sometimes complicated and difficult to spot, especially in adolescents. But the core feature of depression, its defining characteristic, is the cluster of symptoms we call *low mood*.

NORMAL AND ABNORMAL MOODS

Some of life's stresses and the normal human reactions to them are such everyday experiences that common terms have been coined for the associated mood changes—and most people recognize these mood changes as quite normal. Moving to a new community where we don't know anyone often leads to a sense of dislocation and loneliness that we know as *homesickness*, an unpleasant experience that may last for days or even weeks, a mood that everyone has probably experienced at one time or another. When someone close to us dies, we experience a profound sense of sadness and loss that can become temporarily incapacitating—the deep sorrow that we call *bereavement* or mourning.

At the time of various milestones of personal achievement, we experience changes of mood in the other direction. On the occasion of a graduation or winning a championship game or a coveted scholarship, a teenager can be filled with joy and pride and a sense of limitless optimism, feelings that can be nearly overwhelming. We wouldn't call any of these moods "abnormal," even though they can be extreme.

Like many other things we can measure in human beings—body temperature, blood pressure, hormone levels, for example—a person's mood state normally varies within a certain range. People, especially adolescents, are not in the same mood state for long; it is quite normal for everyone to have ups and downs of mood. So, low mood is sometimes *normal*. But there are other times when it is not, when it is the symptom of a *mood disorder*.

THE *SYMPTOM* OF DEPRESSION

Just like physical pain, then, periods of low mood are universal human experiences. People grieve when a loved one dies, are disappointed when an eagerly anticipated trip must be canceled, are heartbroken when a romance ends unexpectedly. In these cases, feelings of depression seem normal. No one would think of low mood in such circumstances as a symptom of anything pathological.

It's not difficult to think of situations when even physical pain can be regarded as almost normal. If the initial lawn mowing in the spring is the first bout of vigorous physical exercise after months of wintry inactivity, waking up the next morning with stiff and sore muscles is no surprise. Spend too much time out in the sun without proper protection, and a painful sunburn results. But no one thinks of after-exercise soreness as a muscle disease or would call the pain from a sunburn an abnormal reaction. Some healing needs to take place in both cases, but neither makes one worry that something in the body isn't working as it should.

But if you woke up one morning after mowing the lawn with achy muscles and joints *as well as* a fever, headache, and scratchy throat and cough, you wouldn't blame these symptoms on unaccustomed exercise. The other symptoms that accompany the sore muscles, especially the fever, indicate that something else is going on—in this case, probably a nasty virus. The *collection* of symptoms points toward a viral infection, even though one of the symptoms—the muscle aches—might be expected after too much physical exertion. A *clinical syndrome* includes a collection of symptoms and clinical findings that point toward a particular illness or group of illnesses.

When depressed mood is accompanied by certain other symptoms (table 1-1), such as disordered sleep and appetite, and includes severe irritability or a severe loss of energy and interest in usual activities, one should suspect that the individual might be suffering from a depressive *illness*—even if there are reasons that would explain one of the symptoms: low mood. Psychiatrists begin to consider the diagnosis of a mood disorder when they find that the patient has the *syndrome* of depression.

THE *SYNDROME* OF DEPRESSION

The core *symptom* of depression, low mood, can show up in many different situations, some of which can be called normal, such as feelings of bereavement during a period of mourning. The *syndrome* of depression indicates the presence of a serious medical problem that requires treatment. A case history will illustrate.

Table 1-1   Symptoms of Depression

Mood Symptoms
    Depressed mood
    Pervasive, constricted quality of mood
    Irritability
    Loss of ability to experience pleasure (anhedonia)
    Guilty feelings
    Loss of interest in usual activities
    Social withdrawal
    Suicidal thoughts
Cognitive (Thinking) Symptoms
    Poor concentration
    Poor memory
    Indecision
    Slowed thinking
    Loss of motivation
Bodily Symptoms
    Sleep disturbance
        Insomnia
        Hypersomnia
    Appetite disturbance
        Weight loss
        Weight gain
    Fatigue
    Headaches
    Constipation
    Worsening of painful conditions

▼ Susan had been thinking for weeks about how to bring it up to her husband. "Tom, I think we made a mistake taking Charlie out of Springfield."

"What do you mean?" said her husband, putting down the newspaper he'd been reading. "Edgemont is the best prep school in Columbia; how could it be a mistake? What makes you think that?"

Susan had closed her book and laid it on her lap. She looked down at its cover, then up at her husband sitting across the den, and said, "I think Charlie's unhappy at Edgemont. He misses his friends at Springfield."

Tom's face, which had frowned with concern briefly, relaxed at this. He picked up the newspaper from his lap and started to scan the columns again. "Is that all you're worried about? He'll get over it, Sue. He had to change schools twice during junior high because of our transfers, and he handled it without any problems." Then Tom lowered the paper again. "Does he talk about missing his friends?"

"Well, I asked him how school was going the other day, and he told me he wasn't sure. He said he felt like he wasn't fitting in, that he's felt disconnected since school started."

"That's not so unusual for a kid starting at a new school at this age. Teenagers are so sensitive about that kind of thing."

"Charlie also said he's worried he might not be as smart as the kids at Edgemont. Tom, that's not like Charlie at all. He's a smart boy, and he's always known it. He's always been so confident about himself."

"Well, I still think it's some kind of adolescent phase. This is only November; give the kid a chance to settle in. Besides, it's not like he was against transferring into Edgemont."

Tom had gotten an important promotion within his company the previous spring—with a hefty salary increase. Tom and Susan could now afford to send their son to a prestigious private school and had asked Charlie what he thought about transferring. "Wow, that would be super!" Charlie had said enthusiastically. "Springfield is a good school and all, but Edgemont Prep! Have you seen their computer labs?"

Tom continued, "Charlie talked all summer about how much he wanted to join some of the computer clubs at Edgemont."

"Well, that's just it. He hasn't."

Tom's face became more serious. "He hasn't?"

"No. He seems to have lost interest in computers altogether."

"Are you sure?"

"Do you remember that computer graphics thing he ordered last month for his PC? So his computer games would work better? It finally came last week, and I put it on his desk in his room." Susan looked down at her closed book again. "I was putting clean clothes in his bureau this morning, and I found it in the bottom drawer."

"Well, maybe it was the wrong piece; maybe it was incompatible or something."

"He hadn't even opened the package. He'd just stuffed it in a drawer."

"Wow, that's not like Charlie at all."

"Another thing," Susan continued. "He goes right to his room when he comes home from school and sleeps. I can't get him to come to dinner at all. I'm sure he's lost weight."

"Well, that's not so unusual, is it? Kids sleep more at this age, don't they?" Tom asked.

"I don't know—not this much, I don't think," said Susan. "Last Sunday, he was in bed most of the day and all night. That can't be normal."

"He has been extra quiet the past few weeks. Let me talk to him and see what I can find out."

"Please do, Tom. I'm worried."   ▲

Let's review the facts of this "case" for a moment. The most significant fact is that Charlie's mother has noticed that Charlie is just not himself. Though you won't find this listed in diagnostic manuals, it's significant and typical of mood disorders. The individual seems to undergo a change in so many aspects of emotional life that those around him, even if they can't quite list details, notice that he is simply different. Sometimes parents have trouble pinning it down, but often, if they think about it, they realize that the activities, enthusiasms, and energy they've come to take for granted in their teenager seem to have drained out of him. Sometimes parents will be tempted to doubt these subtle intuitions that something is wrong and, like Tom in this vignette, ascribe what they notice to "a phase" their teenager is going through. This is usually a mistake. Susan has noticed that her son's energy level, motivation, and interest level have changed. Her intuition that this isn't normal is quite correct and must not be simply dismissed in the face of a contrary opinion, even if that opinion comes from the son himself.

This is a critical point, particularly when it comes to young people. Adolescents are still discovering who they are and how they feel. They may not have the language to describe their feelings, or even be in touch enough with their emotional state to detect such a variation. The official term for this state is *alexithymia*, meaning a lack of awareness regarding one's internal emotional thermometer. Even the *Diagnostic and Statistical Manual of Mental Disorders* (DSM) recognizes this problem, particularly in this age group. Although we don't typically stick to the letter of the DSM criteria unless we are embarking on a scientific study, for the reasons we give throughout this book, these criteria do allow the official, full-fledged diagnosis of depression in children and adolescents even if they deny having a low mood, as long as those around them take notice of the low mood. In fact, this conflict between how adolescents identify feeling and how others perceive them can lead to struggles. When adolescents feel down or low, they can perceive others pointing this out as criticism rather than an observation. They can become defensive, even angry—emotions that, of course, could be amplified if they are in fact depressed. In most cases, attempting to "prove" to them that they are depressed devolves quickly into a power struggle and an argument, so this approach usually isn't that helpful. Agreeing to disagree, and keeping one's eye on the adolescent—prepared to respond should the situation not improve—is usually a better course of action.

But what specifically can point to a low mood, even if those experiencing it don't recognize it themselves? Let's again look at the facts of the case above. Psychiatrists use the word *anhedonia* to designate a loss in one's ability to enjoy things. It is one of the defining features of the depressive syndrome and worth discussing in more detail. Derived from the Greek word for "pleasure," *anhedonia* can be defined as loss of the ability to experience pleasure. One of Charlie's favorite things seems to be his computer—which makes his stuffing a new, unopened piece of hardware into a drawer an indicator of something very wrong. When depressed, adolescents will lose interest in sports, friends and socializing, extracurricular activities, or favorite classes or subjects. They have much more difficulty deriving any pleasure from listening to music, going to a movie, or engaging in the sports or hobbies they usually enjoy. This is an important feature and, at times, can be somewhat deceiving. A depressed adolescent may be able to have something of a mildly pleasurable experience, but the stimulus required to get her that brief moment of sunshine is far higher than what would usually make her happy.

For example, one of us has treated a patient whose parents thought she was not depressed. "She had fun on her birthday. We took her to her favorite place, Disneyland, with all her friends, and she seemed to enjoy herself; she was just a little shyer than usual." This girl was eventually diagnosed with depression. Her old self, her well self, would have been delighted to go to Disneyland. She would have had trouble sleeping due to her excitement, talked constantly in the car on the way there, and run from her parents toward the characters to embrace them. Her last trip, while she was depressed, did bring on a few smiles, and she did seem to enjoy the new ride, but she was far more subdued than would be expected. And this is the difference: depression causes a change in our behavior, in who we are and what we like to do. It is not so black and white as to mean that a depressed person can never, under any circumstances, derive any pleasure from anything. Rather, it means that the amount of pleasure derived from a given task is much lower than usual. Another patient of ours was so depressed that the only thing she found pleasurable was eating doughnuts, though she was simultaneously afraid to gain weight. So she would take an entire box of doughnuts and lick the frosting off them—her only pleasurable experience in an otherwise miserable existence.

Great writers, artists, and musicians who suffered from depression have left us poignant and vivid descriptions of this unresponsiveness to pleasure. In his novel *The Sorrows of Young Werther*, Johann Wolfgang von Goethe has his main character express a loss of responsiveness to the joys and beauty of nature: "Nature lies before me as immobile as on a little lacquered painting, and all this beauty cannot pump one drop of happiness from my heart to my brain."[5] People with depression describe food losing its taste, colors draining away from sunrises and landscapes, flowers losing their textures and perfumes—everything becoming bland, dull, and lifeless. For some, the bright and beautiful things in the world become a source of anguish rather than pleasure. The nineteenth-century Austrian composer Hugo Wolf described a terrible sense of sorrowful isolation during his depressions, a feeling of separation from the world of ordinary pleasures—all the more painful when it occurred in springtime: "What I suffer from . . . I am quite unable to describe. This wonderful spring with its secret life and movement troubles me unspeakably. These eternal blue skies, lasting for weeks, this continuous sprouting and budding in nature, these coaxing breezes impregnated with spring sunlight and fragrance of flowers . . . make me frantic. Everywhere this bewildering urge for life, fruitfulness, creation—and only I . . . may not take part in this festival of resurrection, at any rate not except as a spectator with grief and envy."[6]

Now imagine what it is like when these terrible feelings come over young persons who are just learning to make sense of their feelings, adolescents who are still trying to understand their emotional reactions to the world. Young adolescents, especially, will have difficulty identifying and describing their internal emotional states, and the word *depression* often doesn't mean much to them. This may be one of the reasons that low mood in adolescents sometimes is associated with prominent irritability. Frightened and frustrated by their depressive feelings, young people sometimes lash out at anyone and anything around them. In some adolescents, the irritability can even be the most prominent aspect of their change of mood. This is such a common phenomenon that it is even recognized in the *DSM*. To qualify to enter even the most strict research study, an adolescent can have a purely irritable mood instead of a self-expressed "depressed" mood and still meet full criteria.

Another differentiating factor between a "normal" low mood and the depressive syndrome is that individuals with a mood disorder lose the normal *reactivity* of their mood states. When persons who do not suffer from a mood disorder go through a period of low mood, such as after a romantic disappointment, the loss of a job, or a period of homesickness, they retain the normal *reactivity* of mood, that is, the normal changeability of mood in relation to what is going on around them.

Anyone who has attended a funeral and then returned to the home of the bereaved afterward has probably observed—and perhaps experienced— this normal reactivity of mood. Mourners who might be grief stricken during the funeral service or at the graveside can often relax, reminisce about good times they had with the person who has died, and enjoy catching up with friends and relatives perhaps not seen for a long time. The reactivity of mood is also retained in the lonely or homesick person who goes to the movies, can lose himself in a good film, and forget about his longing for more familiar surroundings. If the depressed mood is a "normal" one, we are able to dispel the feelings of bereavement, isolation, or disappointment—even if it's only for a few hours.

The depressed mood of the syndrome of depression, on the other hand, is frequently *constricted*. Years ago, AM radio stations used to give away free radios, gifts that came with only one catch: they couldn't be tuned to any of the sponsoring station's competitors. These radios were built to receive only the signal of the station that gave them away. The mood state of the person suffering from a depressive disorder is like one of those radios, "set" to receive only one mood signal: depression. The mood of the syndrome of depression is a relentless, pervasive gloom that continues from one day to the next, week after week. As William Styron said of his own depression, "The weather of depression is unmodulated, its light a brownout."[7]

We've just discussed the under-reactive, constricted mood of a true depressive syndrome. It is worth pointing out that, in some cases, the mood state actually appears to be hyper-reactive. An adolescent will suddenly seem touchy and irritable, will explode at the slightest provocation, and will continue a fight against all attempts at amelioration. Though not the most common pattern, we must emphasize that what is lost in a depressive syndrome is the "normalness" of mood reactivity—for most people it diminishes, though for some it seems to be on a hair trigger. However, it is always focused on the negative, sad, or angry aspects of a person's life.

Perhaps the most continuous characteristic of the depressive syndrome is a preoccupation with negative thoughts: depressed individuals often find their thinking dominated by thoughts of inadequacy or loss, regret, and even hopelessness. In depressed adolescents, worries about not "measuring up" in some way that seems out of character for them are not uncommon. Charlie's worry that he's not smart enough to compete in his new school would be a typical kind of negative thought, especially indicative of depression since, as his mother says, he's never been troubled by such a worry. Guilty ruminations are especially characteristic of the syndrome of depression, and psychiatrists often make a special point to ask about guilty feelings when evaluating a person for depression. Unrelenting ruminations on themes of guilt, shame, and regret are common in the depressed states of mood disorders, and they are uncommon in "normal" low mood states. An adolescent who talks about being responsible for his difficulties in some way, who describes himself as "lazy" or "worthless," may be seriously depressed. Individuals experiencing the normal depressed mood that comes after a personal loss usually attribute their bad feelings to the fact that a loss has occurred—only in unusual circumstances will they think they are to blame for the problem and be preoccupied by guilty feelings or feelings of shame. The individual with a depressive syndrome, on the other hand, frequently feels to blame for his troubles, and sometimes for other people's troubles as well. The presence of guilty preoccupations is very significant for making a diagnosis of the syndrome of depression.

ASSOCIATED SYMPTOMS OF DEPRESSION

So far we've concentrated on the mood changes seen in the depressive syndrome. But there are other symptoms as well, changes beyond the change in mood.

Severe depression almost always causes a change in sleeping pattern. Depressed persons frequently suffer from insomnia, but also from its opposite, sleeping too much (*hypersomnia* is the technical term). A peculiar rhythmic pattern of sleep disturbance and mood changes through the day sometimes seen in depressed persons is called *diurnal variation of mood* (*diurnal* is a word used in biology to refer to a twenty-four-hour cycle). Persons with this pattern fall asleep at the usual time and without much difficulty but wake up very early in the morning after only a few hours of sleep. Lying awake hours before sunrise, they experience their lowest mood of the day during this early morning period, and minor problems and regrets seem magnified and overwhelming. They notice a gradual lifting of their mood as sunrise approaches, and when the morning light comes, they can often rouse themselves and start their daily activities despite feeling worn out from fretting for those troublesome hours. As the day goes on, their mood continues to improve little by little until, by day's end, they feel nearly back to their normal self. They typically go to bed and can often fall asleep easily, but several hours later, they awaken depressed, and the cycle repeats itself.

Sleep changes in adolescents can be difficult to identify. Most adolescents go through a period of going to bed later and later, usually in order to stay awake doing fun activities, with subsequent awakening later and later in the day (the technical term is *sleep phase advance,* and it has indeed been shown through research that some adolescents, and adults, have a biological clock that prefers this state). So, how is one to differentiate between the normal changes in sleep pattern that occur as children become more social and focused on fun and those that indicate a depressive episode? Although many adolescents stay awake to enjoy themselves, depressed adolescents do so because it is the only time of the day when they feel good. As fits the diurnal variation discussed above, most persons with depression can only really feel halfway good toward the end of the day, and they want to stay up late to enjoy this period. Nondepressed adolescents will eventually fall asleep, and their body will want to make up for the late hour when they retired by causing them to sleep later. (It is not unusual for an adolescent to sleep past noon if not awakened by an alarm or another person.) Those with the depressive form of insomnia, however, will frequently awaken on their own after only a few hours of sleep and be unable to return to rest despite extreme fatigue.

In depression, as for many adolescents, getting up in the morning is a chore and can result in a transient irritability and grumpiness. For the majority of young persons, however, this quickly dissipates once they arrive at school. In depression, adolescents are persistently irritable or sullen, have trouble attending to class, and may even fall asleep (as opposed to socializing with friends).

But what of hypersomnia? It is true that some people do not experience this early morning awakening when depressed but instead want to sleep seemingly all the time. This holds true for adolescents as well and can be a key defining characteristic of those going through a depression. As we've said, many adolescents enjoy their free evening time and take advantage of it by staying awake. Those with depression will frequently return from school or other activities and either take prolonged and frequent naps or stay up to complete homework but retire unusually early—at times before their parents. In both cases, what is most critical to notice is a *change* from a regular routine. And remember, as with low mood, sleep disturbance is but a single symptom that must be evaluated in conjunction with other symptoms to diagnose the syndrome of depression.

Appetite is usually disturbed in depressed individuals. As with sleep problems, changes occur in both directions: eating too much or too little. Individuals can lose or gain a significant amount of weight during periods of depression. (We discuss the deliberate self-starvation and compulsive eating of *eating disorders* in chapter 13; these behaviors seem to be complex syndromes deserving their own dedicated discussion.)

Of the other bodily symptoms that occur in depression, a sense of fatigue with prominent low energy and listlessness is one of the most striking. Headaches, constipation, and a feeling of heaviness in the chest are common, as are other, more difficult-to-describe uncomfortable physical sensations. Whether these symptoms are caused by depression itself or arise from the lack of restful sleep, lack of exercise, and poor eating habits that depression brings is not clear. Depression seems to lower the pain threshold: depressed individuals seem more sensitive to pain and are more distressed by it.

Even young children can identify a physical pain and are able to describe a headache or a stomachache, but they may not be able to identify and name a painful psychological state. The young adolescent who may not quite understand the concept of low mood may instead complain of headaches that make her want to spend time in bed. In young adolescents who are depressed, uncomfortable physical symptoms may result in frequent physical complaints that overshadow complaints of low mood.

Depression changes thinking as well as mood. Depressed persons can experience slowing and inefficiency in their thinking and often complain of memory and concentration problems. Charlie's complaint that he's not as smart as the other students in his new school might be understood better in this way. It's possible that he is indeed not performing as well as some of the other students in his classes, but his concentration is probably adversely affected by his depression. When concentration is impaired, memory can seem to be affected as well: when we can't concentrate, our ability to register and later retrieve information is also impaired. Falling grades at school are very common in adolescent depression, and though certainly due in part to the energy and motivation problems depression causes, they are probably also caused by what psychiatrists call *cognitive* symptoms. From the Latin *cognoscere*, meaning "to know," this term refers to problems in concentration, thinking, and memory. We know, for example, that in depressed elderly persons, these sorts of thinking problems can be so severe that depression can be misdiagnosed as Alzheimer's disease. In adolescents, on the other hand, these problems may be misconstrued as ADHD (attention-deficit/hyperactivity disorder). We have seen many adolescents whose parents brought them in for an evaluation for "new-onset ADHD" when in fact the adolescent is in the throes of a depressive episode. This type of distinction is why it is absolutely critical to seek help from a qualified psychiatrist when seeking an accurate diagnosis. Analyzing individual symptoms without looking at the larger pattern can easily lead one down the incorrect path. We spend more time discussing the overlap between depression and other psychiatric disorders, like ADHD, later in this book.

MOOD DISORDERS: REAL ILLNESSES

Because everyone has gone through periods of low mood at one time or another, many people think they understand depression. Even the associated symptoms of the depressive syndrome sometimes accompany normal low mood states briefly or in a much milder form: a bit of trouble falling asleep for a night or two or a temporary loss of appetite are not that unusual after a serious disappointment or loss.

These facts can make it tempting to think that serious depressive disorders must follow the same "rules" as ordinary low mood states. They don't. Serious depressions don't get better on their own after a few days. Seriously depressed adolescents can't "shake off" their mood states or get their minds off their troubles by concentrating on school or sports or friends. They can't "get over" whatever preoccupations with loss or failure their depressive illness inflicts on them. They can't "get ahold" of themselves or "shape up," "move on," "lighten up," do something about their situation, pull themselves up by their bootstraps—or any of the things people can often do to get past a period of low mood. Adolescents with mood disorders are in the grip of their illness, and their symptoms stay with them day after day, week after week, relentlessly. It's thought that this is due to real changes of functioning in certain brain "centers" or "circuits."

It is tempting, however, to fall back on our own experiences with low mood as well as our experiences with people in general and to attribute the seriously depressed adolescent's inability to "get over" his depression symptoms to being unmotivated, lazy, stubborn, or simply not trying hard enough. This misunderstanding of what serious depression really is can lead to major problems. At worst, it can lead to the conclusion that there is nothing wrong with the teenager that time, encouragement, or stricter discipline won't solve. It might lead to the conclusion that the seriously depressed adolescent is simply "troubled" and that a few counseling sessions or a few weeks of talking to a therapist will take care of the problem. Although counseling and therapy are certainly important aspects of treating all types of depression, medical intervention, *treatment with medication*, is the mainstay of treatment of serious depressive disorder.

How do we know this?

THE CHEMISTRY OF MOOD

One of the greatest revolutions in medicine occurred during the seventeenth and eighteenth centuries, when physicians began to realize that the workings of the human body followed the rules of science. Indeed, the word *science* came to be used in its modern sense during this time and replaced the older term *natural philosophy*. Today, we take for granted that the heart is a pump and that we can understand a lot about the way it works if we understand how pumps work. After the Frenchman Jean Léonard Marie Poiseuille elucidated the laws of physics that determine the flow rate, pressure, and other properties of liquids flowing through glass tubes, it quickly became apparent that the flow of blood through arteries and veins follows the same principles. Philosophical speculations on the heart as the source of love, loyalty, and other poetic qualities and feelings disappeared and were replaced by cold hard mathematical rules and principles.

It took several hundred more years for us to realize it, but as is now quite clear, the functioning of the brain follows scientific principles as well and depends on processes that follow the rules of biochemistry (the chemistry of living things). We also know that the brain is the organ of emotions and thinking, so it follows that, at some level, thinking and emotions depend on these biological and chemical processes. It also follows that when those processes go awry, abnormalities of thinking and emotions result.

If you think about it for a moment, you'll realize that it really isn't such a new idea. People have used various chemicals to change thinking, emotions, and behavior for thousands of years. Almost as soon as we figured out how to raise crops, we discovered how to ferment some of them and began using ethyl alcohol (the alcohol in alcoholic beverages) to change the way we feel. We found substances that dull the perception of pain (aspirin from the bark of willows, morphine from poppies), substances that boost mood and energy level (caffeine from coffee beans, cocaine from coca leaves), and even substances that induce abnormal mental experiences such as hallucinations (*Psilocybe* mushrooms and the peyote cactus, among others). Ancient peoples attributed these effects to spirits or demons or gods, but during the early part of the twentieth century, biochemists isolated the active ingredients from these natural materials, and several decades later, neuroscientists discovered specific mechanisms of action for some of them (such as the discovery of receptors in the brain to which morphine binds). Our understanding of these mechanisms increased, and today, the number of naturally occurring psychoactive substances (those having an effect on the activities of the brain and nervous system) has now been far surpassed by the number of manufactured ones. We take it for granted now that chemicals, either naturally occurring or synthetic, can alter the biochemical functioning of the brain and thus alter thinking and emotions.

During the middle decades of the twentieth century, researchers discovered that several pharmaceuticals had specific effects on mood. Reserpine is a pharmaceutical extracted from the root of an Indian shrub, *Rauvolfia serpentina*. Ancient Hindu writings mention the use of the plant for medicinal purposes, but not until the 1950s was it discovered to have a potent effect on blood pressure, becoming the first effective agent to treat hypertension (high blood pressure). As was also noted, some patients who took the medication to control their blood pressure developed serious depression. Low mood gradually developed over a period of weeks and soon was accompanied by all the other manifestations of the depressive syndrome—several patients taking this drug committed suicide.

In 1951, several doctors prescribing iproniazid, a pharmaceutical used to treat tuberculosis, noticed an interesting side effect in some of their TB patients: it helped with depression. Patients with low mood, sleep and appetite disturbances, and other symptoms of serious depression had a remission of these symptoms after taking iproniazid for several weeks. Physicians at the time were puzzled by this development, as iproniazid was known to cause sometimes significant and uncomfortable side effects; however, despite the symptoms of the patients' illness and the effects of the treatment, their mood actually improved. The first *antidepressant* medication had been accidentally discovered.

In part II of the book, in the discussions of treatments, you will see that *all* the original medications used to treat mood disorders were discovered more or less accidentally. But accidental or not, the discovery of pharmaceuticals that can cause the depressive syndrome and of others that can make it better unequivocally points to the existence of a *biochemistry of mood*. A mood disorder, then, must be what occurs if something goes wrong with this chemistry.

In this chapter, we've started to give you a picture of adolescent depression, with an emphasis on the most common symptoms and an overview of some approaches to understanding it. In the next chapter, we fill in some details of this complicated picture with some facts derived from research on what is still a poorly understood illness.

Normal Adolescence and Depression in Adolescence

It is not too far off the mark to say that our understanding of serious depressive illnesses in young people is several decades behind our understanding of depressive illnesses in adults. Fortunately, the field is catching up fast. But experts still disagree on many of the most basic facts about depression in adolescence. How frequently does serious depression occur in young people? What exactly are the symptoms? What is the best treatment approach? What are the risk factors for depression in young people? Are there protective factors? How likely is it that depression will continue to be a problem into adulthood for any given individual? Are there common complications of the illness? We go into each of these questions in turn and try to give the best, most up-to-date information regarding the answers as we understand them. But the number one question most people have for us is this: "Is *my* child depressed?" To answer this most perplexing query, it is essential to first give more information on the symptoms of depression, then to cover the changes even nondepressed adolescents go through in this life stage of nearly constant change and development.

MORE ON SYMPTOMS

There was no such thing as a field of child psychiatry before the 1930s, when Adolf Meyer, then the director of psychiatry at the Johns Hopkins Hospital, recognized a need for specialized treatment of children and adolescents. This effort was primarily driven by members of the pediatrics department, who believed themselves somewhat neglected in regard to psychosocial supports for what were obviously suffering children and families. Leo Kanner was recruited to chair the first division of child and adolescent psychiatry in the world. Kanner used his experience to gather information for his book *Child Psychiatry*, published in 1935.[1] He was ahead of his time in his assertions that children could indeed suffer from severe psychiatric abnormalities, an idea that was unfortunately ridiculed and derided by the very people who initially funded his studies—the pediatricians. They despised the idea of pathologizing what they considered the "normal," or reactive, transient depressive symptoms that they believed were a perfectly ordinary part of growing up.

In an article entitled "The Menace of Psychiatry," the famous Chicago pediatrician Joseph Brennemann wrote, "There is a menace in psychologizing the school child, psychiatrizing his behavior and over organizing his habits and his play."[2] Many took his argument to be that children cannot suffer as adults can, furthering an antipsychiatry movement within pediatrics. In fact, Dr. Brennemann clarified later that his ire was directed at the "charlatans" of psychiatry, who claim that every child is suffering from a severe psychiatric illness in need of frequent, extensive (and expensive) treatment that only they are capable of carrying out. He did believe that children can suffer from the same mood disorders as adults, but that careful time and attention must be paid to diagnosing and treating these more significant conditions so that they are neither missed nor overdiagnosed. In that, many psychiatrists would agree. But Brennemann was too late—his message was (mis)heard loud and clear by the pediatric community. Leo Kanner wrote that there "is a tendency among pediatrics to ridicule and resent any psychiatric offerings" in terms of diagnosis and treatment.[3] This unfortunate divide is only recently being mended, primarily by the increasing preponderance of research that has proved that adolescents (and children as well) show the same symptoms of depression as do adults and can develop the full depressive syndrome. In 1987, a study was conducted of 296 children and adolescents between the ages of 6 and 18 years who had been referred to a clinic specializing in child and adolescent depression and were carefully examined for depressive symptoms. A statistical analysis of the pattern of symptoms found that "the similarities across the school age in the [symptoms] of major depressive disorder far outweigh the few differences."[4] The clusters of symptoms included mood symptoms, negative thinking, anxiety symptoms, and appetite problems, and they paralleled the adult symptom pattern in both the children and the adolescents examined. A more recent study, focused on older adolescents (ages 14 to 18), also found that depressed teenagers had symptoms typical of adult depression (table 2-1).

This research also indicates that despite the similarities across age groups, some subtle patterns of symptom differences show up as one looks closely at different ages. Younger adolescents, just like small children, seem to have more in the way of anxiety symptoms: fearfulness and nervousness. They show clinging behaviors, unexplained fears, and physical symptoms of anxiety such as stomachaches and stress headaches. Older adolescents suffer more from loss of interest and pleasure, and they have more in the way of morbid thinking: thoughts of death and suicide. Conversely, they may be more likely to be irritable and angry than either younger children or adults. This special form of depression, present though less common in other age groups, has the danger of being mistaken for other psychiatric diseases (such as bipolar affective disorder, discussed in chapter 3) and can place the adolescent at great risk of misdiagnosis and ineffective treatment.

Another set of symptoms now recognized to occur in some severely depressed adolescents are what are called *psychotic symptoms. Psychosis* is an unfortunately vague term that is nevertheless frequently used in psychol-

Table 2-1   Symptoms of Adolescent Depression

Symptom	Percentage of Adolescents Reporting
Depressed mood	97.7
Sleep disturbance	88.6
Thinking difficulties	81.8
Weight/appetite disturbance	79.5
Anhedonia	77.3
Worthlessness/guilt	70.5
Loss of energy	68.2
Thoughts of death/suicide	54.5

Source: Peter Lewinsohn, Paul Rohde, and John Seeley, "Major Depressive Disorder in Older Adolescents: Prevalence, Risk Factors and Clinical Implications," *Clinical Psychological Review* 18, no. 7 (1998): 765–94.

ogy to describe various symptoms of losing touch with reality, specifically, hallucinations and delusions. Hallucinations are sensory perceptions without actual sensory stimuli: hearing voices when no one is present, or seeing things that no one else can see. Delusions are false beliefs that preoccupy the person with such conviction that he cannot be persuaded otherwise. He may be convinced that he has a terrible incurable illness such as cancer or AIDS or believe that his family has lost all its money, and that he will soon be homeless or institutionalized. In depressive illnesses, the delusional beliefs usually have depressing themes such as these, and the person may believe he has committed some terrible sin or crime and fear severe punishment. The hallucinations seen in psychotic depression are depressing as well: the individual may hear voices calling him bad names or condemning him, telling him he is worthless or a failure. The visual hallucinations are usually frightening and grotesque, of devils or monsters. Delusions or hallucinations in adolescent depression seem to be uncommon, but when present, they signal an especially severe illness.

It is important, however, to distinguish the intersection of what we would call a hallucination with the imaginary world of a child. A true hallucination is, as listed above, a *true* sensory perception without a stimulus. This means that the child actually hears, through his ears, another voice. The child can point to where it is coming from, and in severe cases may try to find the speaker located in his wall. An *imagined* sensory perception, or a *misinterpreted* sensory perception, is another matter entirely and is not necessarily indicative of any malign process at all. We realize that these distinctions are subtle and difficult to tell apart. Who has not known children with imaginary friends they insist are real? Do parents rush to the hospital, fearing their child is psychotic, or instead engage and possibly humor their beloved youngster by setting an extra place at the table? And who themselves has not had the experience of believing they heard their name called only to realize it was either another word entirely or (more eerily but not any more unusual) that no one was there at all? Does this indicate the sort of break with reality with which we usually associate hallucinations? Certainly not, if we experience it ourselves, but if a friend were to tell us about all the invisible people calling her name, would we not begin to worry a bit? Answering these sorts of questions—what is a hallucination and what is not?—is exactly what psychiatrists spend their lives doing and why they must work so hard and spend so much time to reach an accurate diagnosis.

We talk about how to find a skilled psychiatrist, and why it is so important to do so, later in the book. As we go along, however, try not to become overwhelmed as we present these sorts of subtle differences that we as psychiatrists must pay such close attention to. We are not attempting to write a textbook or to teach readers how to become psychiatrists. We do feel it is essential, however, to open the curtain on the world of those who daily diagnose and treat adolescents with depression and to give as clear and as accurate a picture as possible of what this illness looks like, without cutting any corners or softening any of the difficult ambiguities we regularly must face.

MORE ON ADOLESCENCE

The first person to formulate a psychological theory of adolescence was the American psychologist and educator G. Stanley Hall, who believed that emotional turmoil and crisis were always characteristic of this developmental period, something to be endured rather than understood. Writing at the beginning of the twentieth century, Hall proposed that the entire history of the human race had become part of each individual's genetic endowment and that the psychological development of each individual retold the story of human history. Borrowing a German phrase used to describe the sweeping romantic sagas of Schiller and Goethe, Hall characterized adolescence as a period of Sturm und Drang, "storm and stress," a phrase that was used to characterize adolescence for decades afterward. Hall saw adolescence as a recapitulation of the conflicts of preindustrial civilization: a time of crusades and revolutions, great chivalry and great cruelties, self-sacrifice and brutal domination, fervent loyalty and unscrupulous treachery. Adolescents passed through a time of rapidly changing moods and emotions, unbridled optimism giving way to despair, melancholy alternating with youthful exuberance, before a mature, rational adult emerged from the chaos. Even after the genetic and historical components of Hall's ideas had been discredited, his concept of inevitable emotional storminess during adolescence persisted, becoming incorporated into psychological theories that followed and even into popular thinking about adolescence.

It turns out that the "storms" most adolescents go through are fairly minor and short lived—perhaps better thought of as passing cloudbursts. Surveys of teens and their parents through the 1960s and 1970s indicated that adolescents generally tend to have positive self-concepts and place high value on the approval of their parents. A modern study, from 2011, evaluating more than 300,000 high school students, found similar results.[5] It seems, then, that though some bickering between teens and their parents about such everyday issues as what clothing they wear and what time to be in at night is common, serious conflict is not actually the norm. Sir Michael Rutter, a British child psychiatrist who has extensively researched and written about adolescent issues for several decades, puts it this way: "It is evident that normal adolescence is *not* characterized by storm, stress and disturbance. Most young people go through their teenage years without significant emotional or behavioral problems. It is true . . . that there are challenges to be met, adaptations to be made, and stresses to be coped with. However, these do not all arise at the same time and most adolescents deal with these issues without undue disturbance."[6]

A theory of adolescence that has better withstood the test of time is that of the great American psychologist Erik Erikson, who invented the term *identity crisis* in the 1960s to characterize the uncertainty, self-questioning, and existential confusion he believed was inevitable during adolescents' search for their place in the world. Erikson's concept of the identity crisis of adolescence remains one of the best formulations of these issues. Although the word *crisis* conjures up a meaning of danger and even possible catastrophe, Erikson's use of the word is more like that of the Chinese, encompassing a meaning of opportunity as well. "Turning point" might capture the idea better. According to Erikson, the main issue that confronts and preoccupies adolescents is a search for their identity as a person.

Erikson's theory has roots in psychoanalysis but emphasizes the interplay between the individual and society. You may be familiar with the "Eight Stages of Man," which he devised as the outline of his theory (table 2-2). Each of Erikson's stages represents a developmental task that confronts individuals at a particular age as they encounter ever-widening and complex social situations, expectations, and responsibilities. Erikson proposed that each stage has the possibility of a positive or a negative outcome. If individuals are able to manage a positive outcome at any particular step,

Table 2-2   The Life Cycle Stages Proposed by Erik Erikson

Stage	Age	Psychosocial Crisis
I	Infancy	Trust versus mistrust
II	Toddlerhood	Autonomy versus shame and doubt
III	Preschool age	Initiative versus guilt
IV	School age	Industry versus inferiority
V	Adolescence	Ego identity versus role confusion
VI	Young adulthood	Intimacy versus isolation
VII	Middle age	Generativity versus self-absorption
VIII	Old age	Integrity versus despair

they move on to the next with enhanced psychological coping and developmental tools. If the crisis is not well managed, the negative attribute will interfere with the next step in development, and psychological problems are more likely.

Erikson postulated that adolescence is the first time a person begins to ask, in a serious way, "Who am I?" Also pressing for attention are the related questions: "Where did I come from?" "What do I want to become?"

Bodily changes—physical growth, hormonal changes, the onset of menstruation in girls, and voice changes in boys—force the adolescent to come to terms with a new body image. Experimentations with the use of cosmetics in girls, with facial hair and body building in boys, and with clothing and hairstyles their parents don't approve of in both sexes (not to mention piercings and tattoos) are adolescents' efforts to discover their bodies and attempts at self-invention and self-definition.

During this time, greater psychological development allows adolescents to interact in more sophisticated ways with others, and they become much more preoccupied with what others think of them, often comparing these perceptions with how they feel about themselves. This may explain why teens seem determined to be centers of attention but simultaneously complain of feeling as if they are constantly being scrutinized and are "on stage." They crave feedback but at the same time are worried about what they might hear about themselves. As adolescents seek roles and models outside the home, the peer group becomes increasingly important as a reference point and sounding board. Idolization of athletes, musicians, and movie stars is part of this search for self-definition and of developing a vocational identity, the beginnings of thinking about a career.

Sexuality is another aspect of personal identity that adolescents begin to explore, and exploration of the physical aspects of sexuality is only part of the process. Adolescents first begin to feel attraction to specific people, which can be a source of strength and bonding with nonromantic friends, as they discuss their crushes and "likes," or a source of distress, teasing, and torment if those attractions are different from the norm within one's peer group. Adolescents live in an interesting era now, when individual expression is tolerated to an extent never before seen, particularly in America. Adolescents are exploring whole new definitions of sexual and gender expression and feeling supported and cared for while doing so. It is not the place of this book to judge these expressions, merely to point out how disruptive new feelings and new hormones can be to the development of the adolescent mind.

The sexuality most commonly explored through adolescence is more about relationships, about learning to emotionally pair with another and see oneself through that person's eyes, than it is about any simple physical act. Crushes and infatuations with unobtainable partners occur, with inevitable disappointment. The teenager may establish a sense of identity through couple-hood: "Who am I? I'm her boyfriend." The personal feedback of the youthful love affair helps the adolescent reflect on, redefine, and revise his image of himself. As Erikson explained it, "That is why many a youth would rather converse, and settle matters of mutual identification, than embrace."[7]

The adolescent's move toward autonomy and away from parental authority and control also means giving up some measure of parental protection and nurturance, often before secure and comfortable emotional self-reliance is possible. A stage of substituting dependence on a peer group for dependence on parents is not unusual, explaining the intense devotion among friends, cliques, and teams so often seen at this age. Extreme peer group conformity in choice of clothing styles, behavioral norms, and even the heroes and idols of the group provides acceptance and solidarity. Selection of foods and entertainment and use of language and slang expressions are in strict conformity to the peer group. Disdain, intolerance, and even cruelty toward those who act differently are common. This is a time when adolescents can become vulnerable to pathological group allegiances as well: gangs, religious cults, militaristic organizations—all groups that exploit the adolescent's tendency to view the world in terms of black and white. This is even more worrisome today with the boom of the Internet and social media, in that teens can join groups from radically different geographic regions—physical proximity is no longer enough to limit the activities of young persons. Many examples of these phenomena exist, but a particularly striking one is of online groups espousing the ideals of eating disorders, not as life-threatening psychiatric illnesses in need of treatment, but as lifestyle choices equally deserving of respect as vegetarian eating or regular triathlon training, and in the same class of healthy living. These "pro-ana" (pro-anorexia) and "pro-mia" (pro-bulimia) sites describe how much self-control and discipline these lifestyles require, placing their practitioners in a special class of person who is able to achieve "success." Eating disorders are discussed in far greater detail in chapter 13, but we use this example to show the power of social media in connecting people around the globe, at times around ideas that promote negative behavior rather than positive.

For many teenagers, the mental work accomplished in this stage of development results in succeeding in the beginning stages of determining their own identity and learning to trust themselves, balanced with a willingness to take in feedback from others and re-evaluate their values and goals in order to continue growing. The possible negative outcome of this stage, *identity diffusion,* results in an individual who is constantly bedeviled by self-doubt and either morbidly preoccupied with the opinions of others or defiantly indifferent to them. Some adolescents attempt to escape feelings of alienation and anxiety by using alcohol and drugs. In Erikson's most comprehensive consideration of adolescence, *Identity, Youth, and Crisis,* he summed up the dilemma of identity confusion by quoting Biff, a character in Arthur Miller's play *Death of a Salesman:* "I just can't take hold, Mom, I can't take hold of some kind of life."[8]

Like any developmental theory, Erikson's proposals about adolescence should not be taken as a blueprint for every individual. Most important to remember is that psychological development during adolescence is a process, not an event; it proceeds in fits and starts over a period of years (and of course, our search for the answer to the question "who am I?" is never really over at any age). Later theorists expanded and elaborated Erikson's ideas, emphasizing that the process is usually disorganized and erratic and that adolescents inevitably go through at least some period of partial identity diffusion with its accompanying feelings of alienation.

The concept of *developmental foreclosure* has been proposed by American psychologist James Marcia to describe the process whereby the adolescent identifies and commits to some aspect of self-definition by incorporating the goals and values of others without the personal searching and self-examination inherent in true identity exploration.[9] The youth espouses the political or religious views of parents or significant others, sometimes fervently, but without an open exploration and consideration of alternatives. If, for some reason, some aspect of this "foreclosed" identity no longer fits, a temporary crisis can ensue until the adolescent readjusts or perhaps even reinvents this aspect of her identity. An adolescent who has unquestioningly accepted the teachings of the church she was raised in may be forced to question her allegiance to the denomination if she finds her developing political or social ideology at odds with its dogma. A period of questioning, searching, and perhaps stress and confrontation ensues before one or the other jarring element of identity is adjusted.

Inevitably, all this testing, exploring, questioning, and adjusting is psychologically stressful. The adolescent suffers disappointments in relationships, disillusionment with cherished ideas or values, frustration that the answer to "who am I?" keeps changing, anxiety that the answer to "what do I want to become?" isn't as clear as it seemed during childhood. It should not be surprising, then, that anxiety and low mood are common in adolescence.

Michael Rutter and his colleagues studied thousands of children and adolescents on England's Isle of Wight in an attempt to measure the frequency of psychological symptoms and illnesses in the population. They found that more than two-fifths of the 14- to 15-year-old boys and girls they interviewed reported substantial feelings of misery or depression. As Rutter concluded, "It seems that feelings of misery and depression are particularly common during adolescence and are more frequent during this age period than during either earlier childhood or adult life."[10] Many other studies have come up with similar findings.

What can we make of all this "misery" in adolescents? We know from similar studies (discussed below) that only a fraction of these adolescents have severe depression or mood disorders. Rather than depression, it may be more accurate to say that adolescents are prone to periods of *demoralization*.

In his classic book about psychotherapy, *Persuasion and Healing*, Johns Hopkins psychiatrist Jerome Frank states, "A person becomes demoralized when he finds that he cannot meet the demands placed on him and cannot extricate himself from his environment." Demoralized persons are "conscious of having failed to meet their own expectations or those of others, or of being unable to change the situation or themselves."[11] Where could we read a better description of adolescents' dilemma? Repeatedly finding themselves in strange new situations loaded down with expectations from parents, peers, and themselves, and often feeling powerless to affect the outcome, adolescents face big questions.

"In order to function," Frank states, "everyone must impose an order and regularity on the welter of experiences impinging upon him. To do this, he develops out of his personal experiences a set of . . . assumptions about himself and the nature of the world in which he lives, enabling him to predict the behavior of others and the outcome of his own actions."[12] This set of assumptions is called one's *assumptive world*. When something happens that disrupts a person's assumptive world, the environment suddenly seems unpredictable and a little scary. The individual may react with anxiety, feelings of loss of control and of being trapped, powerless, and, yes, miserable and depressed for a time—the state of affairs that Frank calls demoralization.

In the process of identity development, adolescents' assumptive world is constantly being upset and jostled by new experiences that can throw it into doubt. They spend weeks getting up the courage to ask out someone they think is just right for them only to be turned down ("Maybe I'm not as good-looking/popular as I thought"). They fail an exam ("I'm not as smart as I thought"), or don't make the team ("not as athletic . . ."), or lose the audition ("not as talented . . ."). Even positive accomplishments like getting good grades can raise questions about negative identities ("I must be a nerd"). Adolescents often assume that what happens to them indicates something about what kind of person they are. They react strongly to disappointments and setbacks, because they wonder what such events indicate about who they are and what their future will be like. A slight setback that adults would react to with only minor disappointment often causes adolescents to feel much more upset and disappointed and to question themselves in profound ways.

Reading through this, you might wonder why more adolescents don't need treatment for symptoms of demoralization. But as Rutter puts it, these challenges, adaptations, and stresses "do not all arise at the same time"; that is, only under rare and unusual circumstances is the adolescent faced with so many crises simultaneously that they overwhelm psychological resources to cope.

Jerome Frank developed his concept of psychological demoralization in the course of doing research on the effectiveness of psychotherapy. He studied persons with demoralization symptoms such as "depression" (low mood) and anxiety so severe that they sought professional psychological treatment. As Frank discovered, the crucial elements that make psychotherapy effective for these individuals are surprisingly simple: patients must have faith that the therapist cares about them and knows how to help them. Frank's theory was later validated through research into what psychiatrists call *resilience* in young people—that is, their ability to suffer through adverse events in life and come out the other side relatively unscathed. Scientists looked at all sorts of factors in life that could be supportive—other people, religiousness, wealth, social standing, and so on. What they found was elegant and moving in its simplicity. It turns out that the most critical factor in increasing resilience in children is that they have just one person, a single individual, they feel deeply bonded to and can go to in times of crisis. This single individual can make the difference in a person being defeated by life events or growing from them and becoming stronger. Fortunately, most teens have any number of persons in their lives who meet these requirements; they are surrounded by concerned, supportive, and experienced persons, such as parents, teachers, coaches, clergy, even older friends—the list could go on and on—who can help them through periods of uncertainty and discouragement.

All adolescents go through periods of discouragement, suffer from occasional feelings of not fitting in, and are bothered by uncertainty about the future. We must be careful not to "medicalize" this growth process (as Anna Freud is guilty of doing, exemplified by her comment that "to be normal during the adolescent period is by itself abnormal"[13]), and we must remember that a majority of the teenagers in the studies by Rutter and others did *not* report undue depression or "misery."

WHEN IS DEPRESSION "SERIOUS"?

At this point, you may be a little confused. We told you earlier that depression is a serious illness but just spent several pages telling you that adolescent complaints of being "miserable" are not uncommon and do not represent *clinical* depressions—that is, they do not usually warrant medical treatment. The way to understand this better is to recall the discussion in chapter 1 about depression the *symptom* and depression the *syndrome*. In this chapter, we've put an even finer distinction on the issue and have talked about the difference between *depression* and *demoralization*. But how are these related? Can one cause the other? Blend into the other? Where does intense demoralization end and the depressive syndrome begin?

At this point in time, the answers to these questions are not fully known. We know it is not uncommon for adolescents to pass through periods of "miserableness" quite unscathed. But we know that some of this miserableness is a prelude to, or an aspect of, a mood disorder. We also know that adults with mood disorders can have an episode of serious depression triggered by psychological stress and demoralization.

The big mistake that people make in deciding whether to seek treatment for a person with depression is to think that if he seems to have "real" reasons to be depressed, he won't need treatment because he'll "get over it" as soon as he deals with those reasons. A related error is thinking that this individual needs counseling or therapy but not medical treatment. This is not too different from the middle-aged man with chest pains trying to persuade himself that "it's only heartburn" rather than going to the nearest emergency room. When an individual has the signs and symptoms of the syndrome of depression, it's time to get professional help, not to try figuring out whether he has "reasons" to be depressed.

Because we have several ways of understanding depression, one perspective based on biology and the disease model, and a second perspective based on psychology and understanding how people react to events in their lives, it's tempting to think we should be able to categorize depressions in the same way: "biological" and "psychological." We've already led you into this way of thinking a bit, with the discussion of *depression* differentiated from *demoralization*. If only an understanding of people were so easy!

This categorizing of depressions works fairly well in some clear-cut cases at the extremes of the categories. No one would say that a teenage football player who sulks and broods for a day or two after his team misses a chance to be in the state playoffs is suffering from a biologically based mood disorder derived from some misfiring of his physical brain. Similarly, no one would say that Charlie from chapter 1 is simply discouraged, suffering from "normal" teenage angst. This boy is clearly ill.

But there is a large area between these extremes, where differentiation between biological and psychological depressions is not only impossible but also probably meaningless. Another great student of human behavior, Alfred Kinsey, the pioneering researcher on sexuality, said, "The world is not divided into sheep and goats ... Nature rarely deals with discrete categories. Only the human mind invents categories and tries to force facts into separated pigeonholes."[14] Our mental lives involve a complex interplay between biology and psychology that is poorly understood and probably cannot be teased apart. One set of forces affects the other, and there are probably complex feedback loops and an intertwining of influences and processes that make attempts to do so futile.

Michael Rutter, in talking about causes of psychological problems, makes the point that this entanglement of causation is also apparent in physical illnesses as well: we know that a germ called the tubercle bacillus causes tuberculosis. But we also know that genetic factors play a role in resistance to infection and to some extent determine who gets infected. We know, too, that nutritional status is important, that malnourished individuals are much more vulnerable to TB, making it in some ways an illness of poverty. To say that poverty causes tuberculosis isn't quite correct, but to say that tuberculosis is caused by a germ and leave it at that omits a lot of factors that need to be identified in order to treat the illness. Talking too much about what is "biological" and what is "psychological" in depression is simply a waste of time. Serious depression is both.

Not too long ago, psychiatrists and psychologists (more on the differences between these two professions in a bit) made the mistake of relying too much on theories to guide their treatment of depressed patients and not enough on research data and experience. We spent too much time trying to understand depressed persons rather than diagnosing and treating mood disorders. We now know that serious depressive syndromes must be treated medically and that psychotherapy alone will usually not make the patient better. But we also know that people with depressive illnesses are usually demoralized and need support, encouragement, education, and guidance. Adolescents with serious depression should not be denied either kind of treatment just because the details of their symptoms seem to suggest that either depression or demoralization predominates.

So, back to the original question posed earlier: What constitutes *serious* depression? Although you really need a medical or psychology degree and years of clinical training to be able to answer this question for any given individual, you can get some sense of what serious depression is like by rereading chapter 1 for the details of the depressive syndrome. Also, there are some red flags that should always make parents worry that their teen might be seriously depressed:

— *Persistent change in mood*: gloominess, sadness, grouchiness, or irritability that persists over several weeks, on more days than not, such that the teenager seems consistently different from her usual self
— *Loss of interest and enjoyment* in most of the activities that the adolescent usually spends time doing
— *Persistent changes in sleep habits and appetite*: complaints of insomnia, sleeping too much, loss of appetite or increased appetite that results in a weight change of ten pounds or so, persistent complaints of tiredness or low energy, looking tired or haggard all the time
— *Change in self-attitude*, that is, a change in the way the adolescent feels about himself: feeling worthless or useless; self-critical statements about not being as good as other kids; feeling that he is lazy, stupid, ugly, a failure, or good-for-nothing
— *Falling grades*, loss of concentration, complaints that schoolwork is suddenly more difficult
— *Preoccupation with death or illness, especially thoughts of suicide*

The next step in understanding adolescent depression is to learn about the different disorders that exhibit the depressive syndrome. Several decades of research have led to our current classification of the various mood disorders. The depressive syndrome shows up in all of them, but the severity and pattern of the depressive symptoms, their course over time, and some associated symptoms indicate that they are probably different illnesses. Research has also shown that the treatments of these various disorders sometimes need to be very different.

In the next chapter, we discuss the mood disorders of adolescence.

The Mood Disorders of Adolescence

W hen the mental health community started thinking about serious depression as an illness and began to do research on the symptoms of depression, the course of the illness, and its response to various treatments, they found that serious depression shows up in different forms. These forms differ in severity and types of symptoms and in the timing of symptom development. This research has resulted in our current classification system of mood disorders.

PSYCHIATRIC DIAGNOSIS

Diagnosis is just as important in treating emotional problems as it is in treating physical illnesses. Diagnostic classification has two purposes in medicine: (1) to make predictions about the course of an illness and (2) to aid the clinician in selecting the treatment most likely to be effective. In the practice of psychiatry, since the physical basis for most psychiatric illnesses has yet to be discovered, classification systems are largely derived from studying groups of patients with different combinations of symptoms and seeing whether the groups vary in the course of their illness or in their response to medications.

As different types of medications have become available to treat mood disorders, the classification system of mood disorders has continued to evolve. In this chapter, we describe various subtypes of mood disorders. These are the subtypes that currently seem to make sense to clinicians, because they serve one of the two purposes of diagnosis mentioned above: (1) they allow for a better prediction of the course of the illness, and (2) they allow for a rapid selection of effective therapy—saving the patient time that would be wasted trying an ineffective medication. In 2013, the American Psychiatric Association released a new version of their diagnostic manual, the *Diagnostic and Statistical Manual of Mental Disorders*. This fifth edition, often called the *DSM-5*, contains significant changes in the world of adolescent mood disorders for just the reasons mentioned above. It turned out that an increasingly common diagnosis in young persons, bipolar affective disorder, predicted neither the illness course nor the treatment response, as it did in adults. In fact, longitudinal studies of these children diagnosed as having bipolar affective disorder showed that a re-evaluation of their symptoms once they reached adulthood much more closely matched the syndrome of depression, or that of an isolated anxiety. How can such a seeming error be made? How can a child "have" one syndrome at one point in her life and another one later on?

The proliferation of the diagnosis of bipolarity in children helps us illustrate this critical point. No one, neither adolescents nor adults, can be diagnosed in such a way that the diagnostician is absolutely certain that this is and will be the person's underlying syndrome for the rest of his life. Humans, especially adolescents, are evolving and changing creatures, constantly in flux. In medicine, some (though surprisingly few) illnesses remain permanently with individuals in exactly the same way throughout their lives—and these are mainly genetic disorders. In most cases and especially in psychiatry, people need continual re-evaluation to ensure that their condition has not evolved into something else, and that the diagnosis was correct in the first place. In the world of child psychiatry, we know that certain individuals seem to have multiple diagnoses piled on top of them, which can prove confusing to children and parents alike. Much of our time is spent explaining how a child can "have" ADHD at 5, an anxiety disorder at 7, major depression at 12, and then bipolar disorder at 15.

In reality, all of our diagnoses in psychiatry are clinically based—we do not (yet) have the detailed definitive testing, such as a blood test or brain scan, as do so many other fields of medicine. We must think carefully and rationally about what is happening in a person's life at this moment, compared to what has happened before—with no knowledge of what is yet to come. People change, and so with time we are able to see new and more subtle facets of their underlying selves to clarify what we think may be going on in their psyche, including any psychiatric illnesses they may have. It is not so much that an adolescent "used to have" one condition and now "has" a totally different one replacing the first as it is likely that the developmental changes a child goes through are paralleled by changes in the pattern of symptoms, which now more closely matches the description of one syndrome than another.

Take, for example, the symptom of an inability to pay attention. In one snapshot, a child may appear happy and engaged in fun activities but struggle in class and with homework. This child may be given the diagnosis of ADHD. Later in life, as his brain develops and social pressures increase, he may again experience this symptom of difficulty concentrating, but it may be accompanied by frustrations, low mood, a feeling of failure, anxieties about ever succeeding, trouble sleeping, a lower appetite, a withdrawal from friends and fun activities—you get the picture, which now appears to much more closely approximate the depressive episodes we have described.

In this chapter we discuss the various faces of mood disorders in adolescence. Remember that even if someone's symptoms closely match those listed here, this does not mean that this person has a given diagnosis or, more dangerously, has been misdiagnosed. It may merely mean that the person's most recent appearance closely matches a particular description. This is a trap that even experienced clinicians can fall into. Many adolescents have been diagnosed with bipolar affective disorder based on current *symptoms* when they have the *syndrome* of depression with perhaps a greater expression of irritability in that given moment than would be expected. The most recent version of the *DSM*, fifth edition, attempts to clarify these sorts of errors by further emphasizing the long-term pattern of symptoms rather than a simple cross-section. We discuss all of this more as we go through each form of mood disorder in greater detail.

At least once a month, it seems, we see a patient who requests to be "tested for clinical depression," the implication being that a blood test of some type will be able to detect the "chemical imbalance" that underlies serious mood problems. It's not an unreasonable request. Unfortunately, it's not a request that can be satisfied—not just yet. We don't have a blood test or an x-ray or a biopsy that can make the diagnosis of a mood disorder (or, for that matter, that can be used to confirm the diagnosis of most problems that psychiatrists treat).

This is because the biological and chemical basis of mood disorders remains a nearly complete mystery—no one knows what to test for. Despite literally hundreds of years of examining the bodily fluids and brain tissues of individuals with mood disorders, first with the naked eye, then with microscopes, then with x-rays and scanning devices, and more recently with incredibly sophisticated biochemical probes, no one has been able to find any abnormalities that can be accurately and reliably measured in people with this illness and used to aid in the diagnosis of these disorders. Though scientists have certainly tried! In the 1980s, something called the dexamethasone suppression test was employed in patients with low mood to try to differentiate between demoralization and depression. In theory, people who are depressed for a long time begin to produce higher and higher levels of cortisol, a stress hormone. Their bodies become less sensitive to the effects of this stress response and produce more and more. In most persons, if something that looks like cortisol (in this case, a steroid called dexamethasone) is introduced to the body, it senses this increase and relaxes its own production, lowering the cortisol level. The exhausted bodies of depressed persons seem blunted to this response and, perhaps wanting more and more cortisol, don't respond the same way. It seemed to be a good test in theory and was in clinical use for a number of years, but under rigorous study it didn't turn out to be a clinically useful test—the "sensitivity" (a statistical term used to describe the percentage of time the test is right when it comes out positive vs. the percentage of time it's wrong) was 50 percent, so it was wrong half the time.[1]

Today, the work on the genetics of mood disorders holds the promise that genetic markers for the illness may be discovered in the not-too-distant future—suggesting that a blood test might be possible to identify at least some cases of the illness. Although some individuals with mood disorders have been identified as having subtle brain-scan abnormalities—again suggesting a possible diagnostic tool—the clinical applications of these findings are still far off. Modern psychiatrists are left with the same diagnostic tools available to nineteenth-century psychiatrists: their eyes and ears.

We psychiatrists listen to patients and their family members describe symptoms. What has changed? What doesn't feel right? When did it start? Do the symptoms come and go or stay all the time? We observe the patient for the signs of mood disorders described in chapter 1 by performing a *mental status examination,* the psychiatrist's equivalent of the physical examination. This consists of observing speech patterns and behavior, questioning about mood and thinking processes, and evaluating other aspects of mental functioning, such as concentration and memory. In adolescents, information about these aspects of life from other sources (generally parents, sometimes others, such as teachers) can be as important or at times even more important pieces of the puzzle. After this process of history taking and examination, a picture of the person, of her symptoms and the course of her troubles, emerges. We identify a particular diagnostic category that seems a good fit with the clinical information, and once this is done, we can make predictions about the future course of the symptoms and, perhaps more important, select a treatment that has a good chance of relieving them.

MAJOR DEPRESSIVE DISORDER

Major depressive disorder is the name given to the mood disorder characterized by the development of the full-blown depressive syndrome. Research indicates that major depressive disorder is the most common mood disorder of adolescents and young adults.[2]

The illness usually has a fairly definite beginning, and over a period of weeks, the various symptoms of depression gradually come over the adolescent one by one until the full syndrome is present (table 3-1). The symptoms can last for months, with studies indicating that seven to nine months is typical—an entire school year for an adolescent.[3] The symptoms can vary tremendously in severity from fairly mild symptoms that affect the teen's level of functioning only moderately to severe cases in which social, school, and home life are all significantly affected.

In chapter 1 we met the parents of Charlie, who was showing the typical symptoms and course of illness of major depression. Charlie's symptoms included low mood, withdrawal, low energy, sleep and appetite problems, loss of interest in his usual pursuits, feeling bad about himself—symptoms that came on gradually over a period of weeks and basically drained the spark out of this previously energetic, confident boy.

Sometimes, however, major depression can look rather different, espe-

Table 3-1   Symptoms of Major Depression

Mood Symptoms
  Depressed mood
  Dysphoric mood
  Irritability
  Loss of ability to feel pleasure (anhedonia)
  Loss of interest in usual activities
  Social withdrawal
  Feelings of guilt or worthlessness
Cognitive (Thinking) Symptoms
  Poor concentration
  Poor memory
  Indecision
  Slowed thinking
  Thoughts of death, suicidal thinking
Bodily Symptoms
  Sleep disturbance
    Insomnia
    Hypersomnia
  Appetite disturbance
    Weight loss
    Weight gain
  Fatigue
  Headaches
Symptoms of Psychosis
  Delusional thinking
  Hallucinations

cially when the mood change is to irritable rather than low. In these adolescents, the irritable, miserable mood (psychiatrists often use the term *dysphoria*) is so disruptive to the adolescent's social world, especially the family, that other symptoms of major depression are obscured. Another case study will illustrate this.

▼   Heather's mother tried not to worry when her bright and usually bubbly 15-year-old daughter seemed to spend more Saturday afternoons listening to music in her room and fewer with her friends at the mall. But when Heather dropped out of the choral society, Maggie knew something was wrong.

"It's no fun anymore" was Heather's explanation for dropping out of the student choir only a month before the spring concert. "It's really boring; that stuff is for nerds anyway," she said, with a shrug of her shoulders, when her mom asked about it.

This explanation didn't quite sit right with Maggie, but she could guess what the real reason might be. Heather had auditioned to be a soloist in the concert and had been very disappointed that she wasn't chosen to sing any of the solo pieces. The choir director had told her that she wasn't quite ready for solo work yet but urged her to audition again for the fall concert. The director had also started telling the girls who were having trouble with their parts to stand next to Heather on the risers. "Heather has a strong voice and great intonation; she'll help carry you until you get the part down better," she would tell them in front of Heather and the whole group.

Heather had at first seemed to get over her disappointment, but as the weeks went by, it seemed singing was a chore rather than a source of joy and pride. "She didn't mean what she said about my having a good voice," Heather said angrily when Maggie reminded her of her music teacher's encouraging words. "She said that to humiliate me in front of *everyone*." So saying, Heather burst into tears and ran up to her room.

"Heather's just going through a stage," Maggie's sister reassured her one afternoon when they met at the grocery store. "Don't you remember when my Matt dropped off the swimming team with hardly an explanation and started writing poetry at all hours of the night? Kids' interests change all over the place at this age. They're finding themselves, that's all."

"I don't know," Maggie replied warily. "Heather's interests haven't changed. She seems to have lost interest in *everything*. She got lower grades in two subjects on her last report card, and besides she's so . . . oh, I don't know, so *mean* all of a sudden."

"Mean?" her sister asked.

"Well, she's so sarcastic about everything. She has Beth in tears several times a week."

"Big sisters criticize little sisters all the time at this age. It makes them feel grown up."

"I don't know, Fran. Heather and Beth always got along so well. They've never been mean to each other."

"Heather's never been a teenager, either," Fran soothed, patting Maggie's hand on the grocery cart. "And believe me, it gets worse when they're juniors; but you'll get through it somehow. Everyone does!"

Things did get worse. And much worse than Fran had predicted. There were screaming matches between Heather and her mother and father, Phillip, several times a week. Heather's grades continued to drop, and she took to spending most of her time in her room listening to music. Several times, Maggie had awakened in the middle of the night still hearing the music playing softly in Heather's room. She'd gone in to turn it off only to find her daughter still awake, sometimes in tears, but unable to say why she was crying.

Heather started coming in later than her curfew on weekends and often had alcohol on her breath.

Maggie and Phillip got a phone call from one of Heather's teachers warning that summer school might be a good idea if Heather wasn't able to turn her grades around. "I'm worried about Heather, and I think you should be too. Some of the answers on her tests make me think she's not concentrating in class like she should. She doesn't seem to be able to grasp the concepts this semester." But Heather flew into a rage when Maggie and Phillip told her about the call from her teacher. "And I will *not* go to summer school! Don't even think about it! I'll kill myself first!" she hissed ominously through clenched teeth.

Maggie felt alone and bewildered in dealing with her changed daughter. Fran shook her head sympathetically and suggested Maggie and Phillip go to "Tough Love" meetings. Phillip started staying later at the office to avoid the tension at home, and one night had only half-jokingly threatened to leave home "until she's 21 and a normal person again—I'll send you a check every month but you can call me when this part is *over*." Even 12-year-old Beth seemed to be out of the house most nights, needing to "study" with classmates. "I work better with someone else there," she explained sheepishly. "And it's hard to concentrate at home."

And there was no talking to Heather about much of anything. Maggie had made up her mind several times to make an appointment for Heather to see a therapist, but then things would go better for a day or two and she'd hope that the worst was over. And when things seemed to be getting worse, Maggie would become terrified at how Heather might react to the idea of seeing a mental health professional, and she would put the idea off "until she's in a better mood."

Late one evening, the phone rang. Maggie picked up the receiver expecting to hear Heather with her latest excuse for being out later than she should be. Instead, Maggie heard a woman's voice, a woman who seemed to be calling from some crowded place with phones ringing and some kind of beeping sound in the background.

"Mrs. McAllister? This is Ruth calling from the emergency department at St. Luke's Hospital." Maggie felt something in the middle of her chest drop to the soles of her feet. "We have Heather here and—"

"Oh my God, is she all right?"

"Yes, Mrs. McAllister, she's not hurt. There was a car accident, but Heather was not injured. She's fine physically, but—"

"Oh, thank God. We'll come right over to bring her home. Should we—"

"Well, ah . . . yes, you need to come over, but the doctor wants to talk to you about admitting Heather to the hospital."

"I don't understand. I thought you said she wasn't injured."

"No, she wasn't, but the psychiatrist thinks that she needs—"

"Psychiatrist? But what—"

"Heather drove off in her friend's car and ran off the road out by St. Mary's cemetery. The police found her passed out in the driver's seat with alcohol on her breath."

"Oh, God" was all Maggie could say.

"She was pretty alert by the time she got here, but the psychiatrist thinks she's very depressed. She wants to admit Heather at least overnight and see her in the morning, to see if she's still feeling suicidal."

"Depressed? Suicidal? But she's never—"

"Heather had two bottles of over-the-counter pills in her pocket, and we think she was planning to take an overdose. These particular pills probably wouldn't have caused anything serious, but anytime someone tries to hurt themselves we need to—"

Maggie wasn't listening anymore. Depressed? But depressed people are sad and gloomy, Maggie thought, not like this. Why did they think Heather was depressed? She didn't have anything to be depressed about. Could not getting the solo part in the spring concert have caused all this? No, that made no sense at all.

"We'll come right away," she said, and hung up the phone. ▲

Because Heather's problems seem at first glance so different from Charlie's, it doesn't seem possible that they have the same illness: major depression. But when we review Heather's symptoms, they're not really so different.

First, of course, there is the mood change. Heather is mostly irritable and dysphoric rather than suffering what we typically call a low mood. But the mood change is dramatic and pervasive, with her all the time, every day, week after week. Next, she's lost interest in school, in going with her friends to the mall, and she complains that singing is no fun anymore; she's developed a loss of pleasure in things, which you might remember is called *anhedonia*. Heather is in her room alone much of the time and isn't sleeping at night. She's having crying spells frequently. Her teacher has noticed poor concentration, and her grades are dropping.

Heather feels bad about herself and doesn't think she's a good singer after all; she even thinks that the music teacher's compliments were some kind of sarcastic ploy meant to make fun of her. This misinterpretation of the reality of the situation is, in fact, the kind of idea that can become increasingly preoccupying and gradually turn into a *delusion*, a psychotic symptom in which a person has a preoccupying false belief.*

Noting Heather's use of alcohol is also critical in diagnosing her depression. Although substance use and abuse can certainly be stand-alone problems in adolescents or in adults, sometimes substance-abuse problems get started and are sustained by a mood disorder and can be understood as secondary to it. The start of alcohol misuse (and anything that approaches regular use is *misuse* in adolescents) accompanied by the other symptoms are a strong indicator of the seriousness of Heather's problems. And, lastly, the serious attempt to harm herself carries a lot of weight and puts her collection of symptoms squarely into the category of major depression.

---

*Remember that in depressive disorders, the content of delusional beliefs is depressing in some way. In *A Mind That Found Itself*, written in the nineteenth century, author Clifford Beers describes his battle with a mental illness that was almost certainly a mood disorder. In one scene, he describes how, on a train ride to the psychiatric hospital, he noticed people standing on the station platforms reading the newspaper as the train passed through. Beers relates how convinced he was at the time that they were reading about him, about his long history of mental illness, and about what a failure he had been. These themes of shame and failure are typical of a mood disorder.

Because of her mostly irritable rather than depressed mood state, and because of her outwardly directed disruptive behaviors, especially toward her family, a superficial appraisal of Heather's situation might suggest that her problem is being *bad* rather than *sad*. But remember that diagnosing the syndrome of depression requires looking at many aspects of emotional life and behavior in addition to mood, and when this kind of survey is done with Heather, we come up with quite a list: a pervasive mood change, withdrawal from friends and family, low energy, poor concentration, sleep problems, loss of interest in usual pursuits, feeling bad about herself (to the point that she thinks life just isn't worth it and she tries to harm herself)—virtually the same list as Charlie's. Heather's diagnosis is the same as well: major depression.

No one is quite sure why this irritable mood is more common in adolescents than in adults. Irritability can certainly be a part of the picture in adults, but it is rarely the most prominent aspect of the mood syndrome as it can be in adolescents. Research shows that irritability as an expression of severe depression is most striking during adolescence. Though the syndrome of major depression is far rarer in prepubescent children, the symptoms these young ones experience more closely resemble depression in adults, with low mood and energy level. Thus, the mood change that takes place in severe depression before and after adolescence can be different from that seen during adolescence. Why?

It is tempting to speculate that the struggle for independence and separation from family that preoccupies most adolescents somehow makes them more "prickly" and reactive in their interactions with parents and authority figures. Perhaps depression exaggerates the tendency toward defiance that is part of every teenager's drive to find and assert his independence. This theory would state, then, that psychological issues particular to adolescence shape the depressive feelings and result in the prominent irritability. But this is pure speculation, and this very important question remains unanswered.

Onset of depression following a loss or disappointment of some type is not uncommon. In Heather's case, the disappointment was a rather minor one, and this is *not* typical. More commonly, the loss is a significant one, such as the death of someone close, parental divorce, or the breakup of a serious relationship. The exposure to the suicide of someone close has been strongly linked to the development of major depression in adults. One might want to conclude from these sorts of data that loss and stressful events can cause major depression, but this conclusion would not be quite correct, for several reasons. First, some adolescents who get depressed do not seem to have a significant stressful event preceding the development of their depression. Second, many teens who suffer a significant loss do not go on to develop severe depression. A 1995 study compared the occurrences of stressful life events in teenagers with and without major depression. It found no statistically significant difference in the total number of stressful events in the two groups.[4] That said, this is still an active field of research within psychiatry, because it seems like stressful life events should be associated with depression. And they are, but that doesn't mean they *cause* the depression. A 2010 study seemed to show a high correlation between stressful life events and depression but failed to show that these events caused the depression. In fact, this and other studies indicate that the road can go both ways, in that those who experience major depressive episodes are more likely to experience stressful life events because of their condition (failing grades, the end of romance, and similar events).[5] One expert on the relationship between depression and stressful events put it this way: "Undesirable events are ... neither necessary nor sufficient to explain the onset of an episode of depression."[6] It's possible that rather than "causing" depression, stress and especially loss trigger the development of a depression in an adolescent who is vulnerable in some way, perhaps because of genetic factors (more on genetics in chapter 15).

How common is major depression in adolescents? Some of the most recent studies have found that 8 to 10 percent of adolescents will enter a major depressive episode in any given year.[7] This is about the same rate that adults report (7 percent), which has been interpreted to mean that adult major depressive disorder is an illness that starts in adolescence.[8] Girls and women seem about twice as likely to experience major depression than boys and men once they enter into puberty (before that stage, both genders seem to be about equally predisposed).[9]

You may have noticed that we have used two similar-sounding terms: major depressive *episode* and major depressive *disorder*. Is there a difference? The answer to this question takes us into a discussion of the course that mood disorders take. We talk about "episodes" of mood disorders because they are illnesses that usually come and go throughout a person's lifetime. A person with major depressive disorder has an illness that takes the form of periods during which he has all the symptoms that make up the depressive syndrome: these periods are the major depressive episodes. Put another way, major depressive *disorder* is a psychiatric illness characterized by recurrent major depressive *episodes*.

Research has shown that in children and adolescents, a major depressive episode lasts, on average, approximately seven to nine months.[10] But a percentage of these young people have episodes that last longer; a small percentage will still have symptoms one to two years after the beginning of their illness, and in up to 10 percent, symptoms can last even beyond this if untreated.

Another striking fact about adolescent depression is its tendency to recur. In one study of adolescents with major depression, over a period of five years researchers checked in with 196 adolescent patients who'd had an episode of major depression. This study found that 47 percent of the adolescents experienced another episode of depression within the five-year period.[11] Other research suggests that for adolescents who have had major depression, up to 70 percent will go through another period of major depression within the next five years.[12] The patients in these studies are usually from clinics and hospitals, so the results tend to show what the more severe forms of the illness can be like. Also, the researchers often do not take treatment into account. In some of these studies, the teens were getting only psychotherapy, some were taking medication as well, and some were getting little or no treatment. (That many teens with serious depression, even after getting a diagnosis by a professional, either never get into treatment or stop treatment after a short period is a finding in study after study of this type.)

These numbers are sobering. Major depressive disorder in adolescents can cause lengthy periods of symptoms, and once an adolescent has had an episode, the risk for recurrence is high.

DYSTHYMIC DISORDER

Like many words used in the field of medicine, *dysthymia* comes from Greek roots. The prefix *dys-* is from a word that means "bad" or "difficult," and the root *thymia* comes from the Greek word for "mind." In psychiatry, the meaning of this root word has altered a bit and usually refers to "mood." Dysthymia, then, is an illness characterized by "bad mood." How is it different from major depressive disorder?

Persons with dysthymic disorder suffer from a smoldering low-grade depressive syndrome that persists over a period of many months, sometimes for years. It is an illness that can remain undetected and thus untreated for a very long time. These individuals sometimes see a psychiatrist for the first time as adults, when they finally come to realize that the bad feelings they have constantly struggled against are *not* normal. When asked how long they have felt depressed, many of these patients say, "As long as I can remember." Because the symptoms can develop insidiously and smolder on without precipitating a crisis, dysthymic individuals can lose track of the onset of their depressed feelings and eventually seem to forget what "normal" feels like. One of us once treated a young man, whom we will call Max Phelps, with precisely these problems.

▼ Max was the most serious-looking 13-year-old I had seen in a long time. His khakis, white shirt, and blue-striped tie added to this impression, making him look almost like a little college professor rather than a young teenager.

"Max really didn't want to come today, doctor," his mother was saying. "But he said he would as long as he didn't have to miss school to come to the appointment."

"Why was that, Max?" I asked. "Kids don't often mind missing an hour or two of school, even if it is a trip to the doctor's office."

"I don't want to have to explain to people," he answered. "Other kids are too nosy about stuff. I didn't want to have to deal with a lot of questions."

Mrs. Phelps filled in Max's story. She had noticed her youngest son becoming more and more miserable over a period of many months. "He mopes around the house or sits and watches television. His grades have slipped again this year and—"

"No, they haven't," Max said with a bit of irritation showing in his voice.

"Yes, they have, Max," his mom said. "You went from a 3 to a 2 in English in December." Mrs. Phelps looked up at me. "Now I know that's not a bad grade by any means. But it's the pattern we're worried about. He has dropped a grade point in at least one subject every semester for the past two years. Maybe it's not exactly a drastic drop, but his performance has been drifting downward for months." She looked over at her son. "Don't you agree, Max?"

"I guess so," he said, looking down.

"Have you noticed any sleep problems or eating problems?" I asked.

"No, not particularly," Mrs. Phelps replied.

"Max?" I asked.

"Huh?" he said.

"Max, honey, talk to the doctor," his mom said soothingly. She looked up at me. "He doesn't seem to be paying attention half of the time. Do you think this might be why his grades are dropping?"

"I don't know why you have to say that over and over again," Max said. "It really makes me angry."

It turned out that anger was becoming more and more of a problem as well. Max was persistently defiant at home, often about little things. "Max made his bed every day almost from the time he started kindergarten. I don't think he's made it for a year. Now, I know a lot of boys his age don't, but it just doesn't seem right for Max. He's always been so eager to help around the house."

"How is Max getting along with his friends?" I asked.

"OK," Max responded.

I looked over at Max's mom. "Yes?" I asked.

"Well, it's hard for me to tell," she said. "He spends plenty of time with his friends, but he seems to worry a lot that nobody likes him."

"Mom!" Max said a little sharply.

"Max, honey, I'm just telling the doctor what you've told me so he can help you to feel better."

Max peered down at his shoes with a stony look.

"He just seems so miserable all the time," Max's mom said. "I see his friends run up the street yelling and laughing, and then Max comes along after them almost shuffling his feet, like it's almost too much effort. He wasn't this way before." Mrs. Phelps looked over at her son wistfully. "I remember him on his tenth birthday, so full of fun and energy. But something's changed; something has been creeping up on him for a long time now. It's happened so slowly that I didn't realize it for a long time."

The "something" was depression, and the pattern was dysthymic disorder. "You did just the right thing to bring Max in," I said. "I think we can make this 'thing' go away." ▲

We like the word *smoldering* to describe dysthymic disorder. And just as a gust of wind can fan a smoldering fire into flame, stress can inflame the illness and cause symptoms of irritability to flare up. Because the symptoms aren't usually as dramatic as those of major depressive disorder, they may be easier to miss, but dysthymia can be just as dangerous.

Dysthymia, like depression, seems less common in the very young, but is certainly not unheard of—studies have shown that children as young as 5 years old can be affected. These young people have a gloomy, pessimistic, down mood and are often preoccupied with feeling unloved and left out. They feel bad about themselves and worry that they don't measure up in various ways.

In a study that attempted to contrast and compare the symptoms of dysthymic disorder and major depressive disorder, the dysthymic children were younger, had fewer guilty feelings, had less sleep or appetite disturbance, and didn't suffer from the severe loss of pleasure that is characteristic of major depression. Their mood symptoms (depressed and irritable mood) and feelings of being unloved and without good friends were about the same (table 3-2).

One of the most significant findings of this study is that early-onset dysthymic disorder seems to be an indicator for problems with other, often more severe mood symptoms later in life. As with an episode of major depression, a diagnosis of dysthymic disorder is a predictor of increased risk for more problems with depression in the future. In the study, a group of children was observed over a period of up to twelve years, and during that time, 80 percent of the children with dysthymia had another episode of a mood disorder. More than two-thirds of the fifty-five children with early-onset dysthymic disorder went on to have an episode of the more severe collection of symptoms of major depression. Most of the time, these children's symptoms worsened into major depression with no completely well time in between, a phenomenon that has been called *double depression*. In double depression, the more severe symptoms of major depression become superimposed on symptoms of dysthymia. In this group, the second and third years after the beginning of dysthymic symptoms were the period of highest risk.[13]

These findings have been interpreted to indicate that dysthymic disorder might be best thought of as a subtype or a precursor of other mood

Table 3-2 Depressive Symptoms in Children with Dysthymic Disorder and Major Depressive Disorder

| | Percentage of Children Reporting the Symptom | |
Symptom	Dysthymic Disorder	Major Depressive Disorder
Depressed or sad mood	91.7	80.0
Feeling unloved	55.6	48.9
Feeling friendless	41.7	40.0
Irritability	55.6	71.1
Anger	63.9	62.2
Anhedonia	5.6	71.1
Guilty feelings	13.9	31.1
Social withdrawal	8.3	53.3
Impaired concentration	41.7	67.4
Thoughts of wanting to die	16.7	42.2
Reduced sleep	22.2	62.2
Reduced appetite	5.6	46.7
Fatigue	22.2	64.4
Disobedience	58.3	43.2

Source: Maria Kovacs, Hagop Akiskal, Constantine Gatsonis, and Phoebe Parrone, "Childhood-Onset Dysthymic Disorder," *Archives of General Psychiatry* 51 (1994): 365–74.

disorders and may not really be a separate mood disorder after all. These findings also give new meaning to the idea that dysthymia is a "smoldering" type of depression, because in many of these young patients, the symptoms flare up into full-blown major depression.

How common is dysthymic disorder? From studies of large groups of children and adolescents, researchers have estimated lifetime rates for dysthymia of between 0.1 and 8 percent in young people.[14]

PREMENSTRUAL DYSPHORIC DISORDER

There is another, more subtle, form of depression that deserves special discussion. Recall that we earlier discussed how most girls and women are at twice the risk of developing depression than their male peers. This increased risk starts when the woman begins puberty and reverses after menopause. Although the field of psychiatry does not exactly know yet what causes depression, there is no doubt that our hormones play a large role in determining and regulating our mood. This is true for men as well, as can be seen most clearly in older men, as the level of testosterone begins to decline and depression risk increases. But it is also apparent in women who have a regular, cyclical variation of hormones as their bodies prepare for procreation. Premenstrual dysphoric disorder (PMDD) has only recently become an officially recognized entity with the advent of the *DSM*, fifth edition—prior to this, it was discussed in the literature but not officially recognized. (Women with these symptoms had to be given the diagnosis of depression not otherwise specified [NOS], a rather unsatisfying and seemingly contradictory diagnosis.)

Many adolescents report some symptoms, both physical and emotional, within about one week before their menstruation. What we are discussing here is something quite different from these anticipated symptoms. Just as most people have experienced low mood in the past but have not gone through a major depressive episode, the normal premenstrual syndrome and that of PMDD are entirely separate entities. In PMDD, the woman experiences all and exactly the same symptoms as a person with major depressive disorder. What separates PMDD from major depression is not symptoms but timing. A woman in the throes of PMDD suffers only during the week before menstruation (a hormonally tumultuous time known as the *luteal phase* of the menstrual cycle). Outside that time, the woman may be unaffected by depression of any sort, or may suffer from a dysthymia or major depression that seems to significantly worsen during this time. The condition can be serious to the point of impairment in some patients, so that they cannot function at school or work; they may entertain suicidal thoughts. Some have reported experiencing the most severe depressive symptoms, including hallucinations, when at their worst.

We have said all along that the diagnosis of major depression is made not only by the severity of symptoms but also on the symptoms' tenacity, their pervasiveness. The diagnosis of PMDD can be particularly difficult because the symptoms are not consistent—someone incapacitated by her depression can appear to be perfectly fine the next week. What can be examined, however, is a long-term pattern in which an adolescent consistently experiences the same symptoms in the same time frame before her menses. And it can be a critical diagnosis to make, as it nearly always requires biological treatment (that is, medications) rather than psychotherapy. Treatment of depression and its related entities is something we talk more about later, but for now it is important to note that the treatment for PMDD is somewhat different than that for routine major depression, so the distinction between the two can mean the difference between continual suffering and recovery.

PMDD is rare. Although almost 80 percent of women experience some premenstrual symptoms, and approximately 20 percent have symptoms that "interfere with life," only about 1.3 percent experience true PMDD.[15] This disorder is even less common than the other depressive disorders we have been discussing. Rare as PMDD is, we make it a point to routinely ask every female patient we evaluate about any relationship between her depression and her menstruation, because it makes a significant difference when determining what sort of treatment we would undertake.

BIPOLAR DISORDER

Bipolar disorder, or more formally bipolar affective disorder, in children and adolescents is a topic of some debate, even among the most revered experts in the field. The subject has become so extensively argued that it could be the subject of an entire book unto itself. Within these pages, we give an overview of what bipolar disorder is, what it is not, and how it relates to depression. This will necessitate a somewhat lengthy discussion in the midst of a book that is supposed to be devoted solely to adolescent depression, but given the wild increase in diagnosis of bipolar disorder (and a close cousin, mood disorder NOS) in adolescents, we feel it deserves a good amount of thoughtful conversation.

First, according to the *DSM* and the field of psychiatry, what exactly is bipolar affective disorder? The description can be discerned from a careful examination of the name itself: *bi-* (meaning two), *polar* (therefore having two poles), *affective* (relating to mood) disorder. The following case study illustrates these "two poles" of mood as they play out in the life of a teenager whom we will call Kelly.

▼ Finally, finally, thought Anne, the treatment was working! Her daughter Kelly had always been a bit of a bookworm, sure, but so was the rest of the family. Because of Kelly's introverted nature, it had taken Anne some time to recognize that her daughter had started to become depressed. It shouldn't have been that big of a surprise, really, since depression ran in her husband's family, but at first it was hard to believe it had happened to their child. Still, seeing the psychiatrist was the best thing they had ever done. Since starting treatment, her daughter had come back to herself. She found a renewed love of books, her small but close group of friends had gotten back together, and her schoolwork had recovered.

Ever since she turned 16, though, Kelly had started to come out of her shell in a way that no one had expected. She was hanging out with more friends, and Anne's shy, introverted daughter had actually gone out for the school play! In fact, some of the things she was doing were firsts for the whole family. Anne and her husband were quiet people, as was their younger son, Allen, so Kelly joining the cheerleading squad was new to all of them. Anne wasn't all that surprised that Allen was a bit jealous, but some of the things he was saying about Kelly were getting out of control, that she's "so energetic it's like she's on crack." The truth was that both Anne and her husband were really excited to have such a well-rounded child and thought that maybe the psychiatrist had "cured" her.

As Anne was lost in her thoughts, the door slammed open, and Kelly bounded into the room.

"Hi, Mom! How was your day? Mine was great! I got a role in the play, and cheerleading practice was just the best! I can't believe I never got into it before. You know I think I'm the best in the whole squad; I'm teaching other people how to do what I do! Maybe next I'll start that home ec class—I just love cooking lately, and I'm really great at it! I was watching a cooking show the other day, and they were making pizza. That's something we haven't had for a while. Why don't we go out for pizza tonight? My favorite is pepperoni, but I've gotta watch those pounds . . ."

Anne started to lose focus. Her daughter did tend to ramble on lately, but you had to forgive her—she had so many new, exciting things to talk about. It was a little surprising that Kelly was so interested in home ec. Truth be told, she was pretty useless in the kitchen, although she seemed to be working hard at learning to cook. Last week, Anne woke to the sound of pots and pans banging around at three in the morning and found her daughter baking up a storm.

"Are you even listening?!" yelled Kelly.

Anne broke out of her reverie and felt a little shocked. While she had been thinking, Kelly had walked right up to her and was yelling in her face.

"I said I'm going to a party and asked like a billion times for the car keys!"

Now that was strange. Kelly knew she wasn't allowed to go out at night when she had a test the next day.

"Sweetie, you know you have that English—" Anne picked up her purse almost without thinking about it, right as Kelly ripped it out of her hands, so hard Anne lurched forward.

"You can't stop me!" yelled Kelly again, as she took out the car keys, threw the purse to the floor, and ran out the front door.

Anne knew that kids could be moody, but this was ridiculous. Anne reached for the phone and dialed. Her husband picked up after two rings.

"Steven, it's me. Kelly ran out of the house again. No, she grabbed the ones to your car. I still keep mine in the dresser after last time. Look, I know you hate these interruptions. Just please come home. Yes, you told me this is exactly how it started with your brother. That's why I'm worried!" ▲

Some people with severe depressions have other types of abnormal mood states in addition to their depressions, periods that are in many ways quite the opposite. During these episodes, they experience increased physical energy and psychological agitation. Instead of being slowed down and lethargic, they feel sped up and energized. Their thoughts can race so much that their speech can't keep up; they jump from topic to topic, and they don't make sense. Their mood state can be giddy and high, or extremely irritable. But whether the abnormal mood state is pleasantly high or irritable, these individuals are abnormally energized, restless, and activated. These are some of the symptoms of *mania* (table 3-3).

People with bipolar disorder can also have a strange mix of the activation and agitation of mania combined with the negative thinking and mood of depression, a separate mood state called a *mixed affective state*, or simply a *mixed state*. Mixed states are very dangerous, because depressing thought patterns are combined with excess energy, restlessness, and an inner sense of pressure and tension. This negative energy puts these individuals at high risk for hurting themselves with suicidal behaviors.

Originally, the name for the illness characterized by periods of depression and periods of manic symptoms was *manic-depression* (or *manic-depressive illness*, or *disorder*). More recently, the term *bipolar disorder* has come to be used almost universally.

Table 3-3 Symptoms of Mania

Mood Symptoms
- Elated, euphoric mood
- Irritable mood
- Grandiosity

Cognitive (Thinking) Symptoms
- Feelings of heightened concentration
- Accelerated thinking ("racing thoughts")

Bodily Symptoms
- Increased energy level
- Decreased need for sleep
- Erratic appetite
- Increased sexual feelings

Symptoms of Psychosis
- Grandiose delusions
- Hallucinations

Bipolar symptoms can be dramatic and extremely dangerous, but they can be rather subtle as well. Individuals may not have the frenzied, disorganized extreme mood state of mania but may instead have *hypomania* (*hypo-* is the Greek prefix meaning "below"), a less severe "high" in which they are overconfident, tend to be reckless and lose inhibitions, and have a giddy over-optimism that causes them to take unaccustomed risks and to exercise poor judgment.

Many parents might think this sounds precisely like most of the teenagers they have met—a little indestructible, a little overconfident, and somewhat reckless. Remember how we distinguished true depression from more transient and understandable sadness? In mania and hypomania, these characteristics constitute a *change* from someone's normal temperament and way of behaving and feeling. Additionally, they are not usually the result of something that has occurred in the person's life. Every teenager who has a first date may be a little giddy, but for teenagers suffering from mania (yes, it sounds strange to say that someone is "suffering" from excessive happiness, but the same word is used—we get to why later), their high mood descends on them from out of the blue, usually with little or no correlation to what's happening in their lives. Some people cycle through different moods almost daily, feeling gloomy then giddy then irritable for brief periods with hardly any moments of normal mood. This is why we say that someone *suffers* with mania, because that the elevated mood cannot last indefinitely. According to most experts, there is no unipolar manic psychiatric illness, unlike depression, which can be unipolar. We both have experience with patients afflicted with bipolar affective disorder who secretly (or not so secretly) want their manias to last forever and sometimes despise medications for "taking away the highs." But what goes up must, in fact, come down, and people experiencing mania do inevitably enter a depression. It is this wild swing of emotion that brings about the suffering—as, at times, do the activities in which a manic person engages. Persons in a manic state tend to lose all sense of consequence to their actions. They will shoplift, speed, cheat on their loved ones, and so on. Once the mania lifts, only then do they experience the repercussions of their actions and have to face them head on, often while falling into a depressed state, which amplifies their negative feelings tremendously.

CONTROVERSIES SURROUNDING BIPOLAR AFFECTIVE DISORDER IN CHILDREN

The bipolar affective illness and all its variations are well described in adults, but much less so in children. Psychiatry is only beginning to understand how these illnesses show up in younger people. This may seem confusing, because the prevalence of bipolar affective illness in children seems to be exploding. How can there be an exponential increase in the diagnosis of an illness, the symptoms of which even the most revered experts disagree on? This was the challenge facing the committee writing the new version of the *DSM*, the *DSM-5*, and it came up with quite a creative answer to this perplexing question.

From a historical perspective, bipolar disorder was traditionally thought to be extremely rare in young people—even though research data on adults indicated that the first symptoms of bipolar disorder usually appeared before the age of 20. Perhaps because of a reluctance to diagnose children with an illness known to be a lifelong problem, and perhaps because of a hesitation to prescribe for children the powerful medications used to treat its symptoms, bipolar disorder in young children received little attention from researchers until quite recently. At the time of publication of the *DSM-IV* (1994) and the *DSM-IV-TR* ("text revision," 2000), the prevalence of children and adolescents diagnosed with bipolar affective disorder was small. Then, suddenly, something changed. From 1997 to 2003, the number of persons younger than 18 diagnosed with this condition increased forty-fold, from about 0.025 percent of children to about 1 to 2 percent—the same proportion as seen in adults.[16,17] What had been a seemingly rare and mysterious condition had become rather commonplace. When we say that a psychiatric illness is "rare," we mean that the population with a particular illness is small relative to the general, unaffected population. Imagine a room filled with one hundred adolescents—a school lunchroom, for example. In this scenario, in 2004, one of those children would be diagnosed with bipolar affective disorder. This may not seem like all that much, but now imagine a room filled with four thousand young people—a moderately sized liberal arts college, for example. In 1997, only one of those young persons would have been diagnosed with bipolar affective disorder. Quite a difference! And the numbers continue to rise.

There is another, more nebulous diagnosis in the *DSM* called "mood disorder not otherwise specified." It is similar to depression NOS, though even more vague. It is ideally meant to capture all those people who we believe have a mood disorder (something in the depressive or bipolar scales) but who do not meet strict criteria for any specific disorder. Its use, however, has unfortunately grown to describe those adolescents with any sort of extreme emotional state, however transient—among children aged 1 to 17 years old, "mood disorder" was the single most common diagnosis and reason for hospitalization in 2011, edging out even medical diagnoses like asthma and injury.[18]

This extreme increase caught the attention of some of the most renowned experts in the world of psychiatry and invited a number of questions. What was happening? Were children becoming more ill? Was bipolar affective illness occurring earlier and earlier in a person's life? Had the whole of human history missed out on the early development of such a serious condition in the young? Or was it psychiatry's fault—had we lost our way and were misdiagnosing huge swaths of the population? Unfortunately, the last answer seems to be the correct one.

How could this have happened? Essentially, psychiatrists had begun to broaden their definition of what the bipolar syndrome looked like in young people. Some psychiatrists even thought they could predict it.

Recall that mania and hypomania can be characterized by elevated energy, impulsivity, and a giddy or happy mood, *or by those same symptoms combined with irritability*. Some experts felt that the "childhood presentation" of bipolar affective disorder could be different from that of adults, in that it is more frequently characterized by an irritable mood than an elated one (as it is in depression). They reasoned that the combination of wild temper tantrums, disinhibited behavior (such as destroying property), and irritability may be the "bipolar" of childhood.

In bipolar affective disorder of all types, there is a phenomenon known as *kindling*. The name comes from the idea of kindling a fire—what starts off as a small flame can grow to be a large bonfire, given sufficient time. Research has shown that bipolar affective disorder seems to get worse the longer it remains untreated and the more episodes of mania or depression the person has. The episodes become more frequent, more severe, and more difficult to treat. Traditionally, researchers had always been most concerned about the initial "flame"—the first episode of mania. But in the early 2000s, some investigators tried to reach even further back, to find the spark behind the flame.

DISRUPTIVE MOOD DYSREGULATION DISORDER

Though poorly characterized in the literature, there seemed to be a group of children who were angrier and more irritable than their peers. They weren't really depressed, in that they didn't have the other symptoms we typically think of (social isolation, sleep pattern changes, low mood, suicidal thoughts, and so on). In fact, some of their symptoms were a little closer to mania: the children were more likely to act before thinking rather than thinking before acting (called *disinhibition*), seemed to have a restless quality, were aggressive, seemed to need less sleep (as opposed to being unable to sleep but being tired the next day), and so on. These children didn't seem to have discrete "episodes" like adults—in a way, they were like a pilot light yet to turn into a full flame, a little kernel of bipolar affective disorder just waiting to pop. Could this be the precursor to adult bipolar affective disorder? Is this what it looked like in childhood? Early evidence seemed to suggest that, yes, children with this collection of symptoms had family histories of bipolar affective disorder, and yes, some of the same medications seemed to help. The word got out, and psychiatrists expanded their practice to include more and more children with this diagnosis.

Others at the pinnacle of the field disagreed with this theory. As evidence mounted, the explanation that these children had bipolar affective disorder seemed thinner and thinner. One study examined a large cohort of adults with true bipolar affective disorder. Few if any of them had had this constellation of symptoms as children, no more than the nonpsychiatrically ill population, and about 20 percent had had their first true manic episode as an adolescent (none as children). Another study followed a group of children diagnosed with bipolar disorder longitudinally and found that they were far more likely to develop true major depressive or anxiety disorders as adults (with no episodes of mania or hypomania). These experts were concerned by the trend of expanding the bipolar phenotype to include what they saw as normal childhood reactions to life stressors. They took the stance that pediatric bipolar affective disorder should be treated no differently than adult bipolar affective disorder, that a child must meet exactly the same criteria as adults, and that a child who was irritable and throwing tantrums was simply that and was at no higher chance of developing bipolar disorder (and needing medications) than any other child. Irritability, by itself, can be a symptom in several psychiatric conditions and life circumstances—everything from a major depressive episode to simply having a bad day.

Regardless of this undecided debate, many in the field began diagnosing children who experienced an episode of irritability as having mood disorder NOS or bipolar affective disorder. Essentially, psychiatrists had changed their practice from using a quite rigid definition of bipolar disorder to using a looser one that encompassed wider and wider groups of children. Child psychiatrists made this change not out of malice or laziness, but because they had no other way to characterize this population. Unfortunately for the young person, this diagnostic change had dire consequences. As we've said, this diagnosis was the number one reason for hospitalization among this age group, so many children were admitted to a psychiatric hospital. Many others were started on medications to "control their bipolar affective disorder." Although medications can be helpful and at times necessary, they can have side effects, so many of these children may have been exposed to unnecessary uncomfortable physical changes (such as weight gain and fatigue).

Sitting down together, the *DSM-5* committee on mood disorders faced a conundrum. No one would argue that bipolar affective disorder is unheard of in adolescents. There were young persons out in the world who needed to be accurately diagnosed and treated for their sake and the sake of their families. At the same time, this committee had to figure out some way to tease apart more accurately who actually had the *syndrome* of bipolar affective disorder and who may have been having some similar *symptoms* of mania (such as irritability) for another reason. This much larger group of children could not simply be thrown out of the *DSM*. In *DSM-5*, the committee explains its trial between the Scylla of underdiagnosis and the Charybdis of overdiagnosis:

> During the latter decades of the 20th century, this contention by researchers that severe, non-episodic irritability is a manifestation of pediatric mania coincided with an upsurge in the rates at which clinicians assigned the diagnosis of bipolar disorder to their pediatric patients. This sharp increase in rates appears to be attributable to clinicians combining at least two clinical presentations into a single category. That is, both classic, episodic presentations of mania and non-episodic presentations of severe irritability have been labeled as bipolar disorder in children. In DSM-5, the term bipolar disorder is explicitly reserved for episodic presentations of bipolar symptoms. DSM-IV did not include a diagnosis designed to capture youths whose hallmark symptoms consisted of very severe, non-episodic irritability, whereas DSM-5 ... provides a distinct category for such presentations.[19]

How, indeed, does the *DSM-5* accomplish this goal? Here is their solution in their own words:

> Unlike in DSM-IV, this chapter "Depressive Disorders" has been separated from the previous chapter "Bipolar and Related Disorders" ... In order to address concerns about the potential for the overdiagnosis of and treatment for bipolar disorder in children, a new diagnosis, disruptive mood dysregulation disorder, referring to the presentation of children with persistent irritability and frequent episodes of extreme behavioral dyscontrol, is added to the depressive disorders ... Its placement in this chapter reflects the finding that children with this symptom pattern typically develop unipolar depressive disorders or anxiety disorders, rather than bipolar disorders, as they mature into adolescence

and adulthood . . . The core feature of disruptive mood dysregulation disorder is chronic, severe persistent irritability. This severe irritability has two prominent clinical manifestations, the first of which is frequent temper outbursts . . . The second manifestation of severe irritability consists of chronic, persistently ir- ritable or angry mood that is present between the severe temper outbursts.[20]

Disruptive mood dysregulation disorder (DMDD), then, was their solu- tion. They firmly separated this cohort of children into those with a true cyclical, independent syndrome with both manic episodes and depressive episodes and those best described as irritable with temper tantrums out of proportion to, but in response to, life circumstances.

It should be noted that this book is being written mere months after the creation of the *DSM-5*. Change takes time, and many psychiatrists have yet to adopt the practice of using the diagnosis of disruptive mood dysregula- tion disorder. This lag occurs for several reasons—medical billing has yet to figure out where this diagnosis fits in the reimbursement scheme; hospitals and universities have not yet altered their documentation to incorporate it; there is a significant dearth of research on its prevalence and availabil- ity; and, quite simply, old habits die hard. (By the way, a dearth of research always makes practitioners nervous. We like to think we practice based on evidence—in fact, lack of research was what kept premenstrual dysphoric disorder from being officially recognized in the main body of the *DSM* for twenty years.) We believe that the changes made in the *DSM* concerning pediatric bipolar disorder are positive ones that can spare children and their families from unnecessary treatments and hospitalizations while still providing help to those who need it. That said, no one, not even psychia- trists, has a crystal ball, and so we have little idea as to how this diagnosis will be clinically used and how it will evolve over time. Future research may show that disruptive mood dysregulation disorder does not exist as an entity and instead is merely a descriptive term for those children who have trouble controlling their anger. The evidence behind DMDD is in its infancy; but the evidence for bipolar affective disorder, in its traditional form, is decades long, so we can speak about that, at least, with some con- fidence. For the remainder of this chapter, we discuss only those adoles- cents meeting criteria for the bipolar disorder spectrum as defined in the

DSM-5. Along this spectrum, psychiatrists agree that there are three major subtypes of bipolar disorder: *bipolar I, bipolar II,* and *cyclothymia.*

BIPOLAR I

Bipolar I is the designation for the classic variety of bipolar disorder characterized by full-blown manic attacks and deep, paralyzing depressions. A schematic representation of the moods of bipolar I is shown in figure 3-1.

The pattern of abnormal mood episodes seems to vary widely, and the pattern of the illness is almost as individual as the person who has the illness. Symptoms of bipolar I usually begin in the late teens or early twenties, so the diagnosis is important to consider in young people with any type of mood disorder. Like the other mood disorders, bipolar I is what physicians refer to as a *relapsing and remitting illness*—during the course of the illness, its symptoms come and go of their own accord and may disappear, without any treatment at all, for months or even years at a time. Clinical studies on the course of bipolar disorder performed in the years before effective treatments for this disorder were available document and illustrate the pattern of bipolar disorder symptoms that existed when the illness was not treated—what physicians call the *natural history* of the illness.

In a 1942 study, researchers looked at the records of sixty-six patients with "manic-depressive psychosis," some of whom had been under observation for up to twenty-six years. These patients went through what we

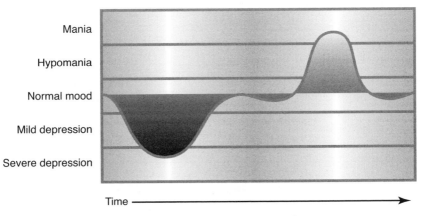

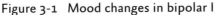

Figure 3-1 Mood changes in bipolar I

now call episodes of the illness, periods of severe depression or mania that lasted for several months (though sometimes much longer) and then went away on their own, with the patient's emotional state returning to normal. Although a few patients seemed to have had only one episode of illness in the period of the study, about one-third had two to three episodes; one-third, four to six episodes; and one-third, more than seven. A few had twenty or more episodes (table 3-4). Unfortunately, when a person is diagnosed with bipolar I disorder, there is no way to know whether the individual will have another two or three episodes during his lifetime or more than twenty.

Bipolar I is the classic manic-depressive illness, with fully developed manic episodes and episodes of severe depression. It is also characterized by long periods of "hibernation," when the symptoms temporarily disappear. The number of episodes varies enormously, but individuals who have only one or two episodes seem to be the exception rather than the rule. Before the availability of effective treatments, the average length of each episode, if untreated, was about six months (in the 1942 study discussed above, the average duration was about six and a half months), but episodes that lasted years and years were not at all uncommon (table 3-5).

Bipolar I disorder seems to be uncommon in teenagers. In 1995, an important study on mood disorders in high school students was published in the *Journal of the American Academy of Child and Adolescent Psychiatry.*[21] To find out how common the various subtypes of mood disorders were in high school students, these researchers interviewed 1,709 boys and girls between the ages of 14 and 17 who attended a high school in western Oregon.

Table 3-4   Episodes of Illness in Sixty-Six Adult Patients with Bipolar Disorder

Number of Episodes	Percentage of Patients
1	8
2–3	29
4–6	26
More than 7	37

Source: Data from Thomas A. C. Rennie, "Prognosis in Manic-Depressive Psychosis," *American Journal of Psychiatry* 98 (1942): 801–14, quoted in Frederick Goodwin and Kay Redfield Jamison, *Manic-Depressive Illness* (New York: Oxford University Press, 1990), 133.
Note: This study was done before the availability of any effective treatment for bipolar disorder.

Table 3-5 Features of Bipolar I Disorder

Mood
    Fully developed manic episodes
    Fully developed depressive episodes
Other Features
    Untreated episodes lasting an average of six months

The students were interviewed twice, about a year apart. Only two cases of bipolar I were identified; that is, two students had a history of a full-blown mania, the main diagnostic criterion for bipolar I. Bipolar affective disorder type I is extremely rare in younger children and should prompt a second opinion evaluation by an expert in the field.

BIPOLAR II

Bipolar II is characterized by fully developed depressive episodes and episodes of *hypo*mania. Figure 3-2 shows a schematic representation of the moods of bipolar II.

When lithium became available in the United States in the 1970s, and researchers were trying to find better diagnostic criteria for bipolar disorder, several noticed a large group of patients who didn't have a history of fully developed manic episodes, but who seemed to have a bipolar disorder nonetheless. These people had severe depressions, but their "highs" never developed into mania. Were they "manic-depressives" who were still early in the course of their illness and simply hadn't had time to have a fully de-

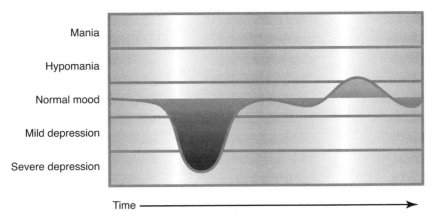
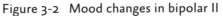

Figure 3-2 Mood changes in bipolar II

veloped manic episode? Several studies attempting to answer this question concluded that these patients did *not* usually go on to have fully developed mania. In one study, less than 5 percent of the patients with recurrent depressions and hypomania eventually became manic.[22] Several studies also showed that many patients with this type of disorder had relatives with a bipolar mood disorder also characterized by major depressions and hypomanias.[23] Although people with bipolar II sometimes have family members who have bipolar I or depressive disorders (without either mania or hypomania), the disorder frequently seems to show up in an identical form in affected families: family members of a person with bipolar II who have mood disorders also tend to have the bipolar II symptom pattern.[24] People with bipolar II disorder also seem to be at higher risk for alcoholism.[25] (See table 3-6 for a list of features characterizing bipolar II.)

Compared with people who have bipolar I disorder, those with bipolar II seem to have more problems with depression—in fact, the depression is sometimes so prominent that many receive a diagnosis of depressive disorder and don't get treatment for bipolar disorder at all. In a study from the National Institutes of Health published in 1995, 559 adult patients diagnosed with a *depressive* disorder were observed over time, some for up to eleven years. Almost 9 percent of them developed symptoms of bipolar II.[26] The first hypomanic episode could usually be documented within several months of the onset of severe depression, but sometimes it took up to nine years for the correct diagnosis to become clear. Some of these 559 "depression" patients also developed a manic episode; that is, they actually had bipolar I, but this was far less common (only 3.9 percent). This study also found that patients with bipolar II disorder had longer depressive episodes (about a year) than those with bipolar I (about six months).

The study of Oregon high school students described above found eleven adolescents (about 0.6 percent) who had had a major depressive episode and had also gone through a period of elevated or irritable mood and other symptoms of hypomania, the pattern of bipolar II.[27] As you might have already figured out, this is about five times the number of students with bipolar I disorder. This finding is consistent with several studies in adults indicating that bipolar II may be more common than bipolar I.

Recall that this study took place prior to the explosion of bipolar affective diagnoses in children. It was undertaken at a time when researchers

Table 3-6 Features of Bipolar II Disorder

Mood
    Fully developed depressive episodes
    Hypomanic episodes
Other Features
    Increased sleep and appetite during depressions
    Depression, sometimes more chronic than with bipolar I
    Family history of bipolar II
    Later age at first hospitalization
    Fewer hospitalizations
    Possible increased risk for alcoholism

still had a more "pure" view of what bipolar affective disorder had to be in children and young adults. Though we do not have access to the actual tools used to describe these young people in their hypomanic states, the states are described as episodes and include distinct periods of elated mood as well as distinct periods of irritable mood that are presumably different from the adolescents' normal mood. Therefore, the results likely encompass those who with some certainty would fit into the bipolar II category. A more recent study may be slightly more suspicious for lumping those with depressed irritability in with the bipolar population.

CYCLOTHYMIC DISORDER

Cyclothymic disorder, or cyclothymia, is characterized by frequent short periods (days to weeks) of mild depressive symptoms and hypomania separated by periods (which also tend to be days to weeks) of fairly normal mood. By definition, the person does not have either fully developed major depressive episodes or manic episodes. A schematic representation of the moods of cyclothymia is presented in figure 3-3.

Individuals with cyclothymic disorder have frequent ups and downs of mood with only comparatively few periods of "normal" mood. Cyclothymic disorder also begins early in life—in the late teens or early twenties. Although many persons with this disorder never develop more severe mood symptoms, a significant number of them eventually have a fully developed depression or manic episode; that is, they develop bipolar disorder. In one study, about 6 percent of patients with the cyclothymic pattern eventually had a manic episode, putting them into the bipolar I category, but a higher

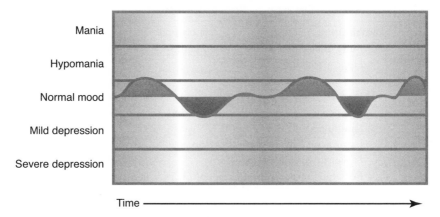

Figure 3-3   Mood changes in cyclothymia

number (25 percent) developed severe depression—they turned out to have bipolar II.[28] Perhaps half of people with the cyclothymic pattern never develop symptoms of "full-blown" bipolar disorder—a finding that makes cyclothymia a true diagnosis in its own right (table 3-7).

Family history studies suggest some relationship between cyclothymia and other bipolar disorders. People with cyclothymia often have relatives with bipolar disorder but rarely have relatives suffering from depressions only. Treatment experiences seem to confirm this relationship—the mood swings of cyclothymic disorder often respond to many of the same treatment approaches as the bipolar disorders do. Cyclothymia was at one time thought to be a personality type, not an illness. Research indicates that this is not true.

In the Oregon study, 5 of the 1,709 students surveyed were diagnosed with cyclothymic disorder. These students had suffered from ups and downs of mood with periods of significant depression but had never experienced the full syndrome of a major depressive episode.[29]

BIPOLAR "SPECTRUM" DISORDERS

If you look at the end of the section on bipolar disorders in the American Psychiatric Association's *Diagnostic and Statistical Manual*, you will see a category titled "Bipolar Disorder Not Otherwise Specified" (also called simply "bipolar NOS"). This odd category exists because the developers of the *DSM* recognized that some patients seem to have a kind of bi-

Table 3-7   Features of Cyclothymic Disorder

Mood
  Frequent alternation between mild depression and mild hypomania
  Short, irregular cycles (days)
  Only short periods of normal mood
Other Features
  Pattern appears in late teens, early twenties
  Frequently mistaken for problems with "personality"
  Sometimes develops into bipolar I or bipolar II disorder

polar disorder but don't really fit the usual picture for bipolar I or II or for cyclothymia.

Psychiatrists have long recognized the existence of many forms of bipolar disorder. For many years, clinicians have described various types of "soft" bipolar disorder, mostly in patients who came to be treated for depression and whose illness seemed related to bipolar disorder.[30] Terms such as *pseudo-unipolar depression* and *bipolar III* have been coined to describe various types of severe depressions that have some features of bipolar disorder but do not fall into traditional categories for bipolar diagnoses. Research into these less defined categories of bipolar disorder are ongoing, but none are officially recognized in the *DSM*.

As more and more treatments for bipolar disorder become available and as more research on the mood disorders is done, we are finding that many patients who suffer from mostly depressive symptoms can benefit from treatment with medications for bipolar disorders and may, in fact, have a type of bipolar disorder. Although we haven't yet figured out how to classify and accurately diagnose these problems, it is becoming clear that they are related in some way to bipolar disorders and that many depressed patients who don't seem to have classic "manic-depressive illness" benefit from medications used to treat those disorders. In the treatment section of this book, we begin to hint at the reasons this may be, but the utter truth is that we simply don't know. From a research standpoint, we do know that people have individual responses to medications: one person's symptoms of depression may respond better to, say, Zoloft (sertraline), while another person with exactly the same symptoms will respond better to Prozac (fluoxetine). The simple fact is that the field of psychiatry has not yet evolved to the point where we can say why this is so (though genetic studies are coming closer to answering the question), any more than we can answer why some individuals with seemingly unipolar depression do much better when a medication for bipolar affective disorder is added to their regimen. This is why having a good psychiatrist who is continually evaluating and reassessing your child's treatment is essential.

MORE ON DIAGNOSIS

As you've probably noticed from the discussion thus far, the boundaries between the various depressive disorders of adolescence are not very clear. Studies indicate that children and adolescents with dysthymia can eventually develop major depressive episodes. Does it make sense to change such a child's diagnosis to major depressive disorder? Did one illness turn into another? Did the child have major depressive disorder all along? If so, why give the problem two different names?

It is useful to remember that modern psychiatry's tendency to split different mood problems into separate diagnostic categories depending on symptom pattern and duration is comparatively new. In fact, the category of mood disorders as a subgroup of psychiatric disorders is only about two hundred years old. Before that, such words as *insanity* and *madness* were used loosely to refer to almost any kind of severe psychiatric problems, even for illnesses we now recognize as medical illnesses that can cause psychiatric symptoms, such as central nervous system syphilis and Alzheimer's disease. The term *melancholia* was used to refer to illnesses we would call severe depression, but this was thought of as a type of "madness" too.

At the beginning of the twentieth century, the great German psychiatrist Emil Kraepelin wrote a new edition of his influential textbook of psychiatry and coined the term *manic-depressive insanity* to encompass *all* the relapsing psychiatric disorders characterized by abnormal mood states. What we now call major depressive disorder, dysthymia, and the various types of bipolar disorder would have been considered forms of manic-depression. Dr. Kraepelin believed that each of these illnesses was a variation of one illness: "In the course of years I have become more and more convinced that all [mood disorders] only represent manifestations of a *single morbid [disease] process*."[31] Kraepelin proposed that seemingly different mood disorders share the same fundamental causes and therefore can never be accurately separated into distinct categories. To modern ears, this makes a certain sort of intuitive sense. What seems to be affected in all the conditions described above is the regularity and integrity of someone's mood state, hinting that a single area of the brain or a single mechanism is affected. Though this may be true, it is similar to saying (and please forgive the analogy), "All cancers represent manifestations of a single morbid process." This is, in a sense, true—in cancer, cells lose the ability to control their own growth and begin to invade surrounding areas. But there are hugely significant differences in the various causes of this change, how it occurs, in which cells, how quickly they grow, how they are treated, and so on. We would argue that mood disorders are similar: they can certainly be grouped roughly together, but in their subtle distinctions, they prove themselves to be different beasts indeed. The *DSM-5* committee seems to be taking a similar view, by separating depressive disorders from bipolar disorders in the fifth edition.

For parents wondering what treatment is best for their depressed child, this discussion might seem a rather useless debate about theoretical matters, the psychiatric equivalent of medieval theologians debating the number of angels that can dance on the head of a pin. But if you remember what we said previously about the importance of diagnosis in predicting the future course of an illness and in helping select treatment, it becomes clearer that this "theoretical debate" has significant practical implications. Research on treatments is meaningful only if the researchers agree on the diagnosis of the individual being treated.

For a time after the first antidepressant medications became available, in the early 1960s, these medications were thought to treat just about any kind of depression. People who suffered from mild, moderate, or severe depressions, with or without the associated symptoms of the depressive syndrome, were often prescribed a "mood elevator," as these pharmaceuticals were sometimes called. The belief then was that antidepressants treated the symptom of depression no matter what the cause, just as aspirin will bring down a feverish person's temperature whether the fever is caused by the flu, pneumonia, or malaria.

Soon it became apparent that antidepressants were of tremendous benefit to some people who complained of depression but seemed to have no effect on others, and that the medications could cause some depressed individuals to develop a manic episode (those who, as we now realize, had a bipolar disorder). By studying the characteristics of patients for whom these medications did or did not work, it became possible to predict with better accuracy which patients antidepressants would help.

Now we have several dozen different antidepressants available, another half dozen or so mood-stabilizing medications, plus several other classes of medications that seem to be helpful in some mood disorder patients. Unfortunately, we are still not very good at predicting precisely which medication will work best for which patient. One of the first steps in getting better at this is improving our diagnostic categories.

Another problem in trying to make a diagnosis in a young person is that mood disorders are, by their nature, relapsing and remitting disorders: symptoms develop, go on for a time, and then may go away on their own, without any treatment. As you have seen, our diagnostic categories are based on how the symptoms fluctuate over time. In a young person who is suffering from depressive symptoms for the first time, an accurate diagnosis may be impossible simply because the course of the illness hasn't had time to play out.

Despite these problems with diagnosis, there are a few facts most psychiatrists agree on. The division of mood disorders into two broad categories based on whether the individual has only depressive symptoms or has depressive as well as manic or mixed symptoms seems to be an important distinction. The terms *unipolar depression* and *bipolar depression* (or *disorder*) describe these two types of depression problems. The bipolar disorders have several subcategories as well, as we've described above. We have already seen that depressive disorders are further subdivided into *major depressive disorder* and *dysthymic disorder*. The foundation for medical treatment of unipolar depressions tends to be antidepressant medications, and treatment for bipolar disorders is usually mood-stabilizing medications. But either type—or both types—of medication may be used in some patients with either type of disorder, because such combinations have been shown to be necessary and effective for some patients.

Some interpret this as proving that Dr. Kraepelin was right after all, that all the mood disorders stem from a "single morbid process." Others insist that we just haven't figured out the right system of categories and diagnostic methods.

So, what is the bottom line here? Psychiatric diagnosis is imprecise and difficult, and the making of a diagnosis must often be tentative. The diagnosis is helpful in predicting the probable course of the illness over time but less helpful in selecting a particular medication.

THE IMPORTANCE OF TREATMENT

Although mental health professionals may disagree about the classification of depressive disorders of adolescence, there is little disagreement about the importance of treatment. Three facts underscore the importance of getting treatment started quickly and making sure the person stays in treatment: (1) depression causes adolescents to suffer significant impairment in many areas of functioning; (2) serious depression is associated with other psychiatric problems, especially substance abuse; and (3) serious depression is a relapsing illness, and adolescent depression can lead to depression in adulthood.

One of the most important reasons for aggressive treatment of depressive disorders in adolescence is the tremendous toll these illnesses take on the functioning and development of teenagers if untreated. As you have seen in this chapter, the symptoms of these disorders can go on for many months, even years, if not treated.

The consequences are far more than repeating classes or being held back a year in school (though these consequences can be significant enough, particularly for adolescents with depleted internal resiliency thanks to depression). These illnesses can essentially shut down the developmental process during a period of very important emotional growth and change. In chapter 2, we reviewed the developmental "tasks" of adolescence, essentially the struggle for differentiation from parents and establishment of a personal identity. Adolescence is a time when important groundwork is laid for mature social functioning and for educational and career development. The adolescent begins to learn to navigate independently in the world and to develop interpersonal skills such as negotiation and compromise. These require a strengthening of self-confidence and healthy independence, exactly the things the adolescent is deprived of by depression. A year of developmental "shutdown" can require several years of "catch-up" to overcome.

In a study that compared the school performance of sixty-two depressed adolescents (average age about 15 years) with thirty-eight adolescents who had no psychiatric illness, the depressed adolescents showed a variety of impairments.[32] In addition to lowered school achievement, these young people were more likely to have behavioral problems in school, they complained that they didn't like their teachers, and their parents received more teacher complaints about them—all illustrating how this illness poisons school life and relationships for the affected adolescent.

There is also evidence that a period of depression has long-lasting effects on adolescents even after they recover from an episode of the illness. The researchers who conducted the Oregon study discussed earlier found that depressed adolescents were "scarred" by the experience of depression in long-lasting ways.[33] They compared a group of students who had never been depressed with a group who had developed and recovered from a major depressive episode. When the adolescents were studied several months after the depressed students had recovered, problems with excess worrying and social withdrawal were found to be more common in the once depressed than in the never depressed group. The formerly depressed students also had less emotional independence and tended to need more emotional support and approval from others. And cigarette smoking was more common among the formerly depressed students. Perhaps the most instructive finding of this study was that only about a quarter of the adolescents who had gone through a depression had received treatment of any kind for their mood problems.

How long does it take to catch up? In 2013, researchers looked at more than one thousand Canadian adolescents (ages 16 to 17) using the national health registry.[34] After two years, those adolescents who had had a depressive episode were more impaired in the realms of educational achievement, employment, social supports, and self-reported health and self-efficacy. At the end of ten years, to some extent the depressed adolescents caught up with their peers in most areas (marital status, employment, financial status). In only two areas were the formerly depressed adolescents behind, but they are two critical areas indeed: level of social support and perceived self-efficacy and health. At least into these individuals' late twenties, the social ramifications of this illness are still evident. It should be noted that this study did not examine those who had been in treatment and those who had not. If more of these teens had gotten treatment and thus been depressed for a shorter time, would depression's "scars" have been milder and perhaps less frequently observed?

Another reason for aggressive treatment of depressive disorders in adolescents is the tendency for depressed adolescents to have other mental health problems, especially behavioral problems. In a study of sixty-seven adolescents with major depression, nearly one in six had behavioral problems severe enough to warrant the diagnostic label "conduct disorder."[35] Young people receiving this diagnosis have serious behavioral problems, such as aggressiveness (bullying others and fighting), destroying property, stealing, truancy, and running away from home. Another study found that these types of severe conduct problems sometimes develop as a complication of the depression and persist even after the depressive symptoms go into remission.[36]

Perhaps the most serious problem associated with depressive disorders is substance abuse. The vignette about Heather illustrates just how dangerous a combination this is. Depressed adolescents, especially girls, are at higher risk than depressed adults for substance abuse, especially as they progress into early adulthood,[37] and the combination of problems puts adolescents at a much higher risk of suicidal behaviors than does either problem alone.

Lastly, the finding that adolescent depressive episodes predict problems with serious depression in adulthood further emphasizes the need for early identification and treatment. Another study looked at the outcome of adolescent major depressive disorder in early adulthood by interviewing young adults who had participated in a study of adolescent major depression about seven years earlier. The results were striking: more than two-thirds of the depressed adolescents had suffered at least one recurrence of major depression. Even more striking was the effect of recurrent depressions on the functional level of the young person. Individuals who had suffered multiple major depressive episodes in the previous years completed less schooling, reported less satisfaction with their lives and more impairment in relationships with friends, and scored lower on a functional rating scale. Also, more had become parents. The individuals who had not suffered a recurrence did not differ from a never depressed control group on any of these measures.[38] These findings show just how important it is to prevent recurrences of depression in adolescents.

Mood Disorders

A *Summary of Diagnostic Categories in the* DSM

Parents who read a diagnosis in their child's medical records or insurance statements often have questions about the diagnostic categories used by mental health professionals and have concerns about the implications of various diagnostic terms. Psychiatry is one of the few medical specialties that have a more or less official list of disorders and diagnoses. In this chapter, we take a closer look at the latest version of this list, the fifth edition of the *Diagnostic and Statistical Manual of Mental Disorders* (the *DSM-5*), developed and published by the American Psychiatric Association. We present here a brief overview of the *DSM* and explain some of the diagnostic terminology for depressive and other mood disorders.

WHAT IS THE *DSM*?

The roots of the *DSM-5* go at least as far back as the United States Census of 1840, which included the category of "idiocy/insanity" in its classification system of American citizens. By 1880, there were seven categories into which persons with mental illness could be placed: mania, melancholia, monomania, paresis, dementia, dipsomania, and epilepsy.[1] In 1917, the American Medico-Psychological Association (the forerunner of the American Psychiatric Association) developed a statistical manual for use in mental hospitals that included various categories of diagnoses. As time went on, other organizations interested in the statistics of mental illness (such as the Veterans Administration and the United States Army) developed their own statistical manuals. The World Health Organization, after the Second World War, included a long section on mental disorders in the sixth edition of its *International Classification of Disease* (the ICD 6).

In 1952, the American Psychiatric Association published the *Diagnostic and Statistical Manual: Mental Disorders*, the DSM-I. This work differed from previous statistical manuals because it contained a glossary that described the symptoms of the different disorders. Thus, in addition to containing an official list of categories of mental illness, the DSM-I provided guidance to the clinician in making psychiatric diagnoses. By the time the third edition of the manual appeared in 1980 (the DSM-III), each category of psychiatric disorders had a list of *diagnostic criteria*—symptoms and other characteristics of each disorder that were thought to define it and to set it apart from other psychiatric disorders. This was a large leap forward in psychiatric diagnoses, as all psychiatrists began to speak the same language. Now, when a patient goes to a new doctor and her medical records indicate a diagnosis of, say, "panic disorder" or "anorexia nervosa," the new doctor knows (if previous psychiatrists did their job well, of course) that the patient has had certain symptoms and not others and that the symptoms have troubled her for a certain period.

The *DSM-III* allowed psychiatric research to flourish. Previously, it was difficult to do a study on a group of "depressed" patients, because (as we've shown) this one word could encompass persons experiencing dozens of varying *syndromes*, all of whom shared the *symptom* of low mood. Use of the DSM in research means that when you read in a study of some particular psychiatric disorder in a professional journal that "the patients met the DSM diagnostic criteria" for that disorder, you can be sure that all the patients in the study had a certain well-defined collection of symptoms and other characteristics in common and that the researchers are not mixing psychiatric "apples and oranges." The *DSM-III* allowed researchers to create a long list of criteria that patients had to meet in order to be included in a study (for example, they must have five symptoms of depression, not merely low mood; must have them for a specific length of time; and so on). The *DSM-III* suffered from the same problems as later versions, in that the checklist of depressive symptoms captured a nonuniform population—one person could have the syndrome of major depressive disorder, while another had just lost a loved one—but still, this advance led to a proliferation of research around these conditions. Sometimes, the research supported the classifications delineated in the *DSM-III*, and other times it suggested that some symptoms needed to be included, or thrown out, of various descriptions. All of this came together fourteen years later to create the *DSM-IV*, which was the pinnacle of psychiatric diagnosis until recently. Now, almost ten years after that edition's release, researchers and clinicians have again come together to update the *DSM*, resulting in the *DSM-5*. Some of these updates were again based on research proving, or disproving, existing classifications. Others were updates to expunge seemingly outdated notions, or to clarify the practice of psychiatry more than the research (recall our discussion of mood disorders and dividing them into two separate chapters in the *DSM*).

A word of warning about the *DSM* is needed here. Because the manual contains a list of psychiatric diagnoses followed by succinct and clearly written criteria for making those diagnoses, it has the unfortunate effect of making psychiatric diagnosis look easy. It is tempting for individuals who do not have any psychiatric training to see the manual as a series of symptom checklists that can be easily applied to make the diagnosis of mental illness. This is not the case, for a number of reasons.

First of all, only with an enormous amount of training and experience can one gain an appreciation for the wide range of *normal* emotions and behaviors and have a sense of what falls outside this normal range. Significant clinical experience and judgment are needed to decide what constitutes an "irritable mood" or an "increase in energy" that is *clinically* significant. The *DSM* is full of diagnostic criteria that use qualifiers—"*clinically* significant," "*marked* impairment," "*excessive* involvement in . . ."—all requiring judgment based on experience. Even some counseling and therapy professionals, if they have not trained in a setting where they have had the opportunity to see very sick patients, may not really have an appreciation for what constitutes *severe*—simply because they have never seen and worked with severely depressed patients. Nonprofessionals, of course, usually have even less experience with the range of normal and abnormal moods. Without the experience of seeing and treating many patients with depressive illnesses, it is impossible to accurately separate normal from abnormal mental experiences or clinically significant mood changes from those that are within the range of normal. In psychiatry as perhaps in no other field, the dictum "a little knowledge is a dangerous thing" holds true.

Second, many *medical* conditions can mimic abnormal mood states. Dozens of pharmaceuticals can cause depressed or euphoric states in some persons, and drugs of abuse can cause all kinds of mood changes and psychoses in almost anyone. Almost all the *DSM* diagnoses contain "exclusion criteria" for medical conditions, such as "the symptoms are not due to . . . a general medical condition." Only a clinician trained in the diagnosis and treatment of physical illness will be able to pick up these sorts of problems.

Third, just as the range of normal experience and behavior is enormous, so is the range and complexity of abnormal mental experiences and behaviors—they cannot be contained in any one book and certainly not all described in a few dozen diagnostic categories.

Last, and perhaps most important, the *DSM* is designed to see the patient in one "plane," rather than three dimensionally. It does not discuss the origin of a syndrome so much as its current symptoms. We discussed earlier how a young person can be diagnosed as ADHD at 5, anxiety at 8, depression at 10, bipolar at 16—to anyone familiar with the *DSM*, it is fairly clear how this can happen. An anxious child, constantly alert to threats in his environment, can certainly have trouble regulating his attention at a young age, as could a traumatized child. Though they may "meet criteria" according to the *DSM* for the diagnosis of ADHD, in reality these symptoms could be the result of their anxiety or trauma. Only through a thorough evaluation, followed by serial examinations and a process of truly getting to know the child and his experiences, can a clinician make such a determination. Filling out a checklist certainly does not suffice and, for inexperienced clinicians, can be the origin of misdiagnosis.

For these reasons, we are not going to list the *DSM* diagnostic criteria for the disorders described in this chapter. We don't want to tempt nonclinicians to engage in self-diagnosis or diagnosis of family members. The *DSM* is easily available in libraries—but it should be considered a reference book for clinicians, not a textbook of psychiatry.

A MULTIAXIAL DIAGNOSTIC SYSTEM

You, the reader, are engaging in this discussion at an interesting time. The multiaxial diagnosis was included in the *DSM* at version III and has been the mainstay of psychiatric assessment for more than thirty years. It can be tremendously useful in dividing up and more clearly thinking about different "types" of diagnoses in separate categories (more on that in a moment). Despite its usefulness, it had the unfortunate effect of setting psychiatry somewhat apart from the rest of the medical fields, because psychiatry is the only specialty that uses its own particular method of discussing diagnoses. As such, the *DSM-5* no longer requires the use of the multiaxial system, though it is still in use by most psychiatrists at the time of this writing. We have already discussed that change takes time, and though the *DSM-5* has only been available for a short while, we expect that the multiaxial system will not go anywhere soon. It is possible, as time marches forward, that fewer and fewer clinicians will choose to employ the multiaxial system in diagnosing their patients, so it is helpful for you to be familiar with, though not attached to, this methodology.

A multiaxial *DSM* diagnosis always lists five types of diagnoses and other pieces of clinical information on patients in five separate categories, each of which is called an *axis*.

Axis I	Clinical disorders
Axis II	Personality and intelligence
Axis III	General medical conditions
Axis IV	Psychosocial and environmental problems
Axis V	Assessment of level of functioning

The reason for this complexity is that, to put it plainly, people are complex creatures, and an understanding of their mental life requires looking at them from several different angles.

On *axis I* is listed the psychiatric illness or condition that is being treated or studied. This is where a mood disorder diagnosis would go, as would diagnoses such as attention-deficit/hyperactivity disorder or panic disorder or alcohol abuse. Because symptoms of a psychiatric illness might be expressed differently depending on a person's personality and intellectual ability, these two factors are also recorded for every patient—on *axis II*. A diagnosis of a personality disorder would be listed here. A person with "avoidant personality disorder," for example, is socially inhibited, hypersensitive to negative comments or reactions from others, and constantly fearful of criticism and rejection. These individuals are so sensitized to criticism that they see it everywhere and avoid making friends or even going to social activities. They withdraw from life and function below their true capabilities because of these fears and preoccupations. This pattern of thinking, relating, and behaving is called a personality disorder because it seems ingrained in the individual's personality from an early age rather than the expression of an illness imposed on him at some point in life. Similarly, personality disorders do not cycle like mood disorders. Rather than being episodic, these conditions are ingrained in every aspect of the person's interactions with the world and are consistent aspects of his being.

Personality disorder diagnoses are not made very often in adolescents, for several reasons. The most important one is that in young persons, personality style is still under development. Personality traits that are present in childhood often do not persist into adult life. Another reason is that prolonged periods of depression can negatively affect adolescents' ways of thinking about themselves and their relationships. You've already seen how depression can adversely affect how young persons relate to others and color their view of themselves and their world. It's not difficult, then, to see how a chronically depressed young person can seem to have the personality style and show the behaviors of avoidant personality disorder briefly described above and thus seem to meet the criteria for this diagnosis. But to make a diagnosis of a personality disorder would be to miss the most important problem: depression. Technically, a diagnosis of personality disorder can be made in someone under the age of 18 if the personality traits have been present and causing problems for at least one year. Nevertheless, for the reasons we've mentioned, most psychiatrists are reluctant (or at least they should be) to make a personality disorder diagnosis in an adolescent, especially an adolescent who is or has been depressed.

Axis III is the place to list any medical problem the individual may have. Examples would be high blood pressure, asthma, kidney failure, or migraine headaches. The axis III diagnosis is sometimes very important in treating a patient with a mood disorder because mood symptoms can be caused or affected by medical conditions, such as thyroid problems or medications being taken for a medical problem. Medication that an adolescent might be taking for asthma, for example, can cause nervousness and anxiety.

On *axis IV* are listed problems in and stresses from the environment that may contribute to the patient's difficulties—parental divorce, serious illness in the adolescent or another family member, a move to a new community, chronic poverty, living in an unsafe neighborhood. These factors can also affect how individuals cope with illness as well as their response to treatment. Axis IV information is especially important in the mood disorders, since environmental stressors can be an important precipitating factor for an episode of illness.

On *axis* V, the clinician records an assessment of the patient's functional level, using a 1 to 100 rating scale called the Global Assessment of Functioning (GAF) Scale. This assessment is a judgment of how impaired (or unimpaired) a patient is by symptoms in everyday life. On this scale, a score of 80 or above indicates basically normal everyday functioning, below 50 indicates serious impairment such as recurrent unemployment due to psychiatric illness, and below 20 indicates a level of impairment that suggests the need for psychiatric hospitalization. This axis is more useful to researchers and statisticians than to clinicians, but it rounds out a picture of the patient, capturing strengths as opposed to afflictions.

MOOD DISORDER CATEGORIES IN THE *DSM*

We've already discussed the two main depressive disorder categories: major depressive disorder and dysthymic disorder. *Major depressive disorder* is the most frequently diagnosed depressive disorder of adolescence. It is characterized by one or more major depressive episodes and periods of recovery between episodes. *Dysthymic disorder* is the smoldering disorder in which symptoms persist for months at a time. According to the *DSM*, symptoms must persist for at least one year in children and adolescents. (Adults must show symptoms for two years.)

In the *DSM*, serious depressive illnesses that don't quite fit the diagnostic criteria for either of these disorders are called "depressive disorder not otherwise specified" (depressive disorder NOS). This is something of a "wastebasket" category and a good example of why the *DSM* should not be considered a psychiatric "bible" when it comes to understanding and treating patients. An adolescent who has had symptoms of dysthymic disorder for 364 days would technically need to be diagnosed with depressive disorder NOS until, on the 365th day, the diagnosis could be changed to dysthymic disorder—obviously not a meaningful distinction for an individual patient. People with severe depression who don't have enough symptoms on a *DSM* checklist also technically need to be put into this category. The *DSM* should be seen as a guide to diagnosis and treatment, not a textbook. It would be wise to repeat our favorite quote from Alfred Kinsey here: "The world is not divided into sheep and goats ... Nature rarely deals with discrete categories. Only the human mind invents categories and tries to force facts into separated pigeonholes."[2] We've already discussed some of the difficulties in separating depressive disorders in young persons into discrete categories and some of the problems with symptom overlap. (Compare table 4-1 to tables 4-2 and 4-3 to see how the mood disorder checklists have changed from the fourth edition to the fifth.)

The *DSM* also provides several other descriptive terms, called *specifiers*, that can be added to the main diagnosis to better describe the current episode of mood problems. The clinician can call the episode *mild, moderate,* or *severe.* If the patient has not had any episodes in two months, the disorder can be designated *in remission (in full remission* if there have been no symptoms for two months, *in partial remission* if only a few symptoms exist or the remission has been for less than two months). In the DSM-IV, if the patient has all the symptoms of major depression continuously for a period of at least two years, major depression is said to be *chronic.*

The specifier *with melancholic features* can be added when the patient's depressive episode is dominated by loss of ability to experience pleasure (anhedonia) and by guilty feelings, loss of appetite, and the classic daily fluctuation of mood (early morning awakening, with the mood lifting slightly as the day progresses)—in short, the "textbook" depressive syndrome so eloquently described by William Styron in *Darkness Visible.*

Another clinical syndrome (more common in pure depressive disorders than in the depressive phase of a bipolar disorder) has been called *atypical depression.* People with this syndrome retain reactivity in their mood (for example, their mood brightens when good things happen). In fact, they seem to have a "hyper-reactive" mood and an especially difficult time with rejection in interpersonal relationships—even when not in an episode of depression. They also tend to have changes in appetite and sleep of the less common pattern: eating and sleeping too much.

The specifier *with psychotic features* can be added if the patient has hallucinations or delusional beliefs during the illness, such as those described in

Table 4-1   Mood Disorders in the *DSM-IV*

Major Depressive Disorder
   Full syndrome of severe depression
      Severity specifiers
         —mild, moderate, severe (with or without psychotic features)
         —in partial or full remission
      Special syndrome specifiers
         —with melancholic, catatonic, or atypical features
         —with postpartum onset
      Longitudinal course specifiers
         —with or without full inter-episode recovery
         —with seasonal pattern
         —chronic
Dysthymic Disorder
   Smoldering, low-grade, long-standing depression
         —early onset (before age 21)
         —late onset (after age 21)
         —with atypical features
Depressive Disorder NOS
Bipolar Disorder I
   Mania and severe depression
Bipolar Disorder II
   Severe depression and hypomania
      Specifiers for bipolar disorders:
      Severity specifiers
      —mild, moderate, severe (with or without psychotic features)
      —in partial or full remission
      Special syndrome specifiers
      —with melancholic, catatonic, or atypical features
      —with postpartum onset
      Longitudinal course specifiers
      —with or without full inter-episode recovery
      —with seasonal pattern
      —with rapid cycling
Bipolar Disorder NOS
   "Soft" bipolar and bipolar spectrum disorders
Cyclothymic Disorder
   Depressive symptoms and hypomanias
Substance-Induced Mood Disorder
   Mood Disorder Due to a General Medical Condition

Table 4-2   Depressive Disorders in the *DSM-5*

Major Depressive Disorder
- Full syndrome of severe depression
  - Severity specifiers
    - —mild, moderate, severe
    - —with mood congruent or incongruent psychotic features
    - —in partial, in full remission or unspecified
  - Special syndrome specifiers
    - —with melancholic, catatonic, or atypical features
    - —with anxious distress
  - Longitudinal course specifiers
    - —with or without full inter-episode recovery
    - —with seasonal pattern
    - —with peripartum onset

Dysthymic Disorder/Persistent Depressive Disorder
- Smoldering, low-grade depression
  - Severity specifiers
    - —mild, moderate, severe
    - —in partial, in full remission or unspecified
  - Special syndrome specifiers
    - —with melancholic, catatonic, or atypical features
    - —with anxious distress
  - Longitudinal course specifiers
    - —with pure dysthymic syndrome
    - —with intermittent major depressive episodes
    - —with peripartum onset
  - Timing modifiers
    - —early onset (before 21)
    - —late onset (after 21)

Premenstrual Dysphoric Disorder
- A time-limited major depressive episode surrounding menses

Disruptive Mood Dysregulation Disorder
- Chronic irritability thought to be related to a low-level depression

Substance/Medication Induced Depressive Disorder

Depressive Disorder Due to Another Medical Condition
- Unspecified Depressive Disorder

Table 4-3   Bipolar and Related Disorders in the *DSM-5*

Bipolar Disorder I
  Mania and severe depression
Bipolar Disorder II
  Severe depression and hypomania
    Specifiers for bipolar disorders:
      Severity specifiers
        —mild, moderate, severe
        —with mood congruent or incongruent psychotic features
        —in partial or full remission
      Special syndrome specifiers
        —with melancholic, catatonic, atypical or mixed features
        —with anxious distress
      Longitudinal course specifiers
        —with peripartum onset
        —with seasonal pattern
        —with rapid cycling
Bipolar Disorder NOS
  "Soft" bipolar and bipolar spectrum disorders
Cyclothymic Disorder
  Depressive symptoms and hypomanias
Unspecified Bipolar and Related Disorder
  "Soft" bipolar and bipolar spectrum disorders
Substance/Medication Induced Bipolar and Related Disorder
  Bipolar and Related Disorder Due to Another Medical Condition

chapter 2. The specifier *with catatonic features* is added if the patient shows symptoms of catatonia, a rare syndrome in which the individual lies (or sometime sits or stands) motionless for long periods staring into space and has other unusual physical mannerisms, such as rigid posturing, grimacing, or meaninglessly repeating whatever is said to him. Both of these problems are unusual in adolescent depressions.

Another set of specifiers describes the course of the illness over time, called *longitudinal course specifiers*. Mood disorders may be *with* or *without full inter-episode recovery*, depending on whether the individual is completely free of symptoms between episodes or not.

Some people have a mood disorder in which they have repeated depressive episodes occurring regularly in the winter and sometimes hypomanic or manic symptoms in the summer. This illness has been called *seasonal af-*

fective disorder. In *DSM-IV*, the specifier *with seasonal pattern* is added to the diagnosis of major depressive or bipolar disorder.

Lastly, patients with a bipolar disorder who have had at least four episodes in twelve months have a disorder *with rapid cycling*.

When drug intoxication or medical problems mimic depressive episodes, the *DSM* diagnoses *substance/medication-induced depressive disorder* or *depressive disorder due to another medical condition* are used. When the mood problem is due to a medical condition, the medical condition and type of mood change are specified in the diagnosis (as in, for example, "mood disorder due to hyperthyroidism, with manic features"). When the problem is due to substance abuse, the type of mood change and whether the symptoms came on during intoxication or withdrawal are specified. (Examples would be "alcohol-induced mood disorder with depressive features, onset during withdrawal" and "cocaine-induced mood disorder with manic features, onset during intoxication.")

CONTROVERSIES IN THE USE OF THE *DSM*

There have been enormous controversies surrounding the use of the *DSM* in the diagnosis of psychiatric problems in children and adolescents. Although these controversies don't touch very directly on the use of *DSM* diagnoses for mood disorders, a brief discussion is still warranted. The misuse of psychiatric diagnosis is, and should be, an important concern for parents.

The problems with the *DSM* arise with the various diagnoses that get applied to children and adolescents with behavioral problems: problems involving high activity levels, defiant behaviors, and disruptive and destructive behaviors. The main criticism usually leveled at the *DSM* is that it "medicalizes" problems in children that are really no more than normal behavioral and developmental variations of one type or another. The parents of a child who is more energetic and less attentive than his classmates get a letter from the teacher recommending that the child be evaluated for attention deficit disorder. When does "inattention" become attention deficit disorder? How does anyone decide what constitutes a "disorder"?

In earlier chapters, we made the point that most of the problems psychiatrists are called on to treat do not have any known physical basis—no abnormalities on brain scans or blood tests (what are called *biological markers* for psychiatric illness). This means that the diagnostic criteria are basically things that the person experiences or does: thoughts, feelings, and behaviors. A problem arises when what are identified as "symptoms" are experiences or behaviors that are not outside the realm of normal except in degree.

There is little disagreement that hearing voices when no one is speaking is not normal. And the frenzied disorganization of mania can't be mistaken for normal high spirits. But what about a childhood diagnosis such as *conduct disorder*, for which the symptoms are behaviors like fighting, setting fires, disobedience, and running away? How does one decide when "bad behavior" becomes "*really* bad behavior," and therefore becomes conduct disorder? Even more slippery is *oppositional defiant disorder*, for which the diagnostic criteria include things like "often loses temper," "often argues with adults," "is often angry and resentful," and "is often touchy or easily annoyed by others." An adolescent who has had these characteristics for six months, to the point where they cause "clinically significant impairment" in her school or family life, would meet the *DSM* criteria for this diagnosis. Now, from what you already know about depression, you can see that a depressed adolescent may be all of these things. Does Heather in the vignette in chapter 3 have both major depressive disorder *and* oppositional defiant disorder? Although, technically, she does not, because the *DSM* diagnosis of oppositional defiant disorder cannot be made when the symptoms occur during an episode of depression, you can see how complicated and difficult the issue of psychiatric diagnosis can sometimes be. For every voice calling for the early identification and treatment of psychiatric problems in young people, there seems to be another one warning that overdiagnosing and, worse, overmedicating young people is the real problem, and a more sinister one at that.

How are these controversies important for the parent of a depressed adolescent? First, they reinforce what we have been saying about the *DSM* being only a guide to psychiatric diagnosis—and a decidedly imperfect one. Second, they should make parents cautious and questioning about the diagnosis of a behavioral disorder in their child if they notice signs of depression. Using the *DSM* criteria for behavioral disorders as a checklist to assess difficult behaviors and assign diagnoses such as conduct disorder and oppositional defiant disorder, while missing a depression or other causes of these clusters of behaviors, happens all too frequently—especially when the *DSM* is in the hands of persons without much training in the assessment of psychiatric illnesses. Third, and perhaps most important, parents should be skeptical of some people's insistence on the opposite view: that the behavioral symptoms of serious depressive illnesses are no more than "bad behavior" and, worse, that punishment rather than treatment is necessary to teach adolescents about the "consequences" of their bad behaviors.

Unlike some other *DSM* categories, depressive disorders in adolescence have a clear demarcation from normal behaviors and need medical treatment. That treatment is the subject of the next part of the book.

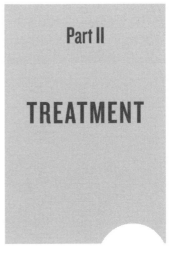

Part II

TREATMENT

IN THESE CHAPTERS, we discuss the available treatments for adolescent depression. We now have a wide range of options, from pharmaceutical and other medical treatments to specific types of psychotherapy that have proved especially helpful in treating depression.

Chapter 5 introduces some of the special considerations that must be given to the use of medications in the adolescent age range. After all, some adolescents are physically more like children, whereas others are close to adults. Are medications given in different dosages to adolescents? Are the medications known to be effective in treating adult depression also effective in adolescents? These are some of the questions answered here. We also present a brief introduction to what we know about the chemical workings of the brain and how the medications used to treat depression work.

In chapters 6 through 8, we talk more specifically about medical treatment, reviewing the various pharmaceuticals used to treat these illnesses. In chapter 8, we include some less frequently used medications, some alternative treatments for depression, and electroconvulsive therapy—still a valuable resource for the treatment of mood disorders. This chapter ends with a discussion of several promising experimental treatments for severe depression. Finally, chapter 9 covers the role of counseling and psychotherapy in treating adolescents with depression.

Medication Issues in Adolescence

We know that the medications used to treat adult disorders don't always work in quite the same way in children and adolescents. Unfortunately, textbooks, research articles, and prescribing guidelines from pharmaceutical manufacturers often provide only limited guidance about the use of medications to treat psychiatric problems in children and adolescents. One reason for this is that far fewer good research studies have been conducted on the use of psychiatric medications in these younger patients than on their use in adults. Pharmaceutical research is more difficult to do in young people, for a variety of reasons. Parents who would willingly volunteer to be in a drug study are often much less willing to volunteer their children for research, making it difficult to recruit research subjects. Issues of informed consent to be a research subject are much more complicated when minors are involved, making researchers reluctant to tackle the issue. Not only are these studies more challenging to do, but the financial returns for pharmaceutical companies are often far lower: children and adolescents usually represent a smaller "market" for medications than do adults.

These factors have added up to a lack of information about the use of psychiatric medications in children and adolescents compared with that available for prescribing to adults. The prescription of psychiatric medication to young people is often what is referred to as "off-label" prescribing, a term we explain below.

PHARMACEUTICALS AND THE FDA

The United States Food and Drug Administration (FDA) is responsible for determining that a pharmaceutical is safe for use in humans and that it is effective for the illness or symptoms for which the manufacturer claims it is effective. The FDA's process of determining the safety of pharmaceuticals is quite thorough, perhaps the most thorough and rigorous in the world. It is credited with preventing an epidemic in the United States of birth defects caused by thalidomide, which occurred in other countries during the 1960s. Thalidomide was widely used in Europe but had not been approved for sale in the United States when it was discovered to cause severe deforming birth defects in children whose mothers had taken it during pregnancy.

A pharmaceutical company performs, sponsors, and encourages research on a drug it wants to sell and then presents the research results to the FDA in support of its request to sell the drug and market it to physicians. Once the drug is approved, the product can be sold in the United States, and the FDA regulates how the drug is "labeled" for use. This "labeling" is the information on the product insert distributed with the drug to physicians and patients. Only the indications for a medication that have been evaluated by the FDA may be listed on the label. For example, antibiotic manufacturers are allowed to list only those illnesses for which the antibiotic has been proved effective by the FDA. Now, doctors may know from research studies and experience that a certain medication works for other illnesses and may legally prescribe it as they see fit. The FDA does not regulate how physicians can prescribe a given pharmaceutical. Doctors can legally prescribe an approved drug for *any* purpose they want to, based on their knowledge of the medical research literature and using their medical judgment—even if the FDA has not reviewed the effectiveness of the drug for that particular use. When a doctor prescribes a pharmaceutical for an illness or symptom that is not covered in the drug's labeling, this is called *off-label* prescribing. There are several reasons that physicians quite frequently prescribe pharmaceuticals for off-label indications. Once a drug has been approved for sale, manufacturers are often very conservative about requesting the FDA to approve a new use for the drug (called the drug's *indication*), even if clinical research shows the new use is an effective one. For example, research had shown quite clearly that antidepressant medications were effective in the treatment of panic attacks for many years before the FDA labeled any antidepressants for treating panic disorder; many antidepressants are still not labeled for this use but are widely and safely prescribed for panic attacks. Research had shown that the antiepilepsy medication divalproex was a safe and effective treatment for manic symptoms for many years before its manufacturer, Abbott Laboratories, requested that its brand of divalproex, Depakote, be approved to treat mania. Off-label prescription of a pharmaceutical for a particular condition often precedes FDA-approved prescribing for that condition by years, even decades. As of this writing, the antidepressant sertraline (Zoloft) is labeled for the treatment of obsessive-compulsive disorder in children 6 to 17 years old but not for the treatment of depression, even though more prescriptions are probably written to treat depression than obsessive-compulsive disorder in this age range.

At other times, the off-label use of medications is driven more by marketing than by medical knowledge. It is obviously in the pharmaceutical company's financial interest to sell as much of its product as possible. To this end, drugs were once "marketed off label" for all sorts of uses that had not been evaluated by the FDA. For many years, the medication Neurontin was used off label as a treatment for bipolar affective disorder, even though later evidence would show that it had no effect on the condition. More recently, Johnson and Johnson has agreed to a $2.2 billion settlement for charges that it was actively pushing the use of medications off label. The manufacturer was accused of creating a misleading marketing campaign targeting aggression in elderly patients, implying that the medication (risperidone, or Risperdal) had been proved safe and effective, when in fact it had not been specifically studied in this population at all and, once it was, was shown to be potentially harmful. Furthermore, they were accused of giving payments and kickbacks to elder care facilities and to physicians for using and promoting the use of the medication in this manner. The federal government was particularly interested in this case as virtually all the medication was being paid for by Medicare, which means in essence that the taxpayers were funding this potentially inappropriate prescribing.

In an effort to minimize extraneous uses of medications, the FDA now strictly regulates how a drug is advertised and marketed to physicians by representatives of pharmaceutical companies. Physicians can still prescribe any medication as they choose, but under the newer legislation, a pharmaceutical company's sales representatives are not permitted to discuss off-label uses of their company's products when they make marketing visits to physicians, nor are they allowed to discuss off-label uses in any of their marketing materials. Some locations have gone a step further. In many major medical centers, pharmaceutical representatives are not even allowed on the grounds except under strictly regulated circumstances, to prevent biased prescribing by the centers' physicians.

As you read this discussion, we worry that you may take our message to be that "pharmaceutical companies are evil, and the FDA is there to prevent their opportunistic parasitism on the ill." This is simply not true. Although they are businesses, they also donate millions of dollars' worth of medications per year to those in need, contribute to charities, and participate in untold billions of dollars in research to help us understand illnesses better. Of course they would prefer that physicians prescribe only the medications that they manufacture, but they also understand that not every medicine works for every patient. In our personal interactions with pharmaceutical representatives, we have never found them to be unnecessarily pushy; nor have they been insulted or affronted when we discuss the use of another company's medications instead. It is true, however, that the FDA takes its job very seriously and wants to ensure that all medications taken by patients are safe, effective, and given for their best interest. This has led the FDA to be exceedingly cautious before approving a new medicine, some may feel overly so.

What are the reasons for the inconsistencies and delays in getting a medication FDA approved? There are several. Perhaps the most important is that once a medication has been approved for one indication, a pharmaceutical manufacturer may decide that it's not particularly advantageous to request a new indication, especially if the new indication is for a less common condition. The expense of going through an FDA approval process may not be offset by the increase in sales that marketing the drug for the new indication would bring about—especially since doctors are able to prescribe the medication off label anyway. This means that the labeling of any pharmaceutical is usually an incomplete guide to the use of a medication and illustrates why a physician must have a familiarity with the clinical research literature to make prescribing decisions. The popular *Physicians'*

Desk Reference (the *PDR*) is *not* a good source of information about medications and prescribing for this very reason: the *PDR* is only a compilation of the FDA labeling for medications. If physicians limited themselves to only FDA-approved uses of pharmaceuticals, many patients would go untreated for conditions for which proven remedies are available.

Just as a pharmaceutical company may decide it's not financially advantageous to ask the FDA to label a drug for a new indication, the company may decide there are no financial incentives to ask the FDA to label a drug for prescription to children and adolescents. If you glance through the *PDR*, you'll notice that for many medications, it makes no mention of uses in children and adolescents and gives only the recommended doses in adults. Many psychiatric medications fall into this category. The FDA is addressing this vacuum, and policy revisions are in the works with new requirements to address the use of medications in young people when approval is sought for new pharmaceuticals.

DOSE ADJUSTMENTS AND OTHER DIFFERENCES FOR YOUNG PEOPLE

The dosing of medications is more complicated for young people than for adults. On the one hand, because children are physically smaller than adults, pediatric doses of medication are often smaller than adult doses. But then again, a healthy 16-year-old who is mature for his age may be physically bigger than many adults and require a dose of medication in the adult range, perhaps even at the top of the adult range. Sometimes a dosing guide is available that calls for a calculation of the appropriate dose of a medication based on body weight—but physical size differences between children and adults are only a part of the story. Many medications are absorbed into fat tissue, and at various ages young people and adults have different proportions of fatty tissue. This factor can be especially important in adolescents, because the distribution of fat tissue can change dramatically during puberty over a short time, especially in girls, requiring more frequent dosage adjustments than in adults.

Young people sometimes absorb medications from the gastrointestinal tract into their bloodstream more rapidly than do adults. This means that after a dose of medication, the level of medication in the blood rises more rapidly and to a higher peak level in adolescents than in adults. This can cause more sleepiness or other side effects immediately after taking the medication. Splitting the dose of medication into several doses throughout the day may help with this problem, but doing so means there are twice or even three times as many opportunities to forget to take a dose.

Young people and adults also eliminate medications differently. The amount of medication active in the body is determined by a balance between how much is going in and how much is going out: the main organ in charge of the "going out" part is the liver, which chemically breaks down most medications into inactive forms, which are then usually eliminated through the kidneys into the urine. In children, the liver is larger in proportion to overall body size than it is in adults. This means that children may eliminate a medication more quickly and may therefore need a surprisingly higher dose than would be expected from their physical stature.

All these differences decrease, of course, as a young person grows from child to adolescent to young adult. But remember that the timing of these physical changes can vary quite a bit from one individual to another. One particular 15-year-old might need to take a pediatric dose of a medication, while another might require an adult dose, because of these differences in physical maturity.

In addition to dosing differences, there may be important efficacy differences between young people and adults. That is, just because a medication is effective in adults for a particular problem doesn't mean it will be equally effective for what seems to be a similar problem in a child or adolescent. The most striking example of this is the difference in efficacy of certain antidepressants. The class of antidepressants called tricyclic antidepressants has been used with great effectiveness to treat depressive disorders in adults for many years, and it was assumed that tricyclics must be effective in childhood depression as well. But in several clinical studies done in the 1980s, tricyclics appeared no more effective than placebo (a sugar pill) in treating childhood depression. (Other types of studies do show some efficacy; we discuss this controversy in the next chapter.) It may be that the different symptoms often seen in younger depression patients are a reflection of variations in the chemical basis of their depression, or perhaps a difference between the developing nervous system and the mature brain makes younger patients respond to some medications differently.

All these issues mean that the dosing rules and guidelines for prescribing most psychiatric medications for young people are still developing. A glance through the *PDR* is *not* a good way to get information about medications. A discussion with the prescribing physician about the reasoning for picking a particular dose of medication *is*.

HOW PSYCHIATRIC MEDICATIONS WORK

A number of years ago, psychiatrist and neuroscientist Nancy Andreason wrote the book *The Broken Brain*, about new discoveries in biological psychiatry.[1] The title makes the point that psychiatric illnesses such as major depressive disorder, bipolar disorder, and schizophrenia are caused by biological and chemical malfunctions of the brain, not repressed memories or traumatic childhoods. Although we still don't know exactly what these malfunctions are, we are getting close to understanding some of the biological mechanisms that might be involved in the symptoms of mood disorders.

To understand the treatment of mood disorders with medications, you should know a little bit about how the brain works. Patients and parents frequently ask, "What does this medication *do*?" The answer to this question turns out to be complicated, so in this chapter, we're going to give a brief overview of the functioning of the human nervous system, just enough to help you understand a little bit about how psychiatric medications work.

Many people imagine that the human brain is a kind of wonderful computer. Although this is a vast oversimplification of the true capabilities of the brain, it's a good place to start in trying to understand how this fantastic organ of the mind works.

Like the computer that we used to write these words, a human brain receives input, processes the information it receives, and then delivers output. Like a computer, it stores information and often uses this stored information to help process the input it receives. The brain receives its input from the sense organs—the eyes, ears, taste buds, touch receptors, and so forth—and delivers output in the form of behavior.

The simplest example of this input-processing-output circuit in our nervous system is the spinal reflex. This circuit is so simple and so automatic in its operation that it richly deserves its label, *reflex*, meaning a simple behavior that requires no "thinking" to be effectively carried out. If you inadvertently touch the hot surface of a stove or a candle flame, a nerve ending detects the resulting tissue damage and fires a message along a nerve fiber (a sensory nerve) that ends in the spinal cord. Here, the first nerve communicates with another nerve, which dispatches a message down again through another fiber (a motor nerve) to activate the arm muscles to pull the finger back from the source of heat (figure 5-1). If you've ever actually had this experience, you may have noticed that your hand pulled away before you even felt the pain. This is because the brain, where consciousness resides, is not yet involved. (The message that is eventually sent up to the brain from the level of the spinal cord responding to the pain signal is more or less an "FYI" message that will be stored in the memory system. Hopefully, this painful memory will lessen the chances of the same thing happening again.)

Let's look at a more complicated example of the input-processing-output circuit—one that is more than a reflex. Say you're walking down the street and pass a florist shop with a sign in the window that reads, "Don't forget, next Sunday is Mother's Day!" You realize with a start that you *have* forgotten, so you go into the shop, pull out your credit card, and order some flowers. This is not really so different a process from the spinal reflex: input (seeing the sign), processing (I forgot!), and output (ordering the flowers). There are a lot more steps (and some very complex ones) this time around: seeing the sign, using the language functions of the brain to draw meaning from all those little shapes we call letters, drawing on memories of what is expected of you on Mother's Day, an emotional tone generated by your feelings for your mother that affects the process—just to name a few. A complex interaction of many, many nervous system functions is going on, some fairly simple (the posture reflexes that let you walk into the shop without falling are nearly as simple as the spinal reflex example above) and others more complex (the arithmetic functions that allow you to answer the question, "How big an arrangement can I buy without going over my credit limit?"). The processes are so complex, in fact, that no computer built today is capable of anything approaching as complex a processing task as this.

You may know that a computer computes by means of many thousands of microscopic switches embedded in its processing chip. The pattern of "on" and "off" in the switches is what stores information, and the flow of input signal through these switches is the processing. The human brain contains about eleven billion nerve cells, or neurons, but as powerful as a computer with eleven billion switches might be, our brain is much more

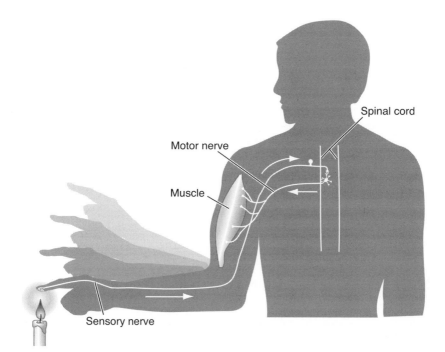

Figure 5-1   Spinal reflex

impressive than that. The neuron is not simply a switch that is either "on" or "off"; rather, it is an impressive microprocessor in its own right. Each neuron receives input from many other neurons, processes this information, and sends output to many others. The brain is not simply a biological computer with billions of switches. It is more like a network of billions of computers, each capable of being individually programmed. Every neuron in the brain may receive input and transmit signals to up to fifty thousand other neurons. This makes the number of *all* the possible connections between neurons in the human brain incomprehensibly huge, a hyper-astronomical number on the order of the number of molecules in the universe. (Even if we could figure out how to build such a computer, there'd be no place on the planet big enough to put it.) This almost unimaginable complexity explains why the capabilities of even the most powerful computers are puny compared with those of the human brain.

Like computers, the human nervous system uses electrical signals to do much of its work, as well as chemical signals called *neurotransmitters*.

Let's go back for a moment to the spinal reflex to examine how these signals do their jobs. Remember that in this reflex, a pain signal from the finger travels up a nerve fiber into the spinal cord. As you might guess, this is an electrical signal, a change in the electrical charge of the nerve fiber that travels as a pulse along the length of the fiber until it reaches a *cell body* that resides in the spinal cord. This cell body is one of the eleven billion tiny computers we mentioned earlier (except that it's in the spinal cord, not in the brain). When a sufficient number of pain signals arrive at the cell body, this microscopic CPU starts communicating with the motor nerve responsible for pulling away the finger, and when the motor neuron computes that it's necessary, this neuron fires its own pulse of electrical energy down the motor nerve to the muscles. The signals by which the neurons communicate with each other are the chemical ones we mentioned above: molecules called neurotransmitters. Most of the medications used in psychiatry work by affecting neurotransmitters in one way or another.

One neuron sends a chemical signal to another at a site called the *synapse*, an area where the two neurons nearly touch, separated only by an ultramicroscopic space called the *synaptic cleft*. The first neuron (the *presynaptic neuron*) releases packets of neurotransmitters that flow across the narrow synaptic cleft and link up with targets called *receptors* on the next cell (the *postsynaptic neuron*); the neurotransmitter molecules fit into their receptors like keys fit into locks. There needs to be some mechanism for this signaling system to be turned off and reset, of course. After neurotransmitter molecules in one pulse link up with receptors across the synapse, they must somehow be removed in preparation for the next pulse. This happens in a variety of ways in different cells, but one of the most important mechanisms is *reuptake* into the cell that released them. A reuptake pump on the presynaptic neuron removes neurotransmitter molecules from the synapse and takes them into the interior of the cell, where they are repackaged for re-release (figure 5-2).

There is a constant level of neurotransmitter release across the synapse, a steady tone of chemical signal that pulses up at times. The neurons are not just "switches" that can be set only to "on" or "off" but rather tiny information-processing units that are constantly communicating with other neurons to which they are functionally linked.

Now let's return to mood disorders. What is "broken" in these illnesses? As you will see, much of what we know about the biological and chemical

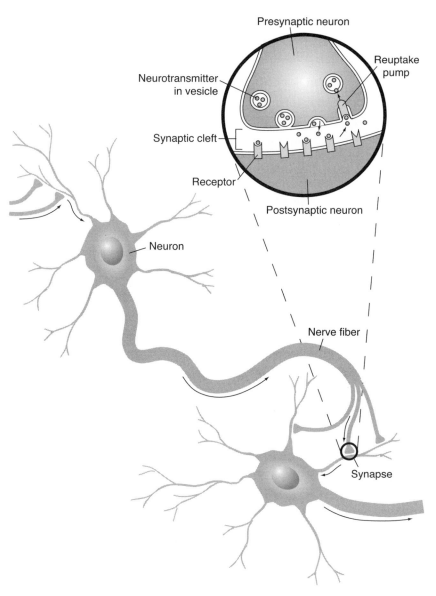

Figure 5-2   Synapse

basis of mood disorders was discovered *after* an effective medication had been accidentally discovered. In a backwards kind of investigative process, by figuring out where in the brain these medications are active and what they do to brain chemistry (usually by observing the effects of these pharmaceuticals on brain preparations in test tubes), we have found clues about the location and function of the "broken" mechanisms in mood disorders.

In chapter 1, we mentioned that the first pharmaceutical to have antidepressant effects, iproniazid, was discovered accidentally when doctors noticed that depressed tuberculosis patients taking the drug for their lung disease had improvement in their mood symptoms. In 1957, another breakthrough in the treatment of mood disorders occurred when Roland Kuhn, a Swiss psychiatrist, discovered that a compound originally developed as an antihistamine also had remarkable therapeutic effects on depressed patients. He reported his results in a Swiss medical journal, in a paper titled "The Treatment of Depressive States with G 22355 (Imipramine Hydrochloride)."[2] Unlike iproniazid, imipramine is still used as an antidepressant medication.

For many years, brain scientists had only vague ideas about the answer to the question, "What does imipramine *do*?" When some of them started to look at the effect of this pharmaceutical on brain chemistry, they discovered that imipramine was a powerful inhibitor of the reuptake of a group of neurotransmitters called *neurogenic amines,* or *neuroamines*, the most important of these being *norepinephrine.*

Remember that neurons turn off their chemical signals (turn *down* is probably more accurate) by scooping up neurotransmitter molecules from the synapse and repackaging them. Just as partially closing the drain in a bathtub while the water is running will cause the tub to begin to fill with water, blocking the reuptake of neurotransmitter molecules has the net effect of *increasing* neurotransmitters in the synapse. This observation, that antidepressants increase the number of neurotransmitters in the synapse by blocking their reuptake, led to the *amine hypothesis* of mood disorders. This hypothesis basically stated that an abnormally low level of norepinephrine caused depression and that, in bipolar disorder, too high a level caused mania.

Further work soon indicated that this explanation was too simplistic. As more antidepressant medications were discovered, it was found that some effective ones seemed to have little effect on the norepinephrine system. Fluoxetine (Prozac) is one of a family of pharmaceuticals that are powerful inhibitors of the reuptake of another neurotransmitter, called *serotonin*, but they have little direct effect on norepinephrine. Some antidepressants also seem to affect other neurotransmitters too, especially one called *dopamine*. As a result of these discoveries, the amine hypothesis was revised, and the proposal was put forward that mood is regulated by a complex interplay of several chemical circuits in the brain. It is now thought that the interplay of activity among all these systems is disrupted in depression and in mania (and actually, it was later discovered that imipramine may be so effective because it has activity in all these chemicals, not just norepinephrine).

Another argument against a simplistic theory involving too much or too little norepinephrine is an observation about the time course of the antidepressant-induced chemical changes in the brain. Antidepressant-induced changes in neurotransmitter levels at the synapse occur almost immediately after the drug is taken—in a matter of hours. But, as is well known, several weeks are required for these agents to start alleviating the symptoms of depression. If the problem were simply too little neurotransmitter in the synapses of certain brain circuits, why would it take several weeks after the drug raised transmitter levels at the synapse for the symptoms of depression to get better? It has been suggested that the neurons respond to these higher levels of neurotransmitters by changing their receptor molecules, either making them more sensitive to the neurotransmitter or putting more of them on the surface of the postsynaptic cell. The idea is that antidepressants work by triggering an "up-regulation" of receptor sensitivity in the neuron. This hypothesis continues to be popular among neuroscientists interested in the chemistry of mood disorders.

This idea fits nicely with some of the work done on the chemical mapping of the brain. Several nuclei of cells (*nucleus* here means a group of neurons) deep in the brain that use norepinephrine as their neurotransmitter project a vast network of fibers that terminate on sheets of cells contained on the convoluted surface of the brain, the cerebral cortex. The cerebral cortex, thought to be responsible for many of our most complex "higher" brain functions, is rich in cells with receptors for norepinephrine. This system seems to be ideally organized to affect the tone of functioning of the entire cerebral cortex—making it a good candidate for the target system of antidepressants. There are serotonin pathways that originate deep in the brain and project widely across the cortex too, as well as pathways that use other neurotransmitters. The balance of activity among these different systems and their interaction with each other are probably very important in the regulation of mood. These neurotransmitter systems are most likely the sites where antidepressant medications do their work.

Because of the uniquely therapeutic effects of *lithium* in bipolar disorder and its important antidepressant effects, a lot of effort has gone into trying to figure out the site of lithium's activity in the brain and its effect on brain chemistry. Lithium doesn't seem to affect neuroamine levels the way antidepressants do, and it doesn't interact with neuroamine receptors or reuptake pumps. In fact, it doesn't have any of the types of direct effects on cells that the antidepressants have (though there is an additional neurotransmitter, glutamate, over which lithium seems to have some pull). Only in the last few years has the probable site of lithium action been found, and it's not at the synapse at all. Lithium (and perhaps the newer mood stabilizers as well) seems to work at a different cellular level: *inside* the neuron.

Although the precise fit between a neurotransmitter and its receptor molecule has often been compared to the precise fit of a key into a lock, it has become apparent that the receptor is much more than just a lock. Starting in the 1970s, scientists were able to elucidate the structure of cellular receptors and discover the details of these complex and elegant mechanisms. Receptors on the surface of the cell are coupled with structures called *G proteins,* which extend through the cell membrane (the outer covering of the cell) and link up with a complex array of other proteins and enzymes within the cell that help regulate various cellular functions (figure 5-3). The G proteins act as transducers, converting data from outside the cell (this data being the presence or absence of neurotransmitters bound to the receptor molecules) into functional changes inside the cell. They don't do this directly but by a complex cascade of chemical events that probably also includes turning genes inside the cell on and off.

There is evidence that lithium has direct effects on G proteins, but scientists have recently started to focus on several other groups of molecules that work inside the cell as *second messengers*. The neurotransmitters, molecules that bring messages from other cells to the neuron, are considered the *first* messengers. The *second* messengers are molecules *inside* the cell

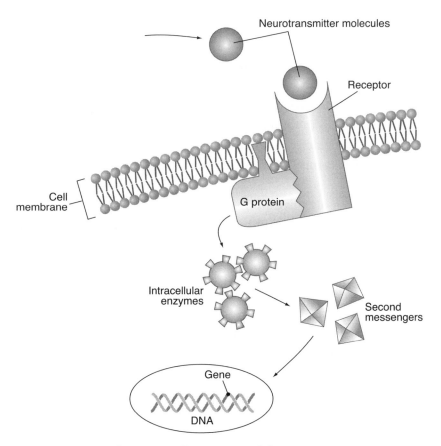

Figure 5-3   Receptors and G proteins

that are activated by G proteins to travel within the neuron to activate various cellular switches in the cell membrane and in the cell nucleus, the main control center of the neuron. Several lines of evidence support the alternative idea that lithium acts by inhibiting enzymes responsible for the manufacture of several second messenger molecules.

One might think of the G protein–second messenger system as a communications and activity-monitoring system for the neuron, constantly assessing the level of neurotransmitter activity and, perhaps by turning genes on and off, constantly altering and adjusting the functioning of the neuron in response to this activity. This process might be a necessary part of maintaining mood within a normal range, and it might control mood by somehow "tuning" the responsiveness of our mood state to experiences and environment. Perhaps mood disorders are the result of a broken G protein–second messenger system in neurons of the norepinephrine and serotonin circuits that regulate mood: the system's sensitivity gets incorrectly tuned too high or too low, and abnormal changes of mood result. (This might explain why the highs and lows of bipolar disorder are *both* effectively treated by lithium. Perhaps the lithium ion fits into and stabilizes the shape of one of the component molecules of this system or in some other way helps the system to work better and to do its job more effectively, thus stabilizing mood.)

This idea may also explain why antidepressants take several weeks to work. One important concept to appreciate is that science is continually discovering more and more actions of the supposedly "selective" serotonin reuptake inhibitors and their counterparts. It turns out that the serotonin receptors are themselves connected to the G protein system and therefore may affect the neuron in a similar way to lithium. Antidepressants may artificially raise neurotransmitter levels in the synapse to very high levels, high enough so that even a "broken" G protein–second messenger system can respond, turning on genes that start making receptor molecules or other cell components necessary to retune the neuron, a process that takes several weeks.

Antidepressants have even more functions. One of their strongest feats is an ability to protect the brain from damage. Some studies have suggested that depression is associated with an area of the brain called the *hippocampus*. In depressed patients, this area seems to be smaller than in those who are not depressed. For a long time, it was thought that the neurons in the brain do not recover in the same way as other neurons do. If, say, one were to have a stroke and some of the neurons died, those neurons would never be replaced. The brain may eventually rewire itself to avoid the broken area, but that area itself would never recover. Researchers were understandably surprised to discover that when depressed patients were treated with antidepressants, the hippocampus seemed to grow. This seemingly astounding feat may be due to the antidepressants' ability to stimulate a particular chemical in the brain that promotes development of brain synapses, called brain-derived neurotrophic factor (BDNF).

It may be a while before we understand how all the molecular and cellular pieces of this complicated story fit together, but the work to unravel the basic cause (or causes) of mood disorders is proceeding rapidly. Adolescent patients and their parents frequently complain that they feel they are guinea pigs when it comes to picking medications to treat mood disorders, because there's no way to know which medication or combination of medications will work best for a particular person. When we understand exactly what is "broken" in these illnesses, the job of treating them will become much easier and also much more systematic.

Antidepressant Medications

A ntidepressant medications have been used for several decades in treating children and adolescents, and the odds are that the first medication to be recommended for your child will be an antidepressant. These highly effective medications are safer than ever, and more and different antidepressants are being introduced every year.

Talking about this group of medications illustrates how the name of a class of medications often doesn't do them justice in describing their true range of efficacy. Medications listed as "antidepressants" have been found to be effective treatments for a whole variety of problems besides depression. In fact, more antidepressant prescriptions may be written to treat problems other than depression than to treat the illnesses for which these medications are named. Tricyclic antidepressants are effective in the treatment of panic attacks, obsessive-compulsive symptoms, and attention-deficit/hyperactivity disorder. Imipramine is effective in treating enuresis (bedwetting).

TRICYCLIC ANTIDEPRESSANTS

Although tricyclics are now prescribed less frequently than other, newer antidepressants, we start with this group because they were the first antidepressant medications developed and because they still provide the standard by which all promising new pharmaceuticals for treating depression in adults are usually judged. As with most psychiatric medications, however, their use in adolescents for the treatment of depression has been mainly based on their proven effectiveness in adults. They are now being used less and less frequently in younger patients because of studies that have thrown significant doubt on the assumption that they are just as effective in children and adolescents. In fact, adolescents who are prescribed these medications tend to be those who have not responded to the more common, newer types of antidepressants. Psychiatrists call these patients *treatment resistant*, or *treatment refractory*. This is by no means intended to imply some sort of fault on the part of the patient—rather, it simply indicates that this individual has a type of depression that for whatever reason does not seem to respond chemically to antidepressants as it should (assuming, of course, that the individual has been thoroughly and correctly diagnosed and treated). In many cases, the switch to a tricyclic is done because these chemicals tend to be involved with more neurotransmitters than the selective antidepressants (the *selective* serotonin reuptake inhibitors, or SSRIs). Table 6-1 shows a list of tricyclic antidepressants. These pharmaceuticals are called *tricyclics* because of the three rings in their chemical structure (figure 6-1).

Although some of these medications have an effect on serotonin systems in the brain, the primary effect of the tricyclics seems to be an inhibition of reuptake of the neurotransmitter norepinephrine by neurons. As we discuss in chapter 5, reuptake of neurotransmitters into the neuron after they have been released into the synaptic cleft and done their work (signaling the next cell) is the means by which the synapse is "reset." Norepinephrine is usually quickly removed from the synapse and pumped back into the cell

Table 6-1 Tricyclic Antidepressants

Generic Name	Brand Name
Amitriptyline	Elavil
Amoxapine	Asendin
Clomipramine	Anafranil
Desipramine	Norpramin
Doxepin	Sinequan
Imipramine	Tofranil
Maprotiline	Ludiomil
Nortriptyline	Pamelor
Protriptyline	Vivactil

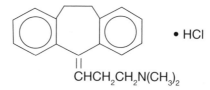

• HCl

CHCH₂CH₂N(CH₃)₂

AMITRIPTYLINE

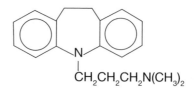

CH₂CH₂CH₂N(CH₃)₂

IMIPRAMINE

Figure 6-1 Chemical structure of two tricyclic molecules, showing their characteristic three-ringed structure

that released it, to turn off and reset the system. By blocking the removal of norepinephrine, tricyclics seem to prolong or intensify norepinephrine's message to the postsynaptic cell.

This effect of tricyclics on norepinephrine in neurons was one of the first chemical effects of a medication active in the brain to be measured in the laboratory. The observation that tricyclics *increased* the amount of norepinephrine in the synapse, along with the discovery that certain other medications used to treat high blood pressure *reduced* norepinephrine—and were observed to cause depression in some patients—led to the early amine hypothesis of mood disorders: the theory that depression was caused by too little norepinephrine (and mania presumably by too much). However, further testing indicated that tricyclics increased amines in the synapse within hours of a person's taking them, whereas the therapeutic effects of antidepressants were known to take several weeks. This led to a search for alternatives to the amine hypothesis.

Following the discovery that tricyclics cause a change in the number and sensitivity of norepinephrine receptors on the postsynaptic neuron, it was suggested that this "down-regulation" of the norepinephrine system by tricyclics was the therapeutic effect of these medications for which researchers had been looking. But other, newer antidepressants don't have this down-regulating effect on norepinephrine.

The fundamental biochemical effect of antidepressants that is actually responsible for their benefits still remains a mystery, though science is getting closer and closer to the answer by looking deeper into the cell itself. It is thought that the change in neuroamine signaling at the synapse caused by antidepressants may set off a cascade of events involving second messenger systems that eventually result in the improvement of the symptoms of depression, likely by altering the genetic expression of the neuron. Unfortunately, how these medications work remains largely unknown.

Although studies show that these medications are far less effective for children than for adults, the principal reason that tricyclics are now infrequently prescribed as antidepressant medications is their many side effects. As with all medications, some patients take these medications easily and without unpleasant side effects, but many have to put up with a few problems to get the benefits. Fortunately, all the side effects are dose related, and most are temporary.

As we mentioned in chapter 5, Roland Kuhn found imipramine, the first tricyclic, among a group of compounds that had some antihistamine effects.[1] It's not surprising, then, that these medications affect some people in the same way antihistamines do, causing mild sleepiness and sometimes what some of our patients have called a "weird" or "spacey" feeling for the first day or two after starting to take them. Tricyclics block another neurotransmitter, called *acetylcholine*, that is used in a part of the nervous system that regulates many automatic functions of the body, such as digestion. The resulting *anticholinergic* side effects include a slowing down of the gastrointestinal tract, causing constipation and dry mouth. This system also controls focusing of the lens of the eye and emptying of the urinary bladder, and tricyclics can cause blurry vision and urination difficulties, although usually only in high doses. Tricyclics also cause weight gain in many patients.

There have been several reports of sudden death in children taking desipramine, one of the tricyclic antidepressant medications, and a more recent sudden death in a child taking imipramine.[2] This appears to be an extremely rare event: fewer than a half dozen such cases have ever been reported. The cause has been presumed to be a sudden heart-rhythm problem, so your doctor should always ask about a family history of abnormal heartbeats (called arrhythmias) or any other sudden, unexplained cardiac death. Additionally, many published guidelines recommend that, before starting to take a tricyclic antidepressant, children and adolescents have an electrocardiogram to make sure there is no undiagnosed heart problem.

Overdoses of tricyclics are very dangerous and are responsible for many of the completed suicides by overdose by people with mood disorders. For adults, the lethal overdose is up to twenty times the normal dose, but children are more sensitive to the toxic effects of these medications, and just a handful of tablets can be fatal in a small child. For this reason, these medications must be scrupulously safeguarded in households with small children.

Accurate blood tests are available to measure tricyclic antidepressant levels in the bloodstream. The level at which these medications have their maximum efficacy, as well as ranges that are associated with side effects and toxicity, has been determined by clinical trials. These blood tests are useful in adjusting the dosage of medication, especially if a usually adequate dose doesn't seem to be helping.

Children and adolescents eliminate these medications more quickly than do adults, perhaps because the size of the liver, the organ responsible for breaking down these medications, is proportionately larger in children than in adults. For this reason, monitoring of blood levels is especially important in adolescents to be sure they are getting the proper dose.

We've referred several times now to studies that have questioned the efficacy of these medications in treating depression in young people. There has been a discrepancy in results between what are referred to as *open* studies and *double-blind* studies of tricyclic medications in young people.

In an open study, the medication under investigation is given to a group of patients with the disorder for which the medication is thought to be effective, and the investigators simply assess how many patients get better and how many do not. Open studies have shown that between 60 and 80 percent of children have a therapeutic response to tricyclics, and significant recovery rates have been found in adolescents as well.[3]

There are two problems with open studies that can trick researchers into thinking a medication is effective when it really isn't. The biggest factor is the *placebo effect*. This is the beneficial effect that comes from taking a medication that is prescribed by a trusted source who is convinced of the effectiveness of the medication and who thus convinces the patient that the medication will help. When a person in a white coat writes a prescription or one in a white uniform gives you a pill, a powerful set of psychological factors is put into action that can make you feel significantly better. In an earlier chapter, we discussed the beneficial effect on demoralization of encouragement from a trusted source. It's easy to see, then, how the placebo effect can be especially powerful with antidepressant medications. The other factor that can mislead researchers in an open study is their own desire to get positive results: no matter how objective the researcher tries to be, there will always be a tendency, perhaps only an unconscious one, to accentuate the positive in measuring improvement in patients. Both these factors can lead to a finding in clinical trials of a medication benefit where there really isn't any.

Double-blind studies eliminate these misleading factors and are the most powerful type of medication trial possible—so much so that this type of study is now pretty much required for all new medications. In a double-blind placebo-controlled study, subjects who are similar in age, diagnosis, severity of illness, and so forth and who agree to be in the study are divided into two groups. One group (the *experimental* group) gets the medication that is being tested, and the other group (the *control* group) gets an identical-looking but inactive tablet, the placebo. The study participants do not know whether they are taking the new medication or the placebo, and neither do the clinicians who are examining them for improvement—hence the term *double*-blind. Only after the trial is over is the group membership of the participants revealed, and the results of the two groups are then compared. Improvement is measured objectively by using checklists of symptoms and various severity rating scales that have been verified as reliable and valid. (In some studies, instead of a placebo, the control group receives a standard medication for the disorder being studied. This allows researchers to study the use of new medications for serious illnesses for which it would be unethical to give patients a dummy pill and not have them receive available treatment for their condition. This type of study would be double-blind, but not placebo-controlled.)

Several double-blind placebo-controlled studies of tricyclic antidepressants in children and adolescents have shown no advantage of the drug over placebo.[4] Critics of these studies have argued that many of the subjects in the studies were only mildly depressed and were perhaps demoralized rather than suffering from a mood disorder, and thus were quite likely to have a placebo response. Some of the studies were of very small groups of patients and thus might not pick up the response for statistical reasons. Other studies have been criticized for not following up on the patients long enough to detect significant improvement and for using measures of improvement that were not sensitive enough.[5]

In cases such as this, when the evidence seems contradictory, scientists will sometimes undertake a vast review of all available research on a particular topic to compare it. This can be done in a couple of ways. In a *meta-analysis,* researchers collect all published (and sometimes unpublished) results of various trials. They then use statistical methods to analyze the studies so that they are comparing apples to apples. This allows them to see which studies had positive results and which had negative results and to look deeper to any possible errors or mistakes that may have skewed the results one way or another. Sometimes the summary of these results is enough to help researchers answer their question of why different studies about the same subject come up with different results. If they wish to take their analysis a step further, they can use this information as part of a *systematic review*. In a systematic review, researchers seek to answer bigger questions, such as "Which patients should we treat with tricyclic antidepressants?" by interpreting and applying the results of the meta-analysis. The review requires a more careful approach in looking at each trial and trying to determine what if any biases might have been present and how they would have affected the results.

In 2013, the Cochrane Collaboration, widely regarded as possibly the best and most thorough research body in existence, completed these procedures to review the treatment of children and adolescents with tricyclic antidepressants. By looking at all available randomized controlled trials to date, Cochrane researchers found no difference between adolescents taking tricyclic medications and those taking placebo in terms of their depression remitting. Despite not fully improving, children taking tricyclics experienced a slight decrease in the severity of some depressive symptoms, based on a particular self-report scale they were given (about 3 percentage points, taking a child from a depression severity of 90 to one of 87—not much of a difference). These children also experienced significantly more side effects (as would be expected). This particular analysis even evaluated whether tricyclic antidepressants may be a good backup option after treatment with an SSRI did not work, and even then these children had no greater response than those given a placebo medication.[6]

It seems reasonable to conclude that tricyclic antidepressants are not as effective in young people as they are in adults—though perhaps unreasonable to conclude that they are completely ineffective. We still have no good way of analyzing a given person's brain chemistry to tell exactly which would be the best medication for her. It is certainly the case that some adults have been depressed for the majority of their lives, and only when they try a particular medication (say, one SSRI versus another) does their depression seem to lift. The research can say that, on a population scale, tricyclic medications don't seem effective for children and adolescents, but the studies can't say that for Shaun sitting in the psychiatrist's office, there is no possibility that a tricyclic might be helpful. Because of this, many psychiatrists have moved tricyclics way down the list of options but haven't crossed them off entirely.

This difference in efficacy between adults and children has yet to be explained. Perhaps there are differences in the biology of depression in younger people; perhaps the chemical pathways that these drugs affect are less developed in the immature brain and thus less responsive to these medications. What is clear, however, is that tricyclic antidepressants must be prescribed with caution in young people and should not be the first choice among antidepressant medications, especially since, as you will see in the next section, safer medications with more clearly proven effectiveness are now available.

SELECTIVE SEROTONIN REUPTAKE INHIBITORS

A new pharmaceutical that had none of the tricyclics' side effects and was not toxic in overdose caused something of a sensation when it was introduced in 1988. That pharmaceutical was fluoxetine (Prozac), and "sensation" sums up the response to this medication quite well. A Prozac capsule showed up on the covers of *Newsweek* and *New York* magazines, the drug was featured in many other magazine and newspaper articles, and for a time it seemed that nearly everyone was either taking Prozac or reading the book *Listening to Prozac* (or *Talking Back to Prozac* or *Prozac Nation*). Prozac was touted by some as a miracle drug that was going to change the world. Many physicians were prescribing Prozac for everything from deep depression to simple mundane sadness, because it was seen as so safe that a mindset of "it can't hurt" started to develop.

The inevitable backlash to this enthusiasm took about another year to fully develop, but once it did, psychiatrists couldn't *pay* their patients to take Prozac. Full-page ads in *USA Today* denouncing the drug appeared for weeks, and various talk show hosts found people who gladly came on national television to swear that Prozac had made their lives miserable. In children, this mindset became especially fixed in October 2004, when the FDA placed a *black box* warning, the sternest warning available to this body, against prescribing selective serotonin reuptake inhibitor (SSRI) medications in adolescents due to a concern about "increased suicidality." This warning was based on the results of a study that seemed to indicate that SSRIs may *double* the rates of suicide in adolescents. Unfortunately, these results were a fairly superficial view of the evidence. First of all, the absolute numbers were miniscule—in the two thousand children in the study, two in the control group expressed suicidal thoughts, whereas four did in the experimental group. More important, these were thoughts only—no suicide attempts or events occurred during the study at all. Finally, subsequent studies have been unable to replicate these results.

Despite these facts, the black box warning remained foremost in the minds (and fears) of doctors as well as parents. For many years, pediatricians and many psychiatrists would not even think of medicating depressed adolescents for fear of "causing" suicidality. In reality, untreated depression is the most important risk factor for suicide, not treatment with an SSRI, so many young people with depression were in a precarious state.

Now, public (and professional) opinion is swinging back toward the middle as more of the facts emerge. Prozac and similar pharmaceuticals that have since been introduced (table 6-2) are extremely safe and have a record of side effects vastly superior to that of tricyclic antidepressants. The most encouraging fact in the treatment of serious depression in young people is that, unlike the tricyclics, this group of medications has shown unequivocal benefits in double-blind placebo-controlled studies in children and adolescents.

Table 6-2 Selective Serotonin Reuptake Inhibitors (SSRIs)

Generic Name	Brand Name
Citalopram	Celexa
Escitalopram	Lexapro
Fluoxetine	Prozac
Fluvoxamine	Luvox
Paroxetine	Paxil
Sertraline	Zoloft

These new antidepressants also differ from tricyclics in that they have little direct effect on norepinephrine in the brain; instead, they block the reuptake of another neurotransmitter into neurons, another amine compound called *serotonin*. The potent and specific blockade of serotonin reuptake by these agents gives this class its name: *selective serotonin reuptake inhibitor*. As with the tricyclics, the effect on serotonin in the synapse seems to occur at the receptors, and there is some evidence that serotonin is actually the more important neurotransmitter in the treatment of depression. Scientists are discovering, however, that despite their name, these medications have more effects on the brain than had initially been appreciated, such as potentially protecting neurons from damage and reducing inflammation in the brain. The development of these new agents, which help with depression but seem to work differently than the tricyclics, has provided more clues to the underlying biology of mood disorders.

Unlike most other psychiatric medications, most of the SSRIs have FDA-approved dosing guidelines for children and adolescents. In many cases, this approval was given several years after the drugs were labeled for use in adults, again proving the point that off-label prescribing is not unusual for psychiatric medications in young people.

The main side effect of the SSRIs is gastrointestinal discomfort. Many patients experience nausea for the first couple of days after starting to take one of the SSRIs, and a few have diarrhea or constipation. We call this a side effect, but it's actually not. In fact, the majority of the serotonin in our bodies, almost 90 percent, is used as a signaling mechanism not in our brains, but in our digestive tract. Scientists are only recently appreciating the complex neurological structure required to maintain our digestive processes, finding an entire neuronal network similar in complexity to our spinal cord residing in and around our gut. So, it is easy to see why medications that affect serotonin signaling would have an effect on this region as well. The gut is remarkably good at maintaining its equilibrium, so once it becomes used to these medications, the gastrointestinal effects are quickly gone (typically within a few days).

These medications (especially fluoxetine) are also somewhat stimulating in some patients, and though this is just what some depressed people need, others feel unpleasantly nervous or "wired" on these medications. In children, this can present as agitation or irritability, which might make prescribing SSRIs for adolescents seem contradictory. We've already said that depression can cause irritability in some adolescents, so why would we give them a medication that could potentially make it worse? The answer is that the irritability of depression and the irritability of SSRI treatment are entirely different. In these medications, this side effect is transient and passes quickly—within a day or two—and is mild. Also, these side effects occur in a small portion of the population taking these medicines. Most important is that once the sufferer of even the most severe side effects is over this brief hump, the benefits of the medication take hold, and the irritability overall lessens substantially.

Unusually, a person may suffer the converse of the side effects described above, such as feeling sleepier than usual, or having slightly less energy. Many patients report that SSRIs seem to curb their appetite a bit, and they also notice some weight loss, especially early on in taking an SSRI. This is, of course, a potential concern in young people who are still growing. Someone who is going to have these side effects usually notices them immediately; none of them sneak up on a person who has been taking an SSRI for weeks or months.

In adults, SSRIs have been reported to cause an unpleasant blunting of emotions; patients complain of being apathetic and indifferent to events, of being unable to get excited or enthusiastic about anything.[7,8] This appears to be a problem only at high doses and does not often trouble patients taking the usual antidepressant dose.

Another side effect that has been described is a change in sexual functioning, specifically a noticeable decrease in sexual interest (loss of libido) or difficulty in reaching or inability to reach orgasm. The frequency of these problems was at first difficult to gauge, because these sorts of side effects were often not asked about during clinical trials. But as more people have been treated with SSRIs since they were introduced in the early 1990s, it has become apparent that this is a significant problem affecting at least one-third of patients. We don't want to get into a discussion of the complicated issue of adolescent sexuality here, but for a young and insecure individual, sexual side effects may be very important. We have had cases of young persons, usually boys, who stop their medications and refuse to restart them but will not tell us why. Through gentle questioning, it eventually became apparent that sexual side effects were behind their sudden departure from treatment. In many cases, the concern was not an inability to perform with a partner but merely how a decrease in sexual desire made them feel separate and different from their peers, further isolating an already depressed individual. Various strategies are available for dealing with these problems when they occur, so it is critical for clinicians to ask about these features with every adolescent started on medications, particularly when an abrupt, unexplained disinterest in further treatment develops. Weekend "vacations" from the medication have been reported to be helpful, as well as the addition of other medications that seem to block these effects, but sometimes a switch to another antidepressant in another class is the only solution (though often an effective one).

Some side effects of SSRI medications may not be noticed outside exceptional circumstances. Some people who stop their medications abruptly (if they, say, forget to bring their pills on a vacation) feel almost as though they have the flu for a day or two—they feel slightly feverish, slowed down, and achy. These symptoms are not dangerous, and they pass fairly quickly, but they can be uncomfortable.

Like most psychiatric medications, SSRIs are metabolized in the liver, and the details of this process have been studied more carefully for this class of medications than for most other psychiatric drugs. Many SSRIs cause a partial blockade of the cellular machinery responsible for breaking down many other medications in the liver, so they can increase the time it takes for the body to get rid of medications. This means that levels of those medications in the body will rise. For example, if an adolescent who is taking theophylline (Theo-Dur and others) for asthma starts taking fluvoxamine (Luvox) for depression, her level of theophylline can rise to toxic levels because the antidepressant slows down theophylline metabolism. For this reason, *all* physicians caring for a patient need to know about any change of medications; they need to pay close attention to drug interactions with SSRIs—and for that matter, with all medications.

OTHER, NEW, ANTIDEPRESSANTS

Since the early 1990s, a whole series of new antidepressants have come on the market that are neither tricyclics nor SSRIs (table 6-3). Most of these pharmaceuticals don't share many common features, so there isn't a good class name for them; you'll sometimes see many of these new agents listed as "atypical" or "second generation" antidepressants. They have a variety of effects on norepinephrine, serotonin, and even other neurotransmitters; some have more than one effect on these systems, so they are thought to provide different ways of manipulating the chemical systems in the brain that are concerned with mood. Their side-effect profiles vary widely: some are more like tricyclics, others more like SSRIs.

SEROTONIN-NOREPINEPHRINE REUPTAKE INHIBITORS

As the 1990s progressed, psychiatrists began to notice a population of patients who had depression that did not respond to the SSRI medications but who were amenable to treatment with the tricyclic antidepressants. By this time, tricyclics were considered a second-line medication, primarily because of the significant side effects and potential lethality in overdose, not to mention the need to get blood drawn for levels periodically. Psychiatrists, and pharmaceutical companies, tried to develop a chemical that had the benefits of the tricyclics but the side-effect profile of the SSRIs. Although the general consensus was that the primary brain chemical responsible for depression was serotonin, this was clearly (as we have discussed) not the full picture. The biggest difference between these two chemicals seemed to lie somewhere in their ability to also target norepinephrine. In 1994, Wyeth introduced the chemical venlafaxine (Effexor), touting it as the perfect antidepressant. This *serotonin-norepinephrine reuptake inhibitor* (SNRI) was active on both serotonin and norepinephrine, like a tricyclic, but had a mild side-effect profile and was nonlethal, like an SSRI.

As it turned out, this description was not strictly true. First of all, at low doses, venlafaxine isn't very active in norepinephrine at all—only at

Table 6-3   New Antidepressants

Generic Name	Brand Name
Serotonin-Norepinephrine Reuptake Inhibitors (SNRI)	
Venlafaxine	Effexor
Desvenlafaxine	Pristiq
Duloxetine	Cymbalta
Dopamine-Norepinephrine Reuptake Inhibitors (DNRI)	
Bupropion	Wellbutrin

higher doses does this benefit become apparent. Furthermore, most patients will tell you that the side effects are indeed more significant than an SSRI, even severe for some. That said, the SNRI was immensely helpful to those patients who did not respond to an SSRI, proving that it did indeed have a place in the pharmacological lexicon of psychiatry. Since its inception, venlafaxine has been placed into an extended release formulation so that it needs to be taken only once a day (as opposed to three times a day). Additionally, other medications in the same class (duloxetine [Cymbalta] and desvenlafaxine [Pristiq]) have been created with more or less the same intent.

In terms of side effects, adding norepinephrine to the equation did add some unanticipated consequences. Norepinephrine is used in the body in a way similar to adrenaline. Patients with too much of this chemical can see a small though significant rise in their heart rate or blood pressure. Also, abrupt withdrawal from these medications can cause a somewhat unusual subjective feeling, almost like small electrical jolts in the muscles, which, though not painful, can be uncomfortable.

Although evidence now shows that SNRIs can be effective for children and adolescents (particularly older adolescents), they have still not been approved by the FDA for these indications and so are typically reserved by psychiatrists for patients who do not do as well on initial treatment with an SSRI.[9] There is some evidence that they may also be helpful for children with attention deficit disorder[10] or chronic pain,[11] so some psychiatrists may use them as a first-line agent for children with these types of problems in addition to depression.

By now, you are probably seeing a pattern in antidepressant medications. Since we do not yet know how exactly these medications do what they do, how they help alleviate depression, researchers are trying to think of every combination possible in helping patients who are suffering with this condition. We have talked about serotonin and serotonin plus norepinephrine, and now we will discuss norepinephrine plus dopamine. Many of you will be familiar with dopamine as the "pleasure chemical" or the "reward chemical" —it is so potent that in particularly susceptible people, it reinforces gambling or drug use to the exclusion of other interests in life. For some, depression constitutes primarily a loss of pleasure in life, so what better way to try to eliminate depression than by stimulating an increase in dopamine? It turns out that dopamine is rather short lived in the brain, so pure dopaminergic drugs don't work the way we would like. But when combined with norepinephrine, dopamine does seem to be helpful. Commonly marketed today as bupropion (Wellbutrin), *dopamine-norepinephrine reuptake inhibitors* (DNRIs) are somewhat different from the antidepressants we've discussed so far.

Bupropion is a widely prescribed antidepressant, popular not so much for what it does do as what it doesn't. Its side effects seem to be quite different from the tricyclics, SSRIs, and SNRIs. It is almost never associated with weight gain and for many leads to a slight weight loss, typically by lowering the appetite. It has few if any sexual side effects, and stopping the medication abruptly does not lead to the same flulike symptoms. Bupropion does have one side effect that can be quite serious, though. In some persons, it has been shown to lower the seizure threshold to the point that epileptic seizures develop. This is a very rare side effect but is notable in people who are already prone to seizures or who have other conditions that may predispose them to this condition (eating disorders, for example, can cause imbalances in the nutritional status of a person, making them more likely to seize).

As an antidepressant, bupropion seems to be about as effective as the other medications. It seems particularly helpful for those depressive symptoms characterized by fatigue, low energy, and sleeping and even eating too much—what was called *atypical* depression at one point. It also helps persons with seasonal affective disorder—a milder depression that seems to come on in the winter, thought to be due to the effect of reduced sunlight. Like the SNRIs, DNRIs have some action in the norepinephrine family of neurotransmitters, so they have been used for people who have both depression and attention deficit disorder. Finally, the dopamine activity seems to blunt the highs and lows of addiction, so DNRIs have been used to help those interested in quitting smoking (when marketed as Zyban). Because bupropion seems to work by a somewhat different mechanism than the SSRIs, it is commonly added to these medications for those patients who don't have full remission of their depression.

Although many SNRIs and DNRIs are used frequently in children and adolescents, they are not approved by the FDA for this purpose and so are, with few exceptions, reserved for young patients who do not respond adequately to one of the first-line medications, typically an SSRI. There are other alternate antidepressants out there, and more are being developed as this is written, so it is important for parents to have open, direct, and potentially lengthy conversations with psychiatrists about why they chose a certain medication, what they are hoping to accomplish with its use, what side effects are possible or can be expected, and how long they expect it to take before the patient and parents see a benefit. More information, in this case, is always a good thing.

MONOAMINE OXIDASE INHIBITORS

You've already heard about iproniazid, the drug developed to treat tuberculosis that caused mood elevation in some patients who took it for their lung disease. In addition to its effect on the tubercle bacillus, iproniazid causes inactivation of an enzyme in the body that metabolizes amine compounds in the nervous system. This enzyme, called *monoamine oxidase*, is responsible for gobbling up molecules of norepinephrine, serotonin, and several other neurotransmitters. Inactivating monoamine oxidase has the effect of increasing the amounts of these compounds in the nervous system, and this effect, in some as yet poorly understood way, may be the mechanism by which these medications alleviate the symptoms of depression. This effect on the enzyme gives this class of pharmaceuticals their name: *monoamine oxidase inhibitors*, or MAOIs (table 6-4).

Monoamine oxidase is also present in the lining of the intestine and in the liver; a number of naturally occurring substances in foods are close

Table 6-4   Monoamine Oxidase Inhibitors (MAOIs)

Generic Name	Brand Name
Phenelzine	Nardil
Selegiline	Eldepryl, Emsam
Tranylcypromine	Parnate

enough chemically to norepinephrine to need deactivation before they are absorbed into the bloodstream. The importance of this becomes clear when we tell you that another name for norepinephrine is nor*adrenaline*. Tyramine, an amino acid that has adrenaline-like effects on blood pressure and heart rate, is present in high enough concentrations in some foods to cause dangerous cardiovascular problems in persons taking MAOIs (table 6-5). A number of pharmaceuticals, including the ingredients of many over-the-counter remedies, also have adrenaline-like effects. Persons taking MAOIs therefore need to observe certain dietary restrictions and, even more important, need to *scrupulously* read the labels of any over-the-counter medication they are considering—or better yet, consult their pharmacist before taking any pharmaceutical bought over the counter.

Medications of this type also interact with other drugs that are prescribed or commonly used in emergency rooms for various problems. Anyone taking an MAOI must be sure to inform all his treating physicians that he is using this medication. He should also consider wearing an alerting bracelet, so that if he is brought unconscious to an emergency room after an accident or a sudden illness, the ER personnel will be aware that he's taking an MAOI.

Other side effects accompany MAOIs too. These medications can be stimulating and cause nervousness, insomnia, and excess perspiration. Dizzy spells, especially when suddenly getting up from lying down, can occur. MAOIs block a blood pressure reflex that usually maintains blood pressure when we stand up, and the sudden drop in blood pressure on standing (called *orthostatic hypotension*) causes light-headedness. Weight gain, water retention, and sexual dysfunction may also occur.

As you might predict from the foregoing discussion, MAOIs are seldom used in the United States unless other antidepressants have failed to be effective, and they are even more rarely used in adolescents. Indeed, taking a medication that would mean not eating pepperoni pizzas seems too much to ask of a teenager. Nevertheless, MAOIs are sometimes uniquely effective

Table 6-5   Foods to Avoid while Taking MAOIs

Fava or broad beans
Aged cheese (cream and cottage cheese permitted)
Beef liver or chicken liver
Orange pulp
Pickled or smoked fish, poultry, or other meats
Sauerkraut
Packaged soups
Fermented bean curd (tofu)
Yeast and protein dietary supplements
Summer (dry) sausage (e.g., pepperoni)
Soy sauce
Sour cream
Draft beer and many wines

Note: This list is not exhaustive, and some items included here are low enough in tyramine that some physicians allow one or two servings per day. Patients, and parents, should get a complete list and discuss the specifics of the diet with a knowledgeable physician, pharmacist, or nutritionist before starting to take an MAOI.

treatments for depression. Almost every psychiatrist we've ever spoken with has had the experience of effectively treating a particular patient with an MAOI after no other antidepressant had helped.

In an attempt to avoid these unpleasant side effects, one company had the idea to bypass the digestive system altogether. It found a way to deliver one type of MAOI, called selegiline (Emsam), through a person's skin. Users place a patch, similar to a nicotine patch, on their body and wear it throughout the day. A small, even dose of selegiline is delivered directly to the bloodstream. In this way, the tyramine in food can still be deactivated. Even the manufacturer admits, however, that you can maintain a normal diet only at the lowest dose of the medication, which is unlikely to be effective for the majority of people; above this dose, you must still maintain a strict tyramine-free diet, difficult for most people and nearly impossible for an adolescent.

ANTIDEPRESSANT THERAPY: SOME GENERAL CONSIDERATIONS

In 2012, the Cochrane Collaboration completed another meta-analysis investigating the use of "newer" antidepressants (the SSRIs and their variations listed above) for the treatment of depression in children and adolescents. They found them to be effective, particularly in adolescents (over 12 years old) rather than children. The majority of the studies used fluoxetine, since it is the only FDA-approved medication for depression and therefore, for multiple reasons, far easier to study than unapproved medications. The study found, however, that "there was no evidence that one particular type of newer generation antidepressant had a larger effect than the others."[12] The safety and effectiveness of the SSRIs are perhaps the most clearly supported by research, but which SSRI (or, in rare cases, other medicine) should be chosen as the first-line drug? What dose should be used? How long does one wait before deciding that a medication isn't working? What then?

When studies have compared antidepressant medications in large groups of (adult) patients for the treatment of depression, no single pharmaceutical has ever been proved to work better or faster than any other. There is no "best" antidepressant. If there were, we wouldn't find several dozen different ones on the market in the United States. Neither is there a "strongest" antidepressant medication. The usual dose of one may be higher, in milligrams, than that of another, but this has nothing to do with effectiveness.

We've already mentioned the evidence for superior efficacy of SSRIs over tricyclics in adolescents, but we have no evidence that one SSRI is superior to another. Considerable evidence suggests that some adult patients who get better with tricyclic medications do not improve on taking SSRIs, and vice versa. The same could well be true for adolescents: there may be a small group of adolescents for whom tricyclic medications are *more* effective than SSRIs, but the proportion of these patients to other patients responsive only to SSRIs is so small that statistical analysis doesn't "see" them in the studies done so far.

Because of this lack of proven superiority of any particular agent, subtle differences in side effects are often used to make a choice among antidepressant medications. An antidepressant that is mildly sedating might be a good choice if insomnia or anxiety is a prominent symptom of depression in a particular patient. A medication that tends to be somewhat stimulating might be a choice if the patient is lethargic and having problems with energy level. One that stimulates appetite might be a major problem for one adolescent but just what is needed for another. Physicians' experience with a particular medication may make it a first among equals in their prescribing for patients. Indeed, a medication that a particular doctor has had a lot of experience with in prescribing for patients probably *is* a better medicine than a similar one that is prescribed less often—for this doctor's patients at least.

We've already discussed some of the problems in deciding on a dose for adolescents. Fortunately, more data are becoming available all the time to help with this. Most of the SSRIs are already labeled for use in young patients (though usually for reasons other than depression, such as panic disorder or obsessive-compulsive disorder). Remember, too, that doses of all medications in older adolescents are usually not so different from those used in adults, and probably little alteration in treatment will be needed from that used for adults. No radical biological shift occurs on an adolescent's eighteenth birthday that makes him suddenly an adult physiologically. Treatment decisions for some 17- and 16-year-olds may be the same as those for adults.

One of the most frustrating aspects of antidepressant therapy is the lag time between starting medication and improvement in symptoms. Most studies of depressed patients first starting to take an antidepressant medication report some improvement of symptoms within two weeks. But it often takes longer for improvement to be noticed. The sequence of events brought about in the brain by antidepressant treatment most likely involves a re-engineering of neurons on some level, probably through turning on genes in these cells. This process takes time. It's not unreasonable to wait four to six weeks before giving up on a medication. Even when a medication is beginning to help, it may take a long time for its *full* benefit to become apparent.

Studies of depressed adults indicate that depressive symptoms continue to improve for up to three months after starting to take antidepressant medications. Unfortunately, this lag time is not usually the same for the side effects as for the efficacy. Most of the bothersome effects of these medications (sedation, appetite changes, sexual side effects) seem to occur through some other, more direct route than genetic manipulation and often appear within days of starting a medication. We often hear parents and patients complain that a medicine "made them worse" than they were before, which can of course seem true if the only effect you are feeling from a medication is a little nausea in the midst of a depression. The best and only counsel we can give is that these side effects do, fortunately, resolve quickly. Patience is the most important virtue when treating depression with a medication, though one that is frequently difficult to find when in the midst of deep suffering.

What options are available if a medication doesn't seem to be helping? Raising the dose is often the first choice. A switch to an antidepressant in a different class is another. At some point, adding another medication is often tried. Some patients respond to combinations of antidepressants or a combination of an antidepressant and another type of medication, such as a mood-stabilizing medication. Use of the maximum dosage has been studied, both in adults and in adolescents. The Treatment of Adolescents with Depression Study (TADS) found that after maximizing the dose of antidepressant, about 60 percent of patients improved significantly.

Within the last few years, a study concerning the Treatment of SSRI Resistant Depression in Adolescents (TORDIA) looked at patients who did not seem to respond well to the first antidepressant tried. The results of this study are still being evaluated, though the initial results seem to show that changing to another SSRI resulted in a further 60 percent of those patients getting better (so, along with the 60 percent who responded to the first medicine, about 15 percent of adolescents in the study still had depressive symptoms). This number was the same as when adolescents were switched to another type of antidepressant (in this study, the SNRI venlafaxine). So, many psychiatrists will first try one or two SSRI medications, then, if there isn't an adequate response, move on to alternate antidepressants. If the child still doesn't seem to be getting better, adding another type of medication, like a mood stabilizer (what we call *augmenting* the antidepressant), can be hugely helpful.

We have no way to know beforehand which patient will respond to which antidepressant. And we have no way to know which, if any, side effects a particular person will develop. Unfortunately, some trial and error is required in the process of finding the medication or combination of medications that works best with the fewest side effects. The clues to how a person will respond to a medication seem to reside within the genetic code of the individual. One of the greatest clues we have lies in the response to medication of a close family member. If we are seeing a patient with, say, an older brother who also had depression but had an excellent response to fluoxetine (Prozac) with no side effects, that would be the first medicine we would reach for, as it is likely that the patient will respond in the same way. In chapter 15, we talk in more detail about how an individual's genes interact with medications, a relatively new field of science known as *pharmacogenomics*. Several commercially available genetic tests aim to take some of the guesswork out of prescribing psychiatric medications by providing the prescriber with information about which medications are more likely to be effective or to cause side effects in a particular patient. Although prescribing antidepressant medications can accurately be described as an art rather than a science, this is changing quickly.

Mood-Stabilizing Medications

True mood stabilizers are medications that have both antimanic and antidepressant effects. They are usually the foundation for the treatment of people with bipolar disorders, and they are used for other problems as well. Mood stabilizers, especially lithium, are often used in combination with antidepressant medications to treat depression that is unresponsive to an antidepressant alone. At the end of this chapter, we discuss how physicians go about making the decision to treat an individual with a mood stabilizer.

LITHIUM

In the second century AD, the Greek physician Soranus of Ephesus recommended that physicians treating patients suffering from mania should prescribe "natural waters, such as [from] alkaline springs."[1] Roman physicians recommended that their patients "take the waters" at various springs for a whole variety of physical and mental ailments. The little town of Spa in eastern Belgium, Bath in England, Wiesbaden in Germany, and dozens of other towns in Italy and Greece that were the sites of natural springs became centers for healing. As the science of analytical chemistry developed, curious chemists and physicians evaluated these various springs and found that the waters of many were rich in lithium.

In the middle of the nineteenth century, lithium compounds were tried as treatments for gout and kidney stones. Unfortunately, the approach was unsuccessful and was soon abandoned. Nevertheless, this work led to formulation of pharmaceutical preparations of lithium compounds and to information on the range of safe doses for lithium preparations in humans.

In the 1940s, lithium came to medical attention again when lithium chloride was introduced as a substitute for table salt (sodium chloride) for people with medical problems, such as heart disease and high blood pressure, that required them to be on a low-sodium diet. But when heart patients were given saltshakers full of lithium salts to sprinkle on their food, the results were catastrophic for some. Because lithium is toxic in surprisingly low concentrations, substituting lithium chloride for sodium chloride turned out to be a disaster. There were many reports of severe lithium poisoning and even several deaths. The use of lithium as a salt substitute ended, and the episode had the effect of giving lithium a bad reputation among physicians.

So it was very much a chance occurrence that led to the discovery of lithium's beneficial effects on mood disorders in 1948. John F. J. Cade, MD, senior medical officer in the Mental Hygiene Department of Victoria, Australia, was working in his laboratory on trying to determine whether some toxin might be present in the urine of individuals with manic-depressive illness. Cade was especially interested in urea and uric acid, by-products of protein metabolism found in urine, and was testing the toxicity of these compounds by injecting small amounts of them into guinea pigs.

One of the technical problems with his work was that uric acid is rather insoluble in water, making it difficult to prepare injectable solutions of higher concentrations. Looking for a soluble urate salt to use instead of uric acid, Cade consulted prior research and discovered that uric acid was easiest to dissolve in water when it was combined with lithium as lithium urate. He injected small amounts of lithium urate into the guinea pigs and noticed that uric acid seemed to be much less toxic in this form. This suggested to Cade that the lithium component of the compound might have some sort of protective effect against urate toxicity. To determine what the effect of the lithium ion might be, he injected lithium carbonate (the carbonate ion is a harmless substance, found, for example, as sodium carbonate in baking soda)* and discovered that "after a latent period of about two hours the animals, although fully conscious, became extremely lethargic and unresponsive to stimuli for one to two hours before once again becoming normally active."[2]

As Cade admitted in his original paper, "It may seem a long distance from lethargy in guinea pigs to excitement in psychotics,"[3] but doctors of the time were desperate for new treatment possibilities. So Cade decided to administer lithium preparations to several patients who were chronically agitated. The effect on individuals with mania was dramatic:

> CASE I—W.B., a male aged fifty-one years, who had been in a state of chronic manic excitement for five years, restless, dirty, destructive, mischievous and interfering, had long been regarded as the most troublesome patient in the ward. His response was highly gratifying. From the start of treatment on March 29, 1948, with lithium citrate he steadily settled down and in three weeks was enjoying the unaccustomed surrounding of the convalescent ward. As he had been ill so long and confined to a "chronic ward," he found normal surroundings and liberty of movement strange at first. He remained perfectly well and left the hospital on indefinite leave with instructions to take a dose of lithium carbonate, five grains, twice a day. He was soon back working at his old job.

> CASE VIII—W.M., a man of fifty years, was suffering from an attack of recurrent mania, the first of which he had had at the age of twenty. The present attack had lasted two months and showed no signs of abating. He was garrulous, euphoric, restless and unkempt when he started taking lithium. Two days later he was reported to be quieter. By the ninth day he was definitely settling down and the following day commenced work in the garden. By the end of two weeks he was practically normal—quiet, tidy, rational, with insight into his previous condition.[4]

At this point, Dr. Cade had treated ten manic patients with lithium, and all ten had shown the same dramatic improvement. One would think the news of Cade's discovery would have spread like wildfire. It did not. In fact,

---

* Many chemicals, including medications, consist of two parts called *ions*, one of which is positively charged (such as lithium or sodium) and the other negatively charged (such as chloride or carbonate). When the two parts exist together as a *compound*, the charges cancel each other out, and the system is stable.

not until several decades later did the United States Food and Drug Administration approve lithium for the treatment of bipolar disorder. Part of the reason for this delay was the state of world psychiatry following the end of the Second World War. Much of European psychiatry, especially German psychiatry, was in ruins, literally and figuratively. In the United States and England, psychoanalytic theories had replaced the traditional medical practices of evaluation, diagnosis, and treatment with the prescription of "the talking cure" for all emotional problems. Accurate psychiatric diagnosis simply didn't exist. Ronald Fieve, the American psychiatrist who would champion the use of lithium in the United States in the 1970s and who was instrumental in getting American psychiatrists to prescribe it for their patients, observed that during the late 1940s and the 1950s in New York, he "rarely met with the diagnosis of manic-depression . . . It had virtually disappeared. Most cases of excitable, talkative, and elated behavior were being diagnosed as schizophrenia."[5]

But a Danish psychiatrist, Morgans Schou, realized that Cade's discovery was a real breakthrough (noting in a 1954 paper that "it is rather astonishing that [Cade's] observation has failed to arouse greater general interest among psychiatrists").[6] Schou quickly became convinced of the effectiveness of lithium in treating acute mania, and he was one of the first clinical researchers to become convinced of another therapeutic effect of the drug: its ability to prevent further episodes of illness (lithium's preventive, or *prophylactic,* effect). Schou had a more difficult time convincing his colleagues around the world that lithium could prevent recurrences of bipolar disorder and that patients should take it even after their acute symptoms had subsided. In 1967, Schou and his colleague Paul Christian Baalstrup reported on eighty-eight patients who had taken lithium for several years and had experienced a dramatic reduction in the frequency and duration of their mood episodes. Several patients who had been sick for several weeks out of every year experienced a complete remission of their illness that lasted for more than five years: their illness had essentially stopped (figure 7-1).[7]

As Schou and his colleagues treated more and more patients with lithium, their findings that lithium favorably altered the course of bipolar illness became so clear that they had ethical qualms about doing a more rigorous placebo-controlled study—one in which patients with bipolar disorder

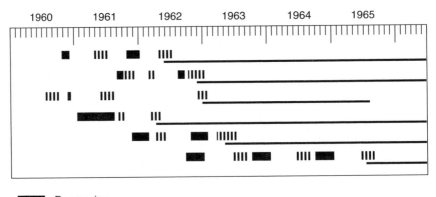

Figure 7-1 This graph illustrates data from six patients in Baalstrup and Schou's early study of the protective effect of lithium against the relapse of bipolar symptoms. Each line represents the symptom course of one patient. In all these patients, when lithium was started, episodes of depression and mania stopped completely. *Source*: Data from Paul Baalstrup and Morgans Schou, "Lithium as a Prophylactic Agent: Its Effect against Recurrent Depressions and Manic-Depressive Psychosis," *Archives of General Psychiatry* 16, no. 2 (1967): 162–72.

would be divided into two groups, some to receive lithium and the others a placebo. Several British psychiatrists scolded the Danes for reporting their results without a placebo-controlled study, so Baalstrup and Schou did a lithium discontinuation study in which they selected patients who had been stable while taking lithium for at least a year, divided them into two roughly equal groups, and in one group substituted a placebo for the lithium. The results were dramatic: of the thirty-nine participants whose lithium was replaced with the placebo, twenty-one relapsed within five months; *none* of the forty-five participants still taking lithium had a relapse.

It took a few more years to show that lithium is an effective antidepressant as well, but by the early 1980s, clinical studies had clearly shown that lithium is also an effective treatment for depressive syndrome.[8] Also clearly proven is that adding lithium to antidepressant medication can benefit people who have had an incomplete response to an antidepressant. This use, often referred to as antidepressant *augmentation*, can effectively turn a poor or incomplete therapeutic effect into a complete one.[9] Its antidepressant properties are thought to come from a completely different mechanism than most traditional antidepressants, which may be one reason it is so effective.

THERAPEUTIC PROFILE

Lithium is a naturally occurring element found in mineral springs, seawater, and certain ores. Like its close cousin, sodium, it is never found in its pure form in nature; it is always combined with other ions as a salt of one type or another. Lithium is mined on an industrial scale for use in the manufacture of ceramics and batteries. Therapeutic lithium preparations usually contain lithium carbonate. (See the therapeutic profile in table 7-1.)

Because it is an element, lithium is not metabolized within the body, and because lithium ions are so similar to sodium ions, the body handles lithium in much the same way it handles sodium. Lithium is rapidly absorbed through the gastrointestinal tract, enters the bloodstream, and is eliminated from the body by being filtered out by the kidneys.

Descriptions of the effects of a pharmaceutical in the body always include a vital statistic called its *half-life*. This is a measure of how quickly the body gets rid of a medication. Specifically, it is the time required for half the amount of the drug to be eliminated or metabolized by the body. Put another way, it is the time the body takes to reduce the level of the medication by half. The half-life of lithium in children and adolescents is about the same as in adults: approximately eighteen hours.[10] Another useful number, which can be derived from the half-life statistic for any medication, is the time required for the level of medication to build up to a constant level in the body—the time required for the amount taken in to equal the amount

Table 7-1 Therapeutic Profile of Lithium

Medication class:	Mood stabilizer
Brand names:	Eskalith, Eskalith CR, Lithobid, Lithonate, Lithotabs
Generic names:	Lithium carbonate, lithium citrate (liquid preparation)
Half-life:	14 to 30 hours
Metabolism:	None
Need for birth control:	Probably mandatory (see text)
Other considerations:	Blood levels extremely important

eliminated: the equilibrium point. By a series of mathematical steps that we don't need to detail here, it can be shown that the equilibrium point is the same for all medications: five half-lives. This means that since the half-life of lithium is roughly one day, it takes about five days for lithium, when first taken, to reach a steady level in the bloodstream. It also means that if the lithium dose is changed, it takes about five days for the blood level to stabilize at a new level.

Because of the toxic effects and even deaths that were reported when heart patients sprinkled lithium salt freely on their food, there was a significant delay in the acceptance of lithium as a therapeutic agent. Lithium is a powerful pharmaceutical, one that must be treated with respect. It has a very low *therapeutic index*, meaning that the difference between the therapeutic dose and a toxic dose is small.* Fortunately, lithium can be measured in the bloodstream accurately and fairly cheaply, and the dosage adjusted accordingly.

Monitoring of lithium levels in the blood is important not only to prevent toxicity but also because clinical studies have clearly demonstrated that, for most individuals, lithium needs to be present in the bloodstream at a certain level to be effective.[†] Clinical studies indicate that the therapeutic range for maximum efficacy is the same in adolescents and adults. But just what that level should be has been a matter of some debate.

An important study from the Massachusetts General Hospital found that a level of between 0.8 and 1.0 meq/L (milliequivalent per liter, a chemical measure of concentration) was most effective. In this double-blind study, adults with bipolar disorder were divided into two groups: a "standard dose" group, whose lithium levels were kept between 0.8 and 1.0 meq/L, and a "low dose" group, whose levels were maintained between 0.4 and 0.6 meq/L. The result was that the relapse rate in the "low dose" group was more than double that in the "standard dose" group (table 7-2).

There is more to these data than may initially meet the eye, however.

------

* To be more precise, the therapeutic index is the ratio of the largest dose producing no toxic symptoms to the smallest dose routinely producing the desired therapeutic effects.

† We speak of a "therapeutic level" in discussing the effective range of lithium in the bloodstream for treatment, not a "normal level." Lithium is a trace element in the body, normally present in undetectable concentrations.

Table 7-2   Comparison of Higher and Lower Lithium Levels in Relapse Rates of Bipolar Disorder

Treatment Group	Any Relapse	Depressed	Mixed/ Manic	Hypo- manic	Withdrew from Study
Standard dose range (0.8–1.0 meq/L)	6 (12%)	3 (6%)	3 (6%)	0	24 (51%)
Low dose range (0.4-0.6 meq/L)	21 (44%)	1 (2%)	17 (35%)	3 (6%)	11 (23%)

Source: Data from Alan Gelenberg, John Kane, Martin Keller, Phillip Lavori, Jerrold Rosenbaum, Karyl Cole, and Janet Lavelle, "Comparison of Standard and Low Levels of Lithium for Maintenance Treatment of Bipolar Disorder," *New England Journal of Medicine* 321, no. 22 (1989): 1489–93.
Note: Percentages are rounded.

Many more patients from the "standard dose" group than from the "low dose" group dropped out of the study because of side effects. The take-home message seems to be that levels closer to 1.0 meq/L are more protective, but that many people have trouble taking such a high dose because of side effects. Many psychiatrists compromise and try to maintain their patients at levels between these two. Dr. Schou, whom many consider the father of lithium therapy, has recommended levels of 0.5 to 0.8 meq/L for the treatment of bipolar disorder in adults.[11] Some people, however, clearly have good control of their symptoms with even lower levels, elderly persons, for example. Lithium levels thus need to be individualized for individual patients, and as Dr. Schou also points out, "Changes in lithium levels as small as 0.1 to 0.2 [meq/L], upward or downward, may substantially improve patients' quality of life during maintenance treatment."[12]

The lithium level rises in the bloodstream after every dose, peaks in about two hours, and then begins to fall again. If a patient takes his lithium two or three times a day, there will be several peaks and valleys. Because the level is rising and falling throughout the day, in checking lithium level it is important that the blood be drawn at a time when the result can be correctly interpreted. The convention that has been adopted is to use a twelve-hour level, making it convenient to draw blood in the mornings. For most people, this means getting to the lab twelve hours after their bedtime dose (for example, at 11 a.m. if the bedtime dose was at 11 the night before), without having taken their usual morning dose.

Lithium is approved for use in treating bipolar disorder in adolescents over the age of 12. Given what we've said about the variability of physical maturity in adolescents, you may wonder why the FDA doesn't label lithium and other drugs as approved for people of a certain height or weight rather than a certain age. The short answer is that this is simply how the FDA decided to do things. Remember that pharmaceutical labeling is a *guide* to prescribing medications, not *rules* for prescribing them.

Clinical research indicates that lithium is as effective for treating bipolar disorder in adolescents as it is in adults.[13] The research on using lithium as an augmentation of antidepressant treatment is more limited for adolescents than for adults, but the results are encouraging. In open trials of lithium as an augmentation of tricyclic antidepressants, about half the adolescents who had not had an adequate response to a tricyclic alone got better when lithium was added. This is about the same response usually seen in adults.[14] There have been case reports of lithium also helping the newer antidepressants to work better.[15] One of the most convincing reasons to consider lithium in certain populations is that it seems to reduce suicide. This has been shown time and again, most recently in a large meta-analysis of more than 6,000 adolescents.[16] No one understands exactly why, but in some way lithium reduces both suicidal thinking and suicide itself. The effect seems to be seen even in patients who continue to have other symptoms of depression that lithium did not reduce.

SIDE EFFECTS

Individuals vary widely in their sensitivity to side effects of lithium (and of all medications, for that matter). Some people have none; others have several. Fortunately, almost all of lithium's side effects can be eliminated or managed (table 7-3).

Many of the side effects are *dose related*: the higher the lithium dose, the more severe the side effect. One management strategy, then, is simply to lower the lithium dose. The advantages of higher levels are clear, as noted above, but most physicians will aim to maintain patients at the lowest possible dose that controls their symptoms.

Because of its similarity to sodium, lithium has some of the same effects that an increased sodium (table salt) intake would have: increased thirst, increased urination, and water retention. These side effects are often tem-

Table 7-3 Treatable Side Effects of Lithium

Side Effect	Remedy
Nausea, diarrhea	Take immediately after meals; switch to a controlled-release preparation
Weight gain	Diet and exercise
Tremor	Cut out caffeine-containing beverages; take beta-blocker medications
Flare-up of preexisting dermatological condition	Dermatological preparations
Hypothyroidism	Thyroid medications

porary and subside as the body adjusts to the medication. If they do not, the judicious use of medications that promote urination and excretion of excess body water (diuretics) can help. DO NOT ALLOW YOUR CHILD TO TAKE DIURETICS WITHOUT CONSULTING A PHYSICIAN! Some diuretics have the effect of raising lithium levels and can cause severe lithium toxicity. The regular lithium dose must usually be lowered and blood levels of lithium must be scrupulously monitored if a patient takes diuretics regularly. There have been reports of persistent and severe increased urination (*diabetes insipidus*, which has nothing to do with *diabetes mellitus*, the common "sugar diabetes") that progresses over time. A few cases of impaired kidney functioning have also been reported. Both these problems are rare and slow to develop. Nevertheless, in addition to monitoring lithium levels, blood tests that measure kidney functioning are routinely ordered for patients taking lithium.

Lithium is irritating to the gastrointestinal tract and can cause nausea or diarrhea; taking it on a full stomach can ease these problems considerably. A fine shaking in the hands (tremor) can occur at higher lithium levels; medications used to treat tremors, called beta-blockers, are frequently prescribed and can be very helpful. Weight gain can be an annoying side effect and unfortunately has an equally annoying remedy: diet and exercise.

Between 5 and 35 percent of people treated with lithium develop depression of thyroid gland functioning (hypothyroidism).[17] A test of thyroid functioning is the third in the battery of blood tests routinely ordered for persons taking lithium.

Lithium can cause flare-ups of preexisting skin conditions, but only rarely causes the new onset of dermatological problems. Individuals with acne, psoriasis, or other dermatological problems may need closer follow-up from their dermatologist.

Because those who start taking lithium for a mood disorder as an adolescent will often continue doing so into adulthood, it's important to note that lithium has been associated with birth defects. By the time a woman misses her period after conceiving, development of many of the embryo's major organs is already well under way. Stopping a medication after a woman *knows* she is pregnant may be too late to prevent a birth defect. Women of childbearing age have usually been advised to practice birth control while taking lithium if there is any chance of becoming pregnant. Some more recent data suggest that children born to women taking lithium have only a slightly increased chance of birth defects. The decision of how to go about lithium treatment during pregnancy is something of a debate, but often the risks of a recurrence of mental illness far outweigh the risks to the developing child, and many practitioners today recommend that patients stable on their medications should continue to take them throughout pregnancy.[18] That said, it is an individual decision, and women taking lithium who want to get pregnant should have a discussion with their psychiatrist and obstetrician about the risks of taking lithium and of stopping it. Lithium is secreted in breast milk, so women taking lithium should not breast-feed.

Another of lithium's side effects that troubles a significant number of people is a noticeable dulling of mental functioning. Patients complain that their ability to memorize and learn is affected and that they have a difficult-to-describe sense of mental sluggishness. A particular complaint is word-finding difficulties. For years, clinicians downplayed these complaints as coming from people who simply weren't used to being "normal," individuals who just missed the mental hyperalertness of hypomania. This view seemed to be supported by research using psychological tests on persons taking lithium for the treatment of bipolar disorder, research that has been basically inconclusive. But when nonpatient volunteers were administered lithium and similarly tested, a small but definite drop in their performance was found,[19] proving that this lithium-induced mental sluggishness is a real problem for some people. This side effect should be checked into for adolescents who seem to be having difficulties in school, even though their mood problem is under better control. This is a dose-related side effect and is another reason to strive for the lowest possible maintenance dose of lithium that still controls mood symptoms adequately.

VALPROATE (DEPAKOTE)

The development of valproate (brand names include Depakote and Depakene) for the treatment of mood disorders is another convoluted study in serendipity. Valproic acid is a carbon-containing compound similar to several others found in animal fats and vegetable oils: a fatty acid. It was first synthesized in 1882 and used as an organic solvent (a liquid in which other substances dissolve) for many years, for various purposes. Many decades ago, pharmacists used it as a solvent for bismuth salts, which were used to treat stomach and skin disorders.

In the early 1960s, scientists looking for treatments for epilepsy were working with a group of new pharmaceutical compounds that appeared promising but were difficult to dissolve. They discovered that valproic acid was an effective solvent for the compounds they were testing, and they started using it to dissolve their test drugs for animal experimentation. As they tested their various new pharmaceuticals, the results they obtained seemed confusing—until someone realized that it didn't matter *which* of the new pharmaceuticals was used. As long as *any* of them was dissolved in valproic acid, the drug was found to be effective in stopping epileptic seizure activity. It soon became obvious that the valproic acid was stopping the seizures, not what was dissolved in it. By 1978, valproate was approved by the FDA for use in treating adult epilepsy,[20] and it is now approved for and widely used in the pediatric population as well.

In the 1960s, there were some reports that valproate might be helpful in mood disorders, and throughout the late 1960s and early 1970s, a French psychiatrist named Pierre A. Lambert published a series of papers about using it to treat bipolar disorders. After the discovery that another antiepilepsy medication, carbamazepine, was effective in treating mania, interest in the possibilities of valproate as a mood stabilizer grew. In the mid-1980s, several studies on the use of valproate in treating bipolar disorder were published by American psychiatrists, and ten years later, valproate had become firmly established as an effective antimanic medication and a mood stabilizer in adults; it is now FDA approved for use in bipolar disorder (in adults only, for now). Less research has been done on adolescents, but the available data indicate that valproate is effective for adolescents with bipolar disorder.[21] Because one of valproate's first uses was for seizure disorders in children and adolescents, there is a large amount of information on dosing, safety, and side effects in young people.

Valproate's therapeutic action in bipolar disorder (or in epilepsy, for that matter) is still largely unknown. We do know that it improves neuronal transmission in the brain that is mediated by the neurotransmitter *gamma-aminobutyric acid* (GABA). GABA seems to have an inhibitory or modulating effect on many brain circuits, and valproate's effect may be through its ability to regulate the amount of GABA in the brain. Valproate is also increasingly recognized as a chemical that alters the gene expression of neurons, protecting them in the brain and making them overall less excitable (and therefore less likely to produce seizures and, potentially, the wide mood swings of bipolar affective disorder).

THERAPEUTIC PROFILE

Valproate is known to be an effective treatment for acute mania. It also appears to be effective in preventing the recurrence, and reducing the severity, of episodes of bipolar disorder. Its effectiveness in treating acute depressive episodes of bipolar disorder has been less impressive, so it may be less likely to help as an antidepressant augmentation agent than lithium in the long run, though a head-to-head study of these medications for this purpose has not yet been completed. (See the therapeutic profile in table 7-4.)

In reading about this medication, you'll notice the many names it goes by: valproate, valproic acid, divalproex sodium, not to mention the brand names, Depakote and Depakene. Valproate is the name of the negative ion. When associated with a hydrogen ion, the result is valproic acid; in combination with a sodium ion, it becomes sodium valproate. Depakote, a preparation manufactured by Abbott Laboratories, consists of a stable combination of sodium valproate and valproic acid called divalproex sodium. (Depakene is Abbott's brand name for their valproic acid preparation.)

Valproate seems to be more effective than lithium for certain subgroups of patients: those with rapid cycling (four or more mood episodes per year) and those with mixed mania, that is, a mixture of manic hyperactivity and pressured thinking and depressed or unpleasant mood.[22] Valproate is also

Table 7-4 Therapeutic Profile of Valproate

Medication class:	Mood stabilizer (anticonvulsant)
Brand names:	Depakote, Depakene
Generic names:	Divalproex sodium, valproic acid
Half-life:	6 to 16 hours
Metabolism:	Affected by other antiepilepsy drugs
Elimination:	By liver and kidneys
Need for birth control:	Probably mandatory
Other considerations:	Blood levels helpful to adjust dose; blood tests for liver inflammation needed

much less toxic than lithium. One big disadvantage of valproate is that it does not seem to be as helpful as lithium in treating acute depression. Nor is it very effective in preventing recurrences of depression.[23] This suggests that valproate may be a better choice for individuals with rapid cycling or with mixed mania, but that those with classic euphoric mania and major depression may have better control of their symptoms with lithium.[24] As with antidepressants, however, overall conclusions about how a medication affects a *group* of patients is at best a guess of how it will affect a *particular* patient. Treatment of yourself or your child can often be a process of repeated trials to find the right medication or combination of medications.

Like lithium, valproate can be measured in the bloodstream; unfortunately, it is more difficult to measure and requires a more expensive test. Blood levels above 45 mcg/mL (micrograms per milliliter) have been shown to be necessary for the therapeutic effect to occur, and side effects become more problematic at levels greater than 125 mcg/mL.[25] Several studies have shown that valproate is helpful in cyclothymia, bipolar II, and "soft" bipolar disorders, and that lower doses and lower blood levels are required than in the treatment of bipolar I.[26] As with lithium, in measuring valproate levels, blood should be drawn twelve hours after the last dose of medication.

Valproate has also been used to treat more general behavioral problems in children and adolescents, specifically impulse problems, aggressiveness, and severe temper tantrums, though evidence for this use is still somewhat controversial, and it has not been approved by the FDA for any of the above.[27] Valproate has significant antianxiety effects and is sometimes prescribed for this reason, especially in Europe.

Valproate has a milder side-effect profile than lithium and is not nearly as toxic in overdose. Side effects that are common as an individual starts taking the medication include stomach upset and some sleepiness. These problems usually go away quickly. Increased appetite and weight gain can occur. Mild tremor also occurs and can be treated with beta-blocker medication. A few patients report hair loss, usually temporary, which resolves even more quickly with vitamin preparations containing the minerals zinc and selenium.[28] Most dandruff shampoos contain selenium, and these help combat this type of hair loss too.

Cases of severe liver problems have been reported in patients taking valproate. These occurred almost exclusively in young children (under age 2) taking the drug for control of epilepsy, most of whom had other medical problems and were taking several different medications. A 1989 review article stated that no fatalities from liver problems caused by valproate had ever been reported for individuals over the age of 10 who were taking only valproate.[29] Just to be on the safe side, however, a blood test that can detect liver inflammation is done for those taking valproate for the first time and is repeated at appropriate intervals while they are taking this medication. Because valproate also, though rarely, causes a drop in blood cell count, a complete blood count is usually done as well. These are very rare problems. Even when they do occur, they develop slowly and usually during the first six months of therapy and thus can be picked up with routine blood tests. Nevertheless, individuals taking valproate should be on the lookout for signs of liver or blood count problems: unusual bleeding and bruising, jaundice (yellowing of the eyes and skin), fever, and water retention.

Valproate has been associated with birth defects, so women in the childbearing years should practice birth control while taking valproate if there is any possibility of becoming pregnant. There is also controversy about the frequency with which valproate causes multiple ovarian cysts (polycystic ovaries) in women who have taken it for many years. A study demonstrated that up to one in ten young women treated with valproate develop this condition.[30] This is an important consideration in prescribing this medication to adolescent girls.

CARBAMAZEPINE (TEGRETOL)

After the introduction of carbamazepine (brand names include Tegretol and Epitol) for the control of epilepsy in the 1960s, several reports appeared indicating that, when taking this medication, people with epilepsy who also had mood problems not only had good control of their seizures but had improvement in their psychiatric symptoms as well. It was a small step to test carbamazepine in patients with mood problems who did not suffer from epilepsy. Much of the earlier work on the use of carbamazepine in treating bipolar disorder was done by Japanese clinicians looking for an alternative to lithium, which was not approved for use in Japan until years after it was available in the United States. In 1980, a study appeared in the *American Journal of Psychiatry* titled "Carbamazepine in Manic-Depressive Illness: A New Treatment."[31] Although carbamazepine has been used to treat epilepsy in children and adolescents for many years, it is currently not labeled by the FDA for the treatment of psychiatric disorders in children or adolescents (or adults, for that matter). Although it seems that carbamazepine may be helpful for children and adolescents with bipolar affective disorder,[32] the effect is smaller than that of either lithium or valproic acid, and it has never been investigated for use in depression.

THERAPEUTIC PROFILE

Carbamazepine is one of those medications that don't seem to have any particular advantage in most studies on groups of psychiatric patients, but it works well—in fact, works when other medications do not—in some individuals. In one well-designed double-blind study, manic patients who took carbamazepine actually seemed to do worse than those taking lithium.[33] But most psychiatrists have had a patient like "Ms. B.," whose case history was reported in a paper from the National Institute of Mental Health in 1983:

CASE 2. MS. B., a 53-year-old woman, had a history of treatment resistant, rapid cycling manic-depressive illness that required continuous state hospitalization from 1956 to her admission to NIMH in 1978. She had been non-responsive to [antipsychotic medications, tricyclic antidepressants] and lithium . . . After institution of carbamazepine, both mood phases improved dramatically and she was able to be discharged...During a subsequent hospitalization her severe mania again did not respond to [antipsychotic medications] and she was not able to leave the hospital until she was treated with carbamazepine.[34]

The authors of this study noted, "Additional improvement appeared to occur when [antipsychotic medications] were used in conjunction with carbamazepine or when lithium and carbamazepine were used in combination." This has become carbamazepine's niche: a second-line mood-stabilizing agent for patients who do not respond to other agents, often used in combination with other agents. (See the therapeutic profile in table 7-5.)

A series of case reports published in 1999 supports carbamazepine's effectiveness in the treatment of bipolar disorder in adolescents. The cases included a 17-year-old girl and a 14-year-old boy who had classic bipolar symptoms with severe depressions and manias. Both had only a partial response to lithium and significant side effects with it. Because of these problems, these children had stopped taking the medication several times and had suffered relapses. Both had excellent remissions of their symptoms on taking carbamazepine, and because they didn't have side-effect problems, they were willing to take it continuously and therefore stayed well.[35]

Like the other mood-stabilizing medications, carbamazepine can be measured in the bloodstream, and the blood levels are used to adjust the dose. Unfortunately, not much work has been done on blood levels of this medication in patients with bipolar disorder, so the therapeutic range used for the treatment of epilepsy is usually the target that psychiatrists aim for in their patients.

Table 7-5   Therapeutic Profile of Carbamazepine

Medication class:	Mood stabilizer (anticonvulsant)
Brand names:	Epitol, Tegretol
Generic name:	Carbamazepine
Half-life:	18 to 55 hours (shortens after time)
Metabolism:	Complex: affects and is affected by other drugs
Elimination:	By liver and kidneys
Need for birth control:	Probably mandatory
Other considerations:	Blood levels helpful to adjust dose; blood tests for liver inflammation and blood abnormalities needed

Carbamazepine is metabolized in the liver, and like some other drugs, it causes the levels of liver enzymes that metabolize it to increase. This means that the longer a person takes carbamazepine, the better the liver becomes at getting rid of it. So after a few weeks, the blood levels of the drug may go down, and the dose may need to be increased. This increase in liver enzymes can also affect other medications that the patient might be taking, including certain tranquilizers, certain antidepressants, other epilepsy medications, and some hormones, including birth-control preparations. It is essential to inform all physicians involved in a person's care that she has started taking carbamazepine, so that dosage adjustments can be made.

SIDE EFFECTS

Carbamazepine can produce the sort of general side effects caused by many medications affecting the brain: sleepiness, light-headedness, and some initial nausea. These problems tend to be short lived and dose related.

As with valproate, there have been rare cases of liver problems, so blood tests for liver inflammation are routinely done. There have also been rare reports of dangerous changes in blood cell counts, so blood counts are also done, especially in the first several weeks of therapy. Some cases of a rare but dangerous skin reaction called Stevens-Johnson syndrome have occurred. Although all these problems are uncommon, patients should be on the watch for the development of a rash, jaundice, water retention, bleeding or bruising, or signs of infection.

LAMOTRIGINE (LAMICTAL)

Lamotrigine (brand name Lamictal) is another antiseizure medication that appears to have therapeutic effects for people with mood disorders. Studies began to appear in the 1980s showing that it was a useful add-on therapy for people with epilepsy who were already taking other antiseizure medications. During the early investigations of this use, researchers noted that patients who took lamotrigine for seizure control reported an improvement in their mood and sense of well-being—even if it hadn't helped much with their seizures. Lamotrigine has several effects on the brain that might explain its efficacy in bipolar disorder. It appears to inhibit release of the neurotransmitter *glutamate*, an amino acid that causes stimulation of various neural circuits. Lamotrigine is also thought to affect at least one of the same second messenger systems that lithium affects, the *inositol triphosphate system.*[36] It is approved as a mood stabilizer for bipolar affective disorder in adults, though not in children.

The most exciting aspect of lamotrigine's profile is its apparent effectiveness in depression, including both bipolar and unipolar depression (table 7-6).[37] One of the first reports on its use in the treatment of bipolar disorder described a patient who had suffered from rapid-cycling bipolar I disorder since he was 14.[38] In the year before starting to take lamotrigine, he had been either depressed or manic continuously with no period of normal mood. When the research team first saw him, he was severely depressed and had not responded to lithium, carbamazepine, or an antidepressant. On taking lamotrigine, his depression symptoms gradually improved, and eleven months later, he hadn't had a recurrence of either depressive or manic symptoms. There are other reports of lamotrigine being helpful in cases of extremely treatment-resistant major depressive disorder in adults.[39]

Other studies indicate that lamotrigine works well with other mood stabilizers in treatment-resistant patients and can sometimes turn a partial medication response into a more complete one.[40] Lamotrigine is a welcome addition to the present array of mood stabilizers—especially in light of its apparent antidepressant effects.

Lamotrigine has a half-life of about twenty-four hours, and the body's ability to metabolize it is affected by taking carbamazepine and valproate. Blood levels are not routinely ordered for lamotrigine because of its low toxicity and because therapeutic effects have not been correlated with a particular blood-level range.

SIDE EFFECTS

Aside from some initial nausea or gastrointestinal upset and the sort of side effects that many medications affecting the brain can cause—sleepiness, light-headedness or dizziness, and headache—lamotrigine has a good side-effect profile. The most serious side effects reported are severe types of skin rashes, Stevens-Johnson syndrome and toxic epidermal necrosis (TED). This last severe rash has the effect of a whole-body third-

Table 7-6   Therapeutic Profile of Lamotrigine

Medication class:	Mood stabilizer (anticonvulsant)
Brand name:	Lamictal
Generic name:	Lamotrigine
Half-life:	15 to 24 hours
Metabolism:	Complex: affected by other drugs
Elimination:	By liver and kidneys
Need for birth control:	Recommended
Other considerations:	Rarely causes severe skin rashes, but has a generally good side-effect profile

degree burn and has been fatal in some cases. The likelihood of this problem developing has been greatly reduced by the practice of starting the medication at a very low dose and raising the dose quite gradually. Although this means it takes a lot longer (several weeks) to get to a therapeutic dose, the technique has greatly reduced the number of serious rashes. Also, the rash problem seems to be more frequently seen in individuals who have had other dermatological reactions to medications. Unfortunately, TED has been reported more often in young people than in adults, so lamotrigine is not recommended by the manufacturer for children under the age of 16. Patients should examine their skin carefully, especially during the first several weeks of therapy, and stop the medication and get in touch with their doctor at any sign of skin rash. Despite this frankly scary though uncommon side effect, lamotrigine can be an excellent option for adolescents who have not responded to other medications.

OTHER MOOD STABILIZERS

Several other agents seemed to show promise for the treatment of bipolar disorder. The evidence for these agents is still in the early stages of development, although unfortunately, it doesn't appear to be as encouraging as the evidence for the medications described above. For the most part, the promise of these medications is based on a few case reports of a therapeutic effect in adults; in some cases, they are medications in the same class as other pharmaceuticals already shown to be helpful.

Gabapentin (brand name Neurontin) is yet another antiseizure medication that initially seemed to be a mood stabilizer as well. As with the others, reports of beneficial effects on mood disorder symptoms in people being treated for epilepsy came first, and a few indicators of effect in bipolar disorder followed. A large study of gabapentin found no difference from placebo in effect on patients with bipolar affective disorder.[41] That said, as is so often the case, for the rare patient who seems to respond to nothing else, it can be a virtual miracle cure. One case report concerned a man with bipolar disorder who refused to take lithium and who had liver disease and low blood counts caused by alcoholism.[42] Because he wouldn't take lithium, and his medical problems made the use of valproate or carbamazepine risky, gabapentin was tried. He had a "dramatic" decrease in manic symptoms, his sleep pattern returned to normal, and best of all, he reported no side effects. Gabapentin is not metabolized in the liver and so does not affect the blood levels of other medications; it doesn't need blood-level monitoring and has a good side-effect profile.

Oxcarbazepine (brand name Trileptal) is an antiepilepsy drug similar to carbamazepine. Several encouraging studies from Germany were published in the 1980s describing its use in treating bipolar disorder in adults, but the drug was not approved for use in the United States until January 2000. The case of a 6-year-old girl with severe bipolar disorder who was successfully treated with oxcarbazepine appeared in the *Journal of the American Academy of Child and Adolescent Psychiatry* in 2001. This little girl had mood symptoms with severe aggression and violent behaviors that included breaking windows and knocking doors off their hinges. She had not benefited from lithium but had "full mood stabilization" after six weeks of taking oxcarbazepine. After three months, her mother reported that she was "fabulous," and her teacher said she was a "little angel."[43] This one case report contrasts with larger studies, which don't seem to show that it is helpful for children or adolescents as a population. Oxcarbazepine has fewer side effects than carbamazepine and has not been associated with the dangerous skin rashes and blood count problems occurring with that drug.

Other antiepilepsy drugs that have attracted the interest of clinical researchers on bipolar disorder are *topiramate* (Topamax) and *tiagabine* (Gabatril). Neither of these has shown any appreciable effect on mania or depression, unfortunately.

Research clearly indicates that lithium, valproate, carbamazepine, and lamotrigine are effective for the treatment of bipolar disorder in adults. The studies on younger patients are more limited, but the results have been encouraging. Adding mood-stabilizing medications, primarily lithium, to an antidepressant medication for adult patients who have treatment-resistant depression is also clearly helpful and can turn a partial remission of symptoms into a complete one. Again, there is less research on this use in adolescents, but what is available supports the view that this is an effective strategy. Thus, mood-stabilizing medications seem to have a place in the management of both bipolar disorders and depressive disorders.

These medications have also been used to treat behavioral problems that have some overlap with the symptoms of mood disorders. It's important that we have a quick sidebar about what exactly a "diagnosis" means in psychiatry, so that it's crystal clear what these medications are treating and how they are supposed to help. Some diagnoses in the *DSM* and in psychiatry refer to conditions that are caused by inborn biological causes over which the person has no control. These diagnoses speak to the *etiology*, the origin, of the condition. Major depression is one such diagnosis, as is bipolar affective disorder.

Other diagnoses are merely descriptive terms used to identify a cluster of behaviors. They don't speak to where the condition comes from or what causes it; instead, they simply are a checklist of different symptoms or characteristics, usually behaviors, that tend to go together. In children, two such diagnoses are *oppositional defiant disorder* and *conduct disorder*. Putting "disorder" at the end of their names may lead some to believe that these diagnoses describe conditions that descend on the poor sufferer without any hope of avoidance. In fact, *conduct disorder* is a diagnosis given to children and adolescents who are aggressive, destructive, and disobedient, and who break the rules and often the law with behaviors such as stealing. There is no description of why they do this, and possibly no underlying neurological cause to begin with; instead, there's a pattern of behavior, of things the person willfully does, that are collected under a single term.

Consequently, when a medication is given to a patient to "treat" one of these disorders, it is not the same as giving an antidepressant to correct the chemical imbalance of depression. Rather, medications used for these conditions usually help the patient with her behaviors in a more roundabout fashion. We have spoken about how the initial trials of lithium in animals showed it to have a sedating, calming effect. In patients with bipolar affective disorder, lithium can reduce impulsivity (or at times creativity) and create a sort of sleepy, lackadaisical mood. In an irritable, angry, disobedient adolescent, this same sort of change may be seen as "treating" her "condition," though in fact it is more likely taking away some of the energy she uses to fuel her negative behaviors.

Now, it is not necessarily the case that an adolescent has either a biological mood disorder or a behavioral conduct disorder. More frequently than not, the two go together. An adolescent develops low mood, irritability, anger, and social isolation, and deals with these feelings by lashing out and having little concern for the consequences. He may begin to develop a behavioral disorder as the result of a mood disorder, or the two may develop independently.

With this caveat in mind, it is worth mentioning that several studies have looked at the effectiveness of mood-stabilizing medications for these behavioral problems; some of the studies have demonstrated beneficial effects, though others have not. Lithium has been shown to help with aggressiveness in children and adolescents in some studies, as has valproic acid.

Based on these sorts of studies on the effects of mood-stabilizing medications on behavioral problems, some child psychiatrists will prescribe a mood stabilizer to a patient whose mood syndrome is complicated by aggressive, irritable, impulsive behaviors, even if the classic bipolar symptoms don't seem to be present. We are not necessarily against this practice, if it is helpful to the child, but we remind patients and parents that the medications are not the path to curing a behavioral disorder. They are useful merely for managing the symptoms while the patient undergoes more targeted treatment, usually psychotherapy, to change behavior patterns and become more positive.

WHY, AND HOW, TO USE MOOD STABILIZERS IN DEPRESSION

Combinations of medications in the treatment of severe mood disorders are becoming the rule rather than the exception. Almost by definition, early-onset mood disorders are severe mood disorders, and when the adolescent has a family history of bipolar disorder, it might be reasonable to add a mood stabilizer to his medication. How should the psychiatrist choose among the different mood stabilizers for a particular patient? It has been suggested that younger children seem to tolerate lithium better than older adolescents, because they are not as troubled by the weight gain and dermatological problems (remember that lithium can worsen acne). That said, children are usually less tolerant of the accompanying blood draws, and parents have to be careful that their child doesn't get dehydrated, as dehydration can increase the blood lithium level. For older adolescents who may have trouble with lithium side effects, valproate may be more appropriate, especially since these teenagers often have more problems with aggressiveness, which valproate has been shown to help.[44]

Even more so than with the antidepressants, the decision to add a mood stabilizer to an adolescent patient's medications and making a choice among the available mood-stabilizing medications is more art than science. The published clinical studies on the use of these drugs for children and adolescents nearly always end with a sentence or two bemoaning the lack of research that proves the pattern of efficacy of these medications in young patients with mood disorders.

All of this makes it crucial that parents understand the target symptoms for which a mood stabilizer is being used, so they can help monitor their child for improvement, or lack of improvement, of these symptoms.

Other Medications and Treatments

Although antidepressant and mood-stabilizing medications are the primary treatment of depression and bipolar disorders, a variety of other medications are often used as adjunctive treatments. Sometimes these medications are used temporarily to relieve severe symptoms of irritability or anxiety, and sometimes they are an ongoing part of the patient's treatment. Only some of the following medications are approved by the U.S. Food and Drug Administration for the treatment of mood disorders in young persons, so their use is still somewhat controversial. Despite this, one class (the atypical antipsychotics) are some of the most frequently prescribed psychiatric medications in this age group and therefore need to be discussed.

As this is written, multiple government regulatory agencies are evaluating how these medications are used. If you recall our discussion in chapter 6 of SSRI medications and how they were being given out like candy for every instance of apparent sadness, you will understand the climate of a few years ago in which some of these medications, considered relatively benign in the short term, were used to treat every type of anger or aggression. An increased understanding of the long-term effects of these chemicals on the developing body is now beginning to curb this practice.

ANTIPSYCHOTIC MEDICATIONS

A difficulty that immediately arises in discussing antipsychotic medications is their unfortunate name. *Psychotic* is an imprecise term at best, and these medications have many more uses than simply treating psychotic symptoms. This group of medications has also been called the *major tranquilizers,* a label that perhaps more accurately describes the usefulness of these pharmaceuticals in treating mood disorders. They can provide substantial and fast relief of the restlessness and mental anguish of severe depression and calm the agitation of mania. We discussed mood stabilizers in the previous chapter. In a large study, antipsychotics were found to be startlingly more effective than any mood stabilizer in acute mania in adolescents,[1] though we have also discussed how some practitioners may misdiagnose "mania." Some may confuse the *symptom* of agitation for the *syndrome* of mania, when in fact the agitation could be due to any number of different causes.

Before we get into the details of antipsychotic medications, a brief explanation about the word *psychosis* is in order. Psychosis can be thought of as a mental state or disorder in which a person's ability to comprehend the environment and react to it appropriately is severely impaired. The layperson's definition of *psychotic* might be "out of touch with reality." The person who is hearing voices (hallucinations) or who has bizarre idiosyncratic beliefs (delusions) is psychotic. The word also has a connotation of a severe disorganization of thinking and behavior, usually with restlessness and agitation. The manic syndrome is a good example of a state of psychosis, and in chapter 4, we talked about "psychotic features" in depression.

In the 1930s, pharmaceutical compounds called *phenothiazines* were synthesized in Europe and were found to have antihistamine and sedative properties. One in particular, chlorpromazine, was found to be useful in surgical anesthesia because it deepened anesthetic sedation more safely than other available agents. In the early 1950s, two French psychiatrists carried out several clinical trials using chlorpromazine to treat highly agitated patients suffering from schizophrenia and mania. They noticed that in addition to its quieting and sleep-promoting effects, chlorpromazine made the hallucinations and bizarre delusional beliefs of many individuals with schizophrenia practically disappear. It also decreased the severity of the disorganization of thinking and agitated behavior seen in patients with acute mania. Chlorpromazine, in other words, had a *specific* effect on the cluster of symptoms usually referred to as "psychotic" symptoms, and thus the name for this group of drugs came about: *antipsychotic medications.* Occasionally, they are still referred to as *neuroleptic* medications (or *neuroleptics*), from *neuroleptique,* the French word coined from Greek roots that means, roughly, "affecting the nervous system." The term *major tranquilizers* was coined to distinguish these medications from *minor tranquilizers,* medications used for sleep problems and anxiety. But because these agents are much more than just "tranquilizers," this term has fallen out of favor too. The far-ranging effects of this group are more than simply "antipsychotic," but until a better term comes along, *antipsychotic medications* is what we're stuck with.

The main chemical effect of all the pharmaceuticals in this class is a blockade of dopamine receptors in the brain. In people with schizophrenia, neural circuits that use dopamine as their neurotransmitter may be dysfunctional in some way, and this may cause the bizarre hallucinations and disorders of thinking typical of that illness. Antipsychotics may work by affecting these systems in some as yet unknown way. Whether these medications alleviate the psychotic symptoms that sometimes complicate bipolar disorder in a similar fashion is also not yet known.

After the development of the original group of antipsychotic medications (table 8-1), the phenothiazines, in the 1960s and 1970s several other potent dopamine-blocking medications were developed. The side-effect profile of these newer medications was marginally better than that of the phenothiazines, but they did not represent much of an advance therapeutically.

More recently, several new antipsychotic medications have been introduced that not only have substantially fewer and less severe side effects but also are more effective for many patients (table 8-2). These agents are called *atypical* or *second generation* antipsychotic medications because although they block dopamine receptors (though not as potently as their predecessors), they differ from the typical antipsychotic medications in that they are also active at serotonin receptors. As you might guess, this effect is thought to explain why these medications might be more helpful in mood disorders. Among these medications, aripiprazole (Abilify), que-

Table 8-1 Traditional Antipsychotic Medications

Generic Name	Brand Name
Chlorpromazine	Thorazine
Fluphenazine	Prolixin
Haloperidol	Haldol
Loxapine	Loxitane
Molindone	Moban
Perphenazine	Trilafon
Thioridazine	Mellaril
Thiothixene	Navane
Trifluoperazine	Stelazine

tiapine (Seroquel), olanzapine (Zyprexa), and risperidone (Risperdal) are approved for treatment of mania in bipolar affective disorder type I.

THERAPEUTIC PROFILE

Antipsychotic medications are effective in reducing the symptoms of delusions or hallucinations that accompany a true psychotic episode. In their role as major tranquilizers, they are strongly sedating and can quickly calm an agitated patient, though unlike the benzodiazepines, they are nonaddicting. Antipsychotics are given primarily for this purpose in such intense environments as the emergency room, and they are rapidly effective and safe. There is good evidence, particularly in adults, that they can be used long term to augment antidepressant effects (particularly the second generation antipsychotics, which seem to affect the serotonin system), as well as reduce the agitation and irritability that tend to accompany the more adolescent forms of depression. Manic patients can find quick relief

Table 8-2 New Antipsychotic Medications

Generic Name	Brand Name
Clozapine	Clozaril
Olanzapine	Zyprexa
Quetiapine	Seroquel
Risperidone	Risperdal
Ziprasidone	Geodon
Aripiprazole	Abilify
Asenapine	Saphris
Lurasidone	Latuda

of their euphoric or irritable states, and these medications can be a helpful augmentation to mood stabilizers for long-term maintenance of a stable mood. Similarly, in a young person with severe symptoms of irritability or aggressiveness, antipsychotic medications may be prescribed temporarily to reduce these symptoms until other medications have time to become effective.

SIDE EFFECTS

The original antipsychotic medications have significant effects on muscle tone and movement, side effects caused by the dopamine blockade these agents cause. The newer agents do not cause these side-effect problems nearly as often, so they are now used much more frequently. In textbook discussions of these medications, you will see these problems referred to as *extrapyramidal symptoms,* or simply EPS. Dopamine is the main neurotransmitter in a complex circuit of brain areas called the *extrapyramidal system,* which coordinates movement. The term *extrapyramidal* contrasts this system with another brain system, called the *pyramidal* system because its main fibers are carried in triangular-shaped bundles into the spinal cord (the *spinal pyramids,* or *pyramidal tract*). The pyramidal system controls the quick, accurate execution of fine muscle movement, and the extrapyramidal system makes sure that the rest of the body moves as needed for the smooth and graceful execution of these movements. Antipsychotic medications, by blocking the dopamine receptors in these extrapyramidal centers, can cause movements to become stiff and slow. *Acute dystonic reactions* are muscular spasms that usually involve the tongue and facial and neck muscles; these spasms are more common in young male patients. People taking antipsychotic medications can also develop an uncomfortable restlessness called *akathisia,* felt mostly in the legs. A person with akathisia often feels the need to walk or pace and can appear agitated though he is in fact merely uncomfortable.

Fortunately, all these side effects are treatable, either by lowering the dose of medication or by adding one of several medications that are also used to treat Parkinson's disease. Although the side effects are uncomfortable, they are not dangerous and usually respond quickly to treatment.

People who took older antipsychotic medications over many years sometimes developed a side effect called *tardive dyskinesia* (TD). This consists of repetitive involuntary movements, usually of the facial muscles: chewing, blinking, or lip-pursing movements. There is no good treatment for TD other than discontinuing the medication. Because TD seemed to persist in some individuals even after they stopped taking the medication, it used to be thought that these problems were permanent. As it turns out, some TD symptoms *do* go away with time.

The great advantage of the newer antipsychotic medications is that most patients who take them have none of these extrapyramidal movement problems. For years, many believed that these medications were hands down safer for children (in some cases, this evidence may have been due to a manipulation of data by pharmaceutical companies, as we discuss below). However, there are several different side effects to consider, and experts are constantly debating which profile is more detrimental to the developing young body.

Although the possibility of movement disorders is significantly lower with atypical antipsychotics, the atypical antipsychotics seem to have a fundamental and unavoidable effect on the way the body metabolizes and uses food. A cluster of conditions, together labeled the *metabolic syndrome*, may develop. In this syndrome, the body's cells become much less sensitive to the insulin we all use to signal that it is time to convert the free sugars floating in our bloodstream into energy. In extreme cases, diabetes develops and requires treatment with additional medications. The way the body uses fats also changes. People begin putting on weight, sometimes in surprising amounts, rather quickly. This is partially an effect of increased appetite but also seems related to a change in how the body stores excess energy. Cholesterol, triglycerides, and lipids all increase. Children develop the cholesterol profiles of 50-year-olds. Most of the time, stopping the antipsychotic can reverse some, but not all, of these effects. Strict diet and exercise are helpful, though difficult for young persons.

Atypical antipsychotics can also alter the way our bodies produce certain hormones. We all have a certain amount of the hormone *prolactin* secreted by our brains. This hormone has many effects, but one of them (as can be deduced by the name) is to signal to a woman's body that it is time to begin producing milk. Antipsychotics, particularly the second generation class, increase this hormone. In some cases, this can cause breast tissue formation (*gynecomastia*) and milk production (*galactorrhea*), even in males.

In 2013, the results of a large study evaluating a second generation antipsychotic indicated that this effect was transient and quickly returned to near normal, and so was clinically negligible.[2] In fact, the study (paid for by the maker of this antipsychotic) had accidentally incorporated a statistical error; the incidence of milk production in boys was actually double what was originally reported. In most men, this is reversible by stopping the medication, but it can take some time to return to normal, which can be an excruciating experience for a young man trying to find his social place in the world.

There are, fortunately, few potentially lethal side effects of second generation antipsychotics, but one deserves further discussion. The first atypical antipsychotic, clozapine, was synthesized in laboratories in the 1960s but was not marketed in the United States until 1990. One of the reasons clozapine took so long to get on the market is that it causes a dangerous drop in the number of white blood cells (a condition called *agranulocytosis*) in about 1 percent of patients.[3] This problem might have meant the end of the line for clozapine were it not found to be highly effective in treating patients with schizophrenia who derived no benefit from traditional antipsychotic medications. Dramatic case studies of patients with chronic treatment-resistant schizophrenia basically "awakening" from years of unrelenting psychotic symptoms after they started taking clozapine sustained the interest of clinicians and pharmaceutical researchers in this medication. Following the discovery that the risk of agranulocytosis could be substantially reduced if the white blood cell count was monitored weekly, clozapine treatment became available to larger groups of patients.

None of the other atypical antipsychotics causes this problem, so weekly blood tests are not necessary with these medications. Clozapine is usually reserved for patients who have not responded to other types of antipsychotics, so it is rarely used in young persons; but it is not an unreasonable possibility if someone has tried two or three other medications with little response.

CONTROVERSIES

A good number of clinical studies have reported on the safety and efficacy of atypical antipsychotics in the treatment of schizophrenia in young people. This is probably because symptoms of schizophrenia often begin in adolescence, and these medications are the foundation of medical treatment of this illness. Until recently, there existed much less clinical research on the use of these medications in adolescents with mood disorders—even less than on the use of antidepressants and mood stabilizers. A 1999 article in the *Journal of the American Academy of Child and Adolescent Psychiatry* titled "Antipsychotics in Children and Adolescents" does not even mention the use of these medications in young people for the treatment of mood disorders.[4]

In the early 2000s, prescribing patterns changed rapidly. We spoke earlier about how, at around the same time, there was an explosion in the diagnosis of bipolar affective disorder in young people (see chapter 3). Accompanying this increase in diagnosis was a rapid increase in the use of atypical antipsychotic medications in an attempt to rapidly and definitively reduce the symptoms of these youth. We didn't know as much about these medications' side effects at the time, so when comparing something like risperidone (a once-daily pill that required no special precautions or monitoring) to something like lithium (with its blood draws and potential for overdose), the choice seemed clear. Between 1993 and 2002, the number of prescriptions for atypical antipsychotics to young people increased six-fold.[5] About one in ten outpatient psychiatry visits of a child or adolescent resulted in the prescription of an antipsychotic, and over half of all children and adolescents admitted to a psychiatric hospital were discharged on one of these drugs regardless of the diagnosis.[6]

In one disturbing trend, the rates of antipsychotic prescribing to children in foster care was found to be much higher than those for children not in foster care. Although about 10 percent of non-foster-care children were on these medications, over 40 percent of foster care children were taking them. It was also found that a high percentage of these children were on more than one such medication at a time (a practice known as *polypharmacy*, which could expose them to more risks of side effects), and that some children were on significantly higher doses than were allowed by the FDA even for adults. Finally, few if any of these children were being routinely monitored for the metabolic effects described above. There was not the same degree of difference in *diagnoses* between foster care and non-foster-care children, seeming to imply that the medications were no longer tied to their intended use. This was all revealed in a congressional report published by the Government Accountability Office.[7] Although no definitive conclusions were drawn, the patterns seemed to suggest that these medications were used to control behavioral outbursts in a fragile and often underserved population.

Among the child psychiatry community, the combined realization that long-term use of these medicines had increasingly harmful effects and that they were seemingly overprescribed, particularly to the underserved, was not a pleasant one. Active discussions are being held within virtually all major academic centers about how to address these trends. In some cases, states are taking up a call to action as well—Maryland, for example, has introduced a peer review program in which physicians will have to submit proof that the proper blood tests and physical examinations are being performed on all children taking antipsychotic medications. This text is being written in the midst of these shifts, though we are certain that psychiatry will settle on an appropriate way to use these critical medications so that those most in need get the help they deserve, while maintaining judicious use and monitoring in all patients.

BENZODIAZEPINES

The benzodiazepines (table 8-3) are widely prescribed for severe anxiety and insomnia in adults, and are used extensively in hospital settings for young people with situational anxiety and worry. They can help relax a child before an invasive procedure, for example, or ease muscle spasms associated with certain illnesses. These uses are time limited, however, so that a young child is exposed to benzodiazepines for only a matter of weeks. For chronic management of anxiety outside the hospital, these medications are probably best avoided. Benzodiazepines can be abused, and it's possible to become psychologically dependent on and even physically addicted to them. (Withdrawal symptoms in persons taking high doses of these medications can include serious problems, including seizures.) Also, their sedating effects decrease over time, and after several weeks of use, their effectiveness as tranquilizers decreases. For these reasons, benzodiazepines are best thought of as temporary measures.

ST. JOHN'S WORT

Hypericum perforatum, commonly known as St. John's wort, is one of about three hundred *Hypericum* species, shrubby perennial plants with

Table 8-3 Benzodiazepine Medications

Generic Name	Brand Name
Alprazolam	Xanax
Chlordiazepoxide	Librium
Clonazepam	Klonopin
Clorazepate	Tranxene
Diazepam	Valium
Lorazepam	Ativan

bright yellow flowers that grow in most temperate regions of the world. Teas and other extracts of St. John's wort (often simply called hypericum) have been recommended by herbalists for centuries to treat everything from insomnia to the painful viral skin infection called shingles. In the late 1980s, hypericum was investigated as a possible treatment for HIV infection, when researchers discovered that it had activity against retroviruses—activity that, unfortunately, did not translate into clinical usefulness against HIV infection. Most of the scientific work so far on hypericum has been done in Germany, where there is intense interest in herbal medicine, and where herbal preparations are more widely available and perhaps more seriously regarded as valid treatment options for major illnesses. Several studies have compared hypericum extracts with placebo and with a standard antidepressant. The results of the earlier studies were generally encouraging, suggesting that hypericum extracts had an antidepressant effect that is clinically significant in some people. A 1996 article in the *British Medical Journal,* which systematically reviewed twenty-three different studies, including a total of 1,757 patients, found that hypericum extracts "are more effective than placebo for the treatment of mild to moderately severe depressive disorders."[8] The review concluded that people taking hypericum preparations generally reported fewer and less severe side effects than those taking standard antidepressants. Hypericum is approved in Germany, and it makes up 6 percent of all prescriptions written to adolescents for depression.[9]

But much work remains to be done to better understand which groups of patients will benefit from hypericum and which should be treated with better-established agents. Problems with the design of many of the original studies (all done on adults, by the way) have made it difficult to draw conclusions about the relative effectiveness of the two approaches, hypericum versus antidepressant medication. For example, in two studies comparing hypericum with the tricyclic antidepressants imipramine[10] and amitriptyline[11] in people with depression, the prescribed doses of the antidepressants in the studies were low—so low, in fact, that they would be considered ineffective by most psychiatrists.* Another problem is that these studies often lump together people with mild depression and people with more severe depression, making it difficult to know what kind of depression hypericum is helpful for: mild depression, severe depression, or both.

One study that avoided all these problems tested St. John's wort against placebo in two hundred patients who had been rigorously evaluated and diagnosed with major depression. This study concluded that "the results do not support significant antidepressant or antianxiety effects for St. John's wort when compared to placebo in a clinical sample of depressed patients" and that "persons with major depression should not be treated with St. John's wort, given the morbidity and mortality risks of untreated or ineffectively treated major depression."[12] Thus, at present, it is difficult to recommend hypericum preparations for anyone with serious depression.

Some proponents of St. John's wort emphasize that it is a "natural" remedy and therefore inherently safer and better than "synthetic" pharmaceuticals. This argument is flawed on multiple levels. It is important to understand that herbal preparations are *not* inherently safer than or superior to chemically synthesized compounds. Toxic substances such as nicotine and strychnine are found in plants, and some of the deadliest poisons we know of, the amatoxins, occur naturally in the death cap mushroom, *Amanita phalloides.*[13] Another important point: the lower incidence of side effects of herbal preparations can often be attributed to the lower concentration of the active compounds in these preparations, an advantage that is easily duplicated by using low doses of synthetic pharmaceuticals. But natural chemicals do not necessarily have fewer side effects. We have already discussed the use of lithium for the treatment of bipolar affective disorder. Although it is a completely natural substance—in fact, one of the most ba-

---

* These studies compared effectiveness of hypericum preparations with doses of 75 mg of imipramine, a dose most psychiatrists would probably consider barely in the effective range, and 30 mg of amitriptyline, a dose that is definitely subtherapeutic for most patients.

sic in nature, an elemental salt—it can have significant side effects and can even be toxic in overdose.

Nevertheless, discovery of a pharmacologically active plant compound has often formed the basis for development of a much larger number of useful new drugs and led to other exciting discoveries. The chemical isolation of opium from the poppy plant led to the development of dozens of safer and more potent pain medications as well as to the discovery of similar compounds in the brain (called *endorphins*)—now the basis for an entire new branch of neurochemistry. As we learn more about hypericum, it may turn out that a whole new class of safer and more effective antidepressants will emerge, derived from the active compounds found in St. John's wort.

OMEGA-3 FATTY ACIDS AND FISH OIL

There are several nutrients that we must consume in our diet, albeit in small quantities, to remain healthy, compounds that our body cannot manufacture but that are nevertheless necessary for normal cellular functioning. The most familiar of these are, of course, vitamins, compounds manufactured by some plants and animals but not by humans. Their name, from the Latin word *vita,* meaning "life," indicates just how important to health they are. Unless we eat foods that contain the vitamins we need, serious illness results. Scurvy, beriberi, and pellagra are three, now thankfully unfamiliar, illnesses that result from deficiencies of, respectively, vitamin C, vitamin B_1, and niacin. All these illnesses have significant central nervous system symptoms, especially B_1 deficiency, which causes severe central nervous system degeneration.

Another group of necessary nutrients is the *essential fatty acids,* a collection of complex molecules found in some vegetables and other plant sources but in much larger amounts in most fish. Nutritionists have long touted the health benefits of diets rich in seafood, and the lower incidence of breast cancer and heart disease in the Japanese population has been attributed to a diet rich in seafood.

There is growing evidence that essential fatty acids, especially a subgroup called *omega-3 fatty acids* (table 8-4), may be useful in the treatment of mood disorders. The particular compounds thought to have the most health benefits have tongue-twisting names typical of complex organic compounds: eicosapentaenoic acid (EPA) and docosahexaenoic acid (DHA).

Table 8-4   Omega-3 Fatty Acids in Fish

High in Omega-3 Fatty Acids
(more than 1,000 mg per serving)
- Salmon
- Tuna
- Trout
- Mackerel
- Anchovies
- Sardines
- Herring

Moderate in Omega-3 Fatty Acids
(500–900 mg per serving)
- Halibut
- Rockfish
- Swordfish
- Yellowfin tuna
- Whitefish
- Smelt
- Sea bass

Low in Omega-3 Fatty Acids
(less than 500 mg per serving)
- Catfish
- Shellfish: shrimp, crab, lobster
- Cod
- Flounder
- Mahi mahi
- Sea trout
- Perch

Several preliminary studies have indicated that omega-3 fatty acids, taken as fish oil capsules, are beneficial for individuals with mood disorders. One study showed that patients who took fish oil capsules in addition to their usual treatments for bipolar disorder had fewer relapses of mood symptoms over a period of four months than patients who took placebo capsules containing olive oil.[14] All subjects in this study were adults with bipolar I or II disorder, and all were taking a number of other medications during the study. Despite these limitations, the results were exciting because they pointed to a whole new approach to the treatment of mood disorders with a new set of compounds. Other than mild gastrointestinal discomfort and a fishy aftertaste, fish oil capsules have no significant side effects.

Unlike bipolar disorder, studies on adolescent depression seem to have more mixed results. One study showed no difference between omega-3 fatty acid supplements and placebo,[15] while others showed almost unbelievably strong effects,[16] in some cases similar to SSRIs.[17]

The possible mechanism of action of omega-3 fatty acids has been described in studies, which show that these compounds are incorporated into cell membranes in association with molecules that are known to be involved in cell signaling. They seem to be active at some of the same points in cellular signaling mechanisms where lithium and valproate are thought to work. Given that valproate is, after all, a synthetic fatty acid, the idea that natural fatty acids might have benefits in mood disorders shouldn't seem strange at all.

Other circumstantial evidence has also been cited to support the importance of omega-3 fatty acids for good mental health. Archeological and epidemiological studies suggest that modern humans consume much less food rich in fatty acids than did ancient peoples, and that, compared with our ancestors, we may be deficient in these important compounds. This fact, combined with the evidence that the prevalence of depression is increasing and the age of onset of mood disorders is decreasing, has been cited as further evidence of a link between these important compounds and mental health.[18]

In most of the studies referred to above, much higher doses of fish oil were used than are generally recommended by nutritionists, who also suggest eating more fish rather than taking capsules. Whether such a high dose of omega-3 fatty acids was a necessary element in the findings of the study is not known. A study that investigated the benefits of eating more fish high in omega-3 fatty acids for preventing stroke found an incremental benefit: the more fish the research subjects incorporated into their diet, the lower their risk of stroke became.[19]

Omega-3 fatty acid therapy is at this point an unproven treatment for mood disorders, so it should not be substituted for proven treatments. One of the best uses of these compounds seems to be augmenting the efficacy of an antidepressant. In a study comparing omega-3 fatty acids to an SSRI, the combination of both was more effective than either by itself.[20] Another study found that patients with recurrent depression maintained on an SSRI had further improvements in their symptoms and fewer relapses in as few as three weeks when omega-3 fatty acids were added to their regimen.[21] Given the apparently low risk of these compounds, supplementation of standard treatments for mood disorders with fish oil capsules, under the supervision of a physician, may be an option some patients will want to explore.

EXERCISE

In recommending a certain treatment for depression, psychiatrists often compare the potential risks of a treatment with their potential benefits. We have endeavored throughout this text to take you through some of that thought process by clearly identifying what symptoms or disorders a certain treatment may be able to help (for example, an atypical antipsychotic may calm the agitation of mania) and what harm it may cause (that same antipsychotic may negatively affect certain features of metabolic functioning in the body). Weighing these risks and benefits for a particular individual is the only reasonable way to arrive at a treatment regimen. There is one treatment, however, that has recently seen a surge of positive evidence with no significant risks—exercise.

Depression can sap one of energy and of joy. Exercise understandably seems like the opposite of what a depressed person wishes to engage in. Psychiatrists see this view of exercise in nearly every depressed patient admitted to the psychiatric hospital. When suffering from depression, even getting out of bed in the morning seems like a struggle, let alone engaging in more strenuous activities. And yet, returning to the normal activities of living can be one of the most powerful and helpful additions to depression treatment. In psychotherapy, the concept of *behavioral activation* means exactly that—introducing a plan to help a depressed individual return to her life activities, such as going to work or simply completing her morning routine.

It's easy to see why this is helpful from a psychological perspective, but are there other factors at play? We know about many of the positive biological effects that exercise has on the body. Could some positive effects also be happening in the brain, to help regulate mood? Some evidence is building that exercise has a neuroprotective effect on brain tissues similar to the effects of lithium or the SSRIs and, if so, may help in depression recovery. Exercise also induces the release of all sorts of chemicals known to improve mood (in extreme cases, this can be the "runner's high" that some athletes achieve).

Analysis of the effects of exercise on depression, particularly in children, is a relatively recent development but is growing in strength. In 2001, over 2,000 British students were interviewed for depressive symptoms and level of physical activity over the course of two years.[22] It turned out that the chance of developing depression was reduced by about 8 percent for each hour of weekly physical activity. So, it seems that activity may have some preventive function against developing depression. But what about children who are already depressed? A more recent prospective study tries to answer this question. Thirty depressed adolescents not on medication were enrolled in an aerobic exercise program or passive stretching (the control group) for three months.[23] Many thought it would be difficult to encourage the adolescents to participate, but about 80 percent of both groups completed the study. At the end, not only had both groups experienced improvement in their depression (the exercise group about twice as quickly as the stretching group), but these improvements continued to hold true up to one year later, regardless of whether the adolescents continued their program. Both groups also had positive effects in other areas of their lives, including school performance and peer relationships.

In general, exercise should be considered in the treatment for any adolescent depression (for those adolescents who are simply not up to the task, even mild physical activity, such as stretching or going for walks, seems to be helpful). This is not to say that exercise can replace medications or dedicated psychotherapy, particularly for those with severe depression, but rather that it needs to be considered as complementary treatment when discussing the management of this illness in a suffering adolescent.

"MEDICAL" MARIJUANA

Some of the readers of this text will think that this section was placed in this chapter by mistake. Indeed, there will be a much more extensive discussion of marijuana in a later chapter on substance abuse. Others of you, in certain states, will know (or know of) persons who are prescribed marijuana for various psychiatric conditions, including anxiety and attention-deficit/hyperactivity disorder (ADHD). During the writing of this text, one of us moved from Maryland to California and was surprised, to say the least, to have young patients being prescribed this substance for these uses. This practice is controversial at best. There is no evidence to our awareness that marijuana has any ability to help ADHD (and in fact, it can mimic many of the symptoms). Although some patients find it relaxing, chronic marijuana use has consequences to cognitive learning and development that make it a poor choice as an antianxiety medication for use in young persons. And given this drug's potential mood-destabilizing properties in some vulnerable individuals, particularly those with mood disorders, the prescription of marijuana to adolescents is unlikely to help in the long term and can in fact be harmful.

ELECTROCONVULSIVE THERAPY

No survey of the available treatments of serious depression is complete without a discussion of electroconvulsive therapy, or ECT. A highly effective treatment for severe depression and also for both phases of bipolar disorder, ECT often provides dramatic and rapid relief of symptoms when other treatments have failed. Unfortunately, patients and their families resist this treatment because of myths and misconceptions about it. A review article titled "Half a Century of ECT Use in Young People" confirms the effectiveness of this treatment in children and adolescents, and the authors conclude that "serious complications [are] very rare."[24]

Too often, the popular media refer to ECT as "shock treatments," with all the unpleasant connotations of that term: *shock* defined as an unpleasant jolt or blow, or reminding one of the pain of an electric shock, such as the painful spark of static electricity that comes from touching a doorknob after crossing a carpeted room on a dry winter day. Calling ECT "shock treatments" is a bit like referring to modern surgery as "knife treatments"—accurate in a crude sort of way, but doing injustice to what is now a safe and effective treatment that can be literally life saving.

Although the effectiveness of ECT in mood disorders was not a completely accidental discovery, the theory originally proposed to explain its benefit has been shown to have no validity, so the development of modern ECT was a kind of happy accident nonetheless. In the early 1930s, the Hungarian physician Joseph Ladislas von Meduna proposed that there was a mutual antagonism between epilepsy and schizophrenia: patients who suffered from epilepsy did not suffer from schizophrenia, and vice versa. Modern research has shown this is not the case, but von Meduna—convinced of this idea based on his examination of the microscopic appearance of the brain of persons with the two conditions—conducted animal experiments attempting to find a way to artificially produce seizure activity. In 1935, he published a paper reporting a dramatic symptom improvement following artificially induced seizures in several patients with schizophrenia. Von Meduna used injections to produce seizures, but several years later, two Italian psychiatrists reported that seizures could be produced by briefly passing a low-voltage electrical current through the skull by means of electrodes applied to the scalp. Ugo Cerletti and Lucio Bini developed their technique in animals and then tried it on several patients with schizophrenia; they also reported remarkable success.

Although individuals with some forms of schizophrenia often did show improvement in some of their symptoms after these treatments, it quickly became apparent that severely depressed patients showed improvement that was little short of miraculous. With "electroshock" treatments, these patients had complete recovery from their symptoms within a matter of days.

One of the first articles to appear in the professional literature on ECT was a 1942 report on the treatment of two adolescents with ECT by two French psychiatrists. The following year, the same clinicians reported on a series of thirty young people with a variety of conditions who were treated with the new procedure. These physicians concluded that ECT was safe in this age group and was most effective in the treatment of "melancholia." Interest in ECT spread quickly around the globe.

Like many seemingly miraculous treatments, ECT was overprescribed at first and probably administered to many hundreds of persons whom it had little chance of helping. It's important to remember, however, that these were desperate times in psychiatry. With the discovery of antipsychotic medications nearly a decade away, and the discovery of antidepressants nearly two decades away, "little chance" of helping was better than no chance at all. Because ECT is a highly effective treatment for mania, some institutions were inclined to use it for any and all highly agitated patients, and sometimes on merely uncooperative ones. Another negative factor was that in the first decade or so after its development, ECT had serious complications. An epileptic seizure is a violent event: all the muscles of the body contract simultaneously for a few moments, sometimes with such force that broken bones result. Also, breathing stops and heart-rhythm irregularities can occur, which can even be fatal when not appropriately monitored.

The nearly indiscriminate overprescription of a therapy that had serious potential side effects led to a backlash against ECT. In the late 1960s and 1970s, although modern anesthetic techniques were making ECT safer, and more careful research was being done to determine which psychiatric disorders the treatment helped with and which it did not, the damage to ECT's reputation was already done. (The film *One Flew Over the Cuckoo's Nest*, awarded the Oscar for best movie in 1975, which depicted ECT as it would have been administered several decades earlier, certainly didn't help ECT's reputation.) State hospitals drew up regulations sharply curtailing its use, and legislation was in effect briefly in California banning the procedure. The prescription of ECT for young people was even more vigorously opposed and even banned completely in several states for various groups of children and adolescents.

Fortunately for those who can benefit from ECT, the pendulum has swung back to center. Modern ECT is safer than most surgical procedures, side effects are minimal, and indications for its use have been clarified. A 1999 survey of twenty-six individuals who had received ECT before the age of 19 reported that "the vast majority considered ECT a legitimate treatment and, if medically indicated, would have ECT again and would recommend it to others."[25] The American Academy of Child and Adolescent Psychiatry recommends ECT for certain adolescents, and notes that "despite misperceptions among the media, patients and families, and even physicians, ECT is a safe and beneficial procedure, and one with a high response rate."[26]

MODERN ECT

Electroconvulsive therapy has been greatly improved by developments in anesthetic techniques. ECT is usually done in the recovery room of the surgical suite of a hospital, the area where surgical patients are taken for observation immediately following an operation. This location is used because ECT treatment is over in about sixty seconds, and most of the "treatment" time is actually the ten minutes or so it takes for the patient to awaken from anesthesia. Some large psychiatric hospitals have their own treatment suites that are equipped like a recovery room.

Patients are usually hospitalized during a course of ECT, although increasingly, ECT is given as an outpatient procedure, just like same-day surgery. Sometimes a patient starts a course of ECT in the hospital and finishes it as an outpatient.

Electroconvulsive therapy is now done under general anesthesia just as safely as is surgery. Because each treatment lasts only a few minutes, intravenous barbiturate is used instead of the inhaled anesthetics used in most surgery. The crucial anesthetic advance for ECT was the introduction in the 1950s of agents called *muscle relaxants*, or more properly, *neuromuscular blocking agents*. These medications, also given intravenously, temporarily paralyze the patient by blocking nervous center transmission to the muscles. This prevents the violent muscle contractions during seizures that characterized early ECT.

Immediately before the treatment, a patient usually receives an injection of a medication that prevents abnormal heart rhythms, an IV is started, and the patient is put to sleep with a barbiturate and then given the muscle relaxant. The patient is asleep and completely relaxed in less than five minutes. Electrode disks similar to those used to take cardiograms are applied to the scalp. Modern ECT equipment, designed specifically for this purpose, delivers a precisely timed and measured electrical stimulus: usually a half-second to several seconds in duration. In *bilateral* treatments, an electrode is applied over each temple; in *unilateral* treatments, where the object is to stimulate only half the brain, one electrode is placed in the middle of the forehead and the other at the temple. (Unilateral treatment causes less post-ECT confusion and memory problems—side effects discussed below—and is now used almost exclusively. Occasionally, unilateral treatments don't work as well, and some patients must therefore receive bilateral treatments.)

The "seizure" in modern ECT is pretty much an electrical event only, with few or none of the jerking movements that usually characterize seizures. Most ECT machines used today also record an electroencephalogram (a measurement of the electrical activity of the brain) through the same electrodes used to deliver the stimulus, so the physician can see how long the induced "seizure" lasts—usually twenty-five to forty-five seconds.

A few brief muscle contractions might be observed during this time, but the muscle relaxant keeps the patient nearly motionless. There is usually a brief quickening of the heart rate and increase in blood pressure, which also signal that the "seizure" has occurred. The anesthetist applies a facemask breathing device to deliver oxygen to the patient until he wakes up five or ten minutes later and the treatment is over.

The only patients who absolutely can't receive ECT are those with medical conditions so severe that even ten to fifteen minutes of general anesthesia is too dangerous, for example, patients with severe cardiac or lung disease.

Typically, when the decision is made to give a course of ECT, most or even all psychiatric medications are stopped. (Sedative medications often shorten and otherwise interfere with the ECT "seizure," as do the antiepilepsy mood stabilizers. Lithium seems to make patients more prone to episodes of confusion after treatments.)

Patients awakening from anesthesia are a bit groggy, of course, and often are also slightly fuzzyheaded and feel "spacey" for another hour or so. This is probably related to the treatments themselves, not just the anesthesia, and resembles the mild postseizure confusion sometimes experienced by people with true epilepsy. Occasionally, a more severe period of confusion called delirium is seen, especially after bilateral treatments and especially toward the end of a course of treatments. Sedatives can treat this problem quickly, but when it occurs, consideration should be given to stopping the treatments or giving them less often.

The most troublesome possible side effects of ECT relate to its effect on memory; about two-thirds of patients report that ECT affects their memory in some way. The most common memory loss is for events occurring during the several weeks of the ECT treatments. Treatments are typically given three times a week, and a patient usually needs six to twelve treatments for complete recovery, so a course of ECT will last two to four weeks. Patients commonly lose memory for some events that occurred during those weeks. Some also suffer *retrograde amnesia*: memory loss for a period before they started receiving ECT. This is thought to occur because ECT somehow disrupts the process by which shorter-term memories become incorporated into longer-term memory. (If you've ever lost an hour's worth of computer work because you didn't save your work before something untoward locked up your computer, you get the idea. The short-term memories that are still in the brain's memory "buffer" seem to be lost due to ECT.) Patients who have successfully completed a course of ECT may not remember checking in to the hospital, or may not recollect a home visit or trip they took with their family during the treatments. This problem seems to be worst just after receiving ECT. In a study of forty-three patients interviewed about their memory a few weeks after completing ECT, some reported difficulty remembering events from a period of up to two years before their treatment. But when the subjects were tested again seven *months* after their treatment, these more distant memories were almost completely recovered.[27] One explanation for this finding is the known effect that severe depression has on memory. Several studies indicate that complaints of memory problems after ECT correlate better with the severity of patients' depression than with how they do on memory tests.[28] Unilateral ECT appears to sharply reduce the number of memory complaints.[29]

We should be clear about the effects of ECT on memory. Although there is an associated short-term memory loss for the period before or during ECT, many studies have shown that ECT has a *protective* effect on long-term memory. It seems to prevent the development of dementia and other conditions of long-term memory loss when patients who have received ECT reach an older age. This may be due to the remission of their depression to the ECT itself—the reason is not yet clear. What is certainly clear is that there are no negative effects of ECT on memory in the long run.

Data on the effect of ECT on memory in young people are scarcer than for adults, but one study of a group of adolescent patients who received ECT for bipolar disorder found that only 2 percent of them complained of any memory problems.[30] A more rigorous study of the longer-term effects of ECT on thinking and memory in adolescents—ten patients who had received ECT before the age of 19—involved testing learning ability and short-term memory and asking questions about their subjective sense of their memory ability. The testing was done an average of two years following the course of treatment. No differences were found in learning, short-term memory, or complaints about memory between the subjects who had received ECT and a similar group of subjects who had also been depressed but had never received ECT.[31]

The mechanism by which ECT works continues to be profoundly mysterious. During seizure activity, the neurons of the brain fire simultaneously and rhythmically, and there is a massive discharge of many neurotransmitters. We used to compare ECT to cardiac defibrillation: just as applying a current to the heart can "reset" abnormal rhythms in cardiac muscle, perhaps ECT "resets" rhythmic discharges in the brain in some way. But newer work seems to indicate that, as with other treatments for bipolar disorder, the effect occurs at the level of the individual neurons. Animal experimentation indicates that ECT, like lithium, affects G proteins within the neurons. It may be that ECT, like lithium, works on the neuronal "tuning" mechanisms: the G protein–second messenger system discussed in chapter 5.

PRESCRIPTION OF ECT FOR ADOLESCENTS

Electroconvulsive therapy is perhaps the most effective treatment there is for severe depression and severe mania and often works more quickly than medications. Naturally, it should be a treatment consideration whenever a person continues to be severely depressed despite antidepressant medication treatment. It is *rapidly* effective: many patients have dramatic improvements after three or four treatments, that is, after five to seven days. Severely suicidal individuals, or those who have stopped eating and drinking and are in danger of malnutrition and dehydration— any patients for whom profound depression has become an imminently life-threatening illness—are candidates for ECT. For these individuals, the effectiveness of ECT can seem truly miraculous, as this account shows:

> On February 10, 1977, electroconvulsive treatment was administered for the first time to a 16-year-old female who had not eaten, spoken or walked unaided for the past four months . . . The first treatment produced an unclenching of the fists . . . The second treatment produced consumption of small amount of fluids . . . The fifth was productive of eating and talking normally . . . She was allowed to go home two days after the [seventh] treatment and for the past three months has been getting along nicely and doing all things previously done in a satisfactory fashion.[32]

Electroconvulsive therapy is also a highly effective treatment for mania. A review in the *American Journal of Psychiatry* of fifty years' experience of the use of ECT for treating mania found that it provided complete symptom remission or marked improvement in 80 percent of the manic patients studied. Many of the patients in these studies had failed to respond to many other available treatments—making this success rate all the more impressive.[33] ECT seems to work more quickly in mania than in depression. One study found that patients with mania recovered after an average of six treatments, about half the usual requirement for the treatment of depression.[34] Severely manic patients whose highly agitated state becomes physically dangerous are obvious candidates for ECT.

Although ECT can quickly interrupt an episode of depression or mania, the effect of the treatment doesn't usually last more than several months. Thus, medication treatment will still be necessary to sustain the benefit of ECT and keep the patient's mood state stable after the treatments are finished. Some experts are now recommending that medication be started before the treatments are finished. Depressed patients with bipolar disorder who receive ECT can become slightly hypomanic. Obviously, it's time to stop the treatments when this occurs. Unlike antidepressants, however, ECT does not seem to increase the cycling of the illness.[35]

A survey of adolescents who had received ECT and of their parents illustrates how difficult and frightening it is for parents to give consent for ECT for their children. Most of the parents volunteered, even before being asked by the researchers, that the decision was very difficult and the prospect of the treatment frightening at the time they were asked to agree to it for their child. The use of electricity and the induction of seizures was the scariest part for them. But once the treatments were over, attitudes about them were positive. All the parents (and the adolescents too) said they thought ECT had been a helpful treatment that should be available to treat severe depression in young people.[36]

Your child's psychiatrist should be up to date on the most recent recommendations regarding use of ECT in children and adolescents. The American Academy of Child and Adolescent Psychiatry recommends the treatment "when there is a lack of response to two or more trials of [medication] or when the severity of symptoms precludes waiting for a response to pharmacological treatment." That said, each of us has had many experiences of patients for whom ECT was not only effective but life saving.

OTHER NEW TREATMENTS

TRANSCRANIAL STIMULATION

Repetitive transcranial magnetic stimulation (TMS, or sometimes rTMS) is a new therapeutic technique similar to ECT that has been shown to be effective in treating mood disorders, with several devices receiving FDA approval for treating adults with depression. TMS is still in the early phase of research with adolescents, but preliminary results are encouraging, particularly when TMS is used as an adjunctive treatment for patients for whom antidepressants help but are not fully effective.[37] The great advantage of TMS over ECT is that TMS is much simpler to administer: no seizure activity is induced by the treatment, and therefore no anesthesia is necessary.

This technique takes advantage of a principle of electromagnetism called *induction* (in which a magnetic field induces an electrical current in a nearby conductor) to deliver an electrical stimulus to the brain without applying electrical energy to the scalp (as in ECT). During TMS treatments, a magnetic coil is held against the scalp, and the magnetic field that develops in the coil causes electrical current to flow through nearby neurons under the skull (figure 8-1). No electricity passes through the skull as in ECT, only magnetic waves. Because the electrical current that is generated in the brain tissue by TMS is so small, a seizure does not occur—which is why no anesthesia is necessary. Pulses of magnetic energy are delivered over a period of about twenty minutes while the patient simply sits in a chair. The patient is awake and alert through the whole procedure. Other than some soreness from muscle stimulation, there appear to be no side effects of any kind.[38]

Transcranial magnetic stimulation has been used for a number of years to do brain mapping. Mapping of the motor areas of the brain involves stimulating a brain area and measuring for electrical activity in muscles controlled by that area. Stimulating sensory areas of the brain can cause a person to feel tingling in the part of the body that sends sensory messages to that brain area. Sophisticated TMS techniques are also being used to study language functions, as well as the organization of complex movements.

It is possible to give a placebo TMS treatment, allowing valid research on the efficacy of TMS in depression. When the TMS coil is applied to the

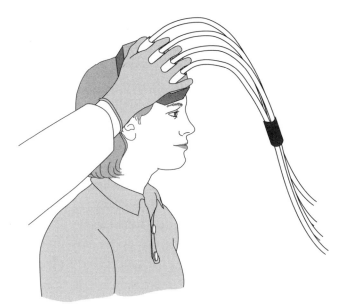

Figure 8-1 Transcranial magnetic stimulation

scalp at a slightly different angle from that used to give treatments, it does not cause electrical current to flow through the brain tissue and thus will not have the usual TMS effect. Because the muscles are still stimulated, the slight muscle soreness associated with the treatment still occurs, and research subjects have no way of knowing whether they are getting a sham treatment or the real thing. This makes the all-important double-blind placebo-controlled studies fairly easy to do.

Several studies indicate that the brain areas known as the left prefrontal lobes are less active than normal in depression. This finding has led researchers to try TMS treatments on depressed patients by stimulating the left prefrontal lobes. Early results have been very promising. In one of the first studies on TMS in the treatment of depression, twelve patients received twenty TMS stimulations of two seconds each over a period of twenty minutes every weekday for two weeks.[39] Either before or after the two weeks of therapy, the subjects were given two weeks of sham treatments (the placebo), during which the TMS coil was held at an angle that would not cause brain tissue stimulation. The patients were tested for depressive symptoms by trained investigators using a standardized questionnaire. Neither the subject nor the investigator giving the mood questionnaire knew whether the patient was receiving real or sham TMS (making the study double blind). The study found statistically significant mood improvement after TMS treatments but not after the sham treatments. Several patients continued TMS after the completion of the study and experienced even further clinical improvement in their depressive symptoms. Another study found similar results in a group that included some individuals with bipolar disorder.[40] In several studies, patients with drug-resistant depression showed improvement after TMS.[41]

Transcranial magnetic stimulation is in its infancy. All indications are that it will be safe, but its efficacy remains untested in the young. The strength of the magnetic stimulation that is most beneficial, the exact placement of the coil, the number of treatments, and the duration of therapy are all under investigation at various centers around the world. Will TMS, like ECT, be effective in bipolar depression as well as in unipolar depression? How about in mania? These and many other questions remain to be answered. Perhaps the biggest unanswered question is, How does TMS work? It has always been thought that the seizure is the necessary therapeutic factor in ECT. Does TMS work in a different way? Or is it some kind of "gentler" ECT that works by a similar mechanism but without causing a seizure? (If the TMS coil is made to generate a strong enough magnetic field, a seizure can indeed be triggered with this technique, perhaps supporting the latter explanation.) As with so much of the science of psychiatry, these questions remain unanswered. What is known, however, is that this safe, effective treatment is more and more available and may find a home in helping treatment-resistant adolescent depression when medications don't seem to be enough.

VAGAL NERVE STIMULATION

Vagal nerve stimulation (VNS), another experimental approach for severe treatment-resistant depression, is also currently under investigation. Because it is sometimes discussed in the media, a brief description is in order. The vagal nerve (or *vagus*) is a long nerve that emerges from the base of the human brain and travels down the neck and into the chest and abdomen; it regulates several vital bodily functions, such as digestion and heart rate. Its connections in the brain are through important centers thought to be involved in emotional regulation, specifically mood regulation. VNS is done by means of a pacemaker-like device that must be surgically implanted to deliver the tiny electrical signals that stimulate the vagus.

Animal studies done as early as the 1930s demonstrated that electrical stimulation of the vagal nerve produced changes in the electrical activity of the brain. In the 1980s, it was demonstrated that VNS could control epileptic seizures in dogs. By the 1990s, VNS had become available for the treatment of intractable epilepsy in humans, first in Europe and then in the United States. And by the end of 2000, about six thousand patients worldwide had received VNS, almost all of them for the treatment of epilepsy. As with antiepilepsy medications that later turned out to be effective mood stabilizers, VNS was noted to have beneficial effects on mood in several of the patients who received it to treat their seizures. Several epilepsy patients had substantial antidepressant effects from VNS, even though the treatment didn't improve their seizure control.

In one of the first studies of VNS treatment in depression, thirty adults received VNS for severe, treatment-resistant depression; some of these patients had taken up to five different medications and received ECT, with little benefit. About half of the patients benefited from VNS.[42] This is still an experimental treatment, and as of this writing, there are no reports of its use in young people for depression, though it has been used extensively to combat seizures in all ages and has been fairly safe. Given the invasive nature of placing the device, VNS is not likely to find a place in treating depression in a younger age group for some time, if ever.

Counseling and Psychotherapy

Medical treatments such as pharmaceuticals often form the foundation of the treatment of serious mood disorders, but counseling and psychotherapy are important, perhaps indispensable, additional therapeutic interventions for these illnesses. Parents are often interested to know the answers to two very different questions about the treatment of depression with counseling and psychotherapy: first, whether this form of treatment is *necessary,* and second, whether it is *sufficient.* Put another way, these questions become "If medications are going to make the depression better, why bother with psychotherapy?" and "Is it possible that psychotherapy alone will successfully treat depression and make medication treatment unnecessary?" We hope to persuade you that the "medication *versus* therapy" perspective is not a good way to think about the treatment of depression.

THE "BIOLOGY-PSYCHOLOGY" SPLIT IN PSYCHIATRY

In the early twentieth century, after the discovery of the biological causes of mental illnesses such as general paresis (central nervous system syphilis) and cretinism (mental retardation due to thyroid deficiency), psychiatric illnesses were divided into two categories: *organic* and *functional.* Organic psychiatric illnesses were "real" illnesses, caused by germs, or abnormal hormone levels, or something else that could be seen under a microscope or measured in a blood test. In functional illnesses, on the other hand, it was assumed that nothing was wrong with brain functioning, at least not in a physical sense. Patients with severe depression, manic-depressive illness, and even schizophrenia were having some kind of abnormal reaction to life events.

The question then became, Why do some people have these abnormal kinds of reactions while others do not? It was at this point that the attempt to understand and treat these illnesses turned away from medicine and toward psychology. Sigmund Freud spent his lifetime treating and trying to understand people who were unhappy in their relationships, disappointed in themselves for choices they had made, perhaps confused and anxious about life decisions they were facing. Freud and his followers developed a large and sophisticated system of understanding human behavior based on understanding childhood development. They developed the "talking treatment" for psychiatric problems: psychotherapy. This basically consisted of helping patients understand themselves better: let go of grudges, resentments, and fears triggered by traumatic experiences and learn better, more mature coping mechanisms. This approach has come to be called *dynamic* psychology or psychiatry and is based on the belief that mental life is best understood as a dynamic interplay between emotions and intellect, present circumstances and unconscious memories of past experiences, and many other psychological factors.

Although this approach was extremely successful in helping people with a wide variety of problems and symptoms, practitioners of dynamic psychotherapy soon discovered that it didn't make much of an impact on the symptoms of persons with major psychiatric illnesses such as schizophrenia or bipolar disorder. The explanation given was that these individuals were too disturbed or too immature or that their families were too dysfunctional for patients to benefit from therapy. Then a revolution occurred: imipramine, lithium, chlorpromazine, and other effective medications for "functional" illnesses were developed. Persons with depressive disorders, bipolar disorders, and schizophrenia, along with their families, started leaving the therapists who often seemed to be blaming them for their illnesses for a new kind of doctor: the biological psychiatrist, the pharmacotherapist, someone who would treat them for a "real" illness.

For a time there was a kind of schism in American psychiatry between those who believed that dynamic psychology best explained mental illnesses and those who believed that biology was the key that would unlock the mysteries of psychiatric disorders.

In the mid-1970s, this biological psychiatry–dynamic psychiatry split was in full swing. Many departments of psychiatry in university medical centers proudly identified themselves as either "biological" or "psychodynamic" in their approach. Usually each camp denigrated the other: psychodynamic psychiatry was "touchy-feely" soft science based more on nineteenth-century literary theory than medicine; biological psychiatrists were "pill pushers" who didn't even talk to their patients and had no appreciation for the human experience.

But a few departments of psychiatry taught their students and resident physicians that mental experiences were not just a series of chemical reactions or simply a collection of dynamically interrelated thoughts and feelings, but both. People with mood disorders are still people, still subject to disappointments and loss and relationship problems and blows to their self-esteem. To see their moods as just the expression of so many chemicals to be fine-tuned with more chemicals was to do them a great disservice. This schism has now healed for the most part, and even the most ardent biological psychiatrists understand that a psychodynamic understanding of the patient is *always* important.

Although there is certainly a place for dynamic psychotherapy in modern psychiatry—*including* traditional Freudian psychoanalysis and the psychoanalytic couch—the variety of available psychological treatments has broadened tremendously in the past twenty-five years or so. Sophisticated techniques have been developed that work for particular kinds of problems. Some involve individual sessions with a therapist, others a group setting. Some are focused on a particular problem, such as family problems; some are symptom-focused, such as on depression or panic attacks; some are designed to last only a few sessions, while others are more open ended. Some are not therapy in the traditional sense at all but are support groups made up of individuals who offer guidance and support to each other and don't even include a "therapist." Research is also being done to determine which psychological treatments work best for which problems. The prescription of a certain kind of counseling or therapy for a particular kind of problem is often backed up by as much research as the prescription of a particular medication.

IS PSYCHOTHERAPY ALONE SUFFICIENT?

A number of reasonably well-designed clinical studies show that some forms of psychotherapy are by themselves effective treatments for many cases of adolescent depression. It's difficult, however, to decide from these studies which cases of adolescent depression can be successfully treated with psychotherapy alone. It seems clear from this work that psychotherapy alone is *not* effective for the treatment of *severe* depression.

Some studies showing that psychotherapy is successful in treating adolescents with depression have recruited their research subjects from schools by means of screening questionnaires that identified students with symptoms of depression. Often, comparisons are made between a group of adolescents who receive treatment and a group who are put on a waiting list, that is, those receiving no treatment at all. Given that it would be unethical to identify individuals with a serious medical problem and then not get them into treatment quickly, we can assume that the adolescents in many of these studies were, by and large, not severely depressed.

Some studies have actually excluded severely depressed adolescents right up front. A 1996 study titled "A Controlled Trial of Brief Cognitive-Behavioral Intervention in Adolescent Patients with Depressive Disorders" (*cognitive-behavioral* therapy is a specific type of psychotherapy that we discuss later in this chapter) found that psychotherapy had a "clear advantage" in a group of depressed adolescents.[1] In this study, research subjects were chosen from individuals applying to an outpatient clinic specializing in adolescent depression. Although this would suggest that a group of more seriously depressed young people was being studied, a closer reading of this paper reveals that any adolescent "taking or likely to require antidepressant medications" was excluded from the study. Almost always, studies of children and adolescents exclude severe symptoms (psychosis, suicidality), which are usually associated with more severe depressive episodes.

Rather than focusing entirely on which patients psychotherapy can help, several studies of the treatment of adolescent depression with psychotherapy have tried to figure out why this treatment *doesn't* help some patients. One such study attempted to compare the efficacy of several different types of therapy in 12- to 18-year-olds with major depression.[2] It found that therapy was not very helpful for 21 percent of the adolescents who had been recruited into the study. These subjects had chronic depressive symptoms during 80 percent of the time the study was conducted—over a period of about two years. (This study had already eliminated more difficult to treat and severely ill patients by excluding adolescents with bipolar disorder, substance abuse, and other complicating factors.) The researchers reported that the subjects who did not respond to psychotherapy treatment had been assessed at the beginning of the study as being more severely depressed.

A study titled "Which Depressed Patients Respond to Cognitive-Behavioral Treatment?" also found that the nonresponders were the subjects who were more depressed at the beginning of the study.[3] This study also measured "impairment" in the subjects at the beginning of the treatment and found that adolescents who were having more trouble functioning in school and at home were less likely to benefit from psychotherapy. Perhaps the most interesting finding was that no particular pattern of individual symptoms predicted which subjects would benefit—that is, there weren't any "red flag" symptoms that seemed to predict that psychotherapy wouldn't work, symptoms such as suicidal thinking or significant weight loss. Subjects who had more symptoms and were functioning poorly didn't do as well with psychotherapy as did subjects with fewer symptoms who were functioning more normally. (This study had already excluded adolescents who were taking antidepressant medications.)

These studies would seem to indicate that psychotherapy alone can be sufficient to treat adolescents with less severe depression—but just what *less severe* is has not been defined very well. Clinical judgment and experience are still the requirements for successfully prescribing treatments for depression, whether medication or psychotherapy.

An important last note to add is that psychotherapy alone is *never* sufficient to adequately treat bipolar disorder. Adolescents with bipolar disorder are uniformly excluded from such studies, and a large clinical literature on adults with bipolar disorders indicates that medication must always be their primary treatment.

IS PSYCHOTHERAPY ALWAYS NECESSARY?

The related question of whether psychotherapy is always required for treating depressed adolescents is also an important one to try to answer. If medication is the more effective treatment for severe depression, why bother with time-consuming and expensive psychotherapy treatment? The TADS trial, which we spoke about in discussing SSRI treatments, looked at this question.[4] One of the major findings in the study was that regardless of the origin of the depression (whether a biological major depressive disorder or a more moderate low mood due to life circumstances), psychotherapy was helpful. This was true both for the group taking medications and for the group taking a placebo. The combination of medications and psychotherapy was the most effective intervention in the study, possibly suggesting that psychotherapy should always be considered in the treatment of depression.

One of the problems with doing this kind of research, and in making any specific recommendations, is that the term *psychotherapy* can cover a lot of territory. It might be helpful to stop for a moment and explore exactly what *psychotherapy* means. Dr. Jerome Frank, who spent his career researching the techniques and effectiveness of psychotherapy, defines it as any technique that attempts "to heal through persuasion" and characterizes the process as one of "employing measures to restore self-confidence and help [the patient] find more effective ways of mastering his problems." Frank emphasizes that psychotherapy works insofar as it can "clarify ... symptoms and problems, inspire hopes, provide [the patient] with experiences of success or mastery, and stir him emotionally."[5]

Psychotherapy, then, is not just giving advice and encouragement (though these are certainly important constituents of the process); it also helps people to make sense of their negative feelings, understand the source of these feelings, and make the changes necessary to relieve them. Part education and part inspiration, psychotherapy tries to help the patient step outside herself and see her situation objectively, in order to identify changes in thinking and behavior that will make things better for her. Frank's research indicates that a crucial ingredient is the ability of the therapist to persuade the patient that things *can* get better.

MATCHING THE PSYCHOTHERAPY TO THE PATIENT

Different therapists use different theories to help their patients make sense of their situations. Freud and his followers emphasized a person's early childhood experiences as the most important issues, and other theories after Freud have focused on communication, changing thinking patterns, or family dynamics. The healing power of psychotherapy depends on the patient's being able to make use of new ways of thinking about his situation. This means that the type of therapy needs to be matched to the patient's problems and to his way of looking at them. This is important because each family of psychotherapy takes a different view regarding most aspects of how to make this improvement happen and places different demands on the patient, the therapist, and the systems surrounding both. We'd like to briefly discuss each broad type of therapy so that you and your family can have some concept of which type might be helpful to your situation and understand what you can expect when beginning a psychotherapeutic journey.

COGNITIVE-BEHAVIORAL THERAPY

In the 1960s, Dr. Aaron Beck and his colleagues developed a theory of depression, and a psychotherapeutic treatment, called *cognitive therapy*.[6] This type of psychotherapy has been researched more thoroughly than most others and has a proven track record in helping with symptoms of depression; in some studies, it has been found to work as well as, or even better than, antidepressant medication for some patients.[7]

The theory of cognitive therapy maintains that people who are chronically or frequently depressed have developed a distorted view of themselves and of the world and have adopted certain patterns of thinking and reacting that perpetuate their problems. This emphasis on thinking, or *cognition,* lends the theory and the therapy their name. Research has shown that depressed adolescents tend to (1) think negatively about themselves, (2) interpret their experiences in a negative way, and (3) have a pessimistic view of the future. Cognitive theory calls this the *cognitive triad*.[8]

The theory further proposes that all this negative thinking causes a person to develop a repertoire of mental habits called *schemas,* or *negative automatic thoughts,* that spring into action and reinforce the negative thinking.

▼   John was a 17-year-old high school junior whose application to enroll in a summer creative-writing seminar at the local university had just been turned down. He came to his therapy session and brought along a lengthy critique of the short story he had included with his application, a critique handwritten by the seminar's director, a well-known local author.

"You see, I should have known better than to apply for this seminar. Phillip Preston, no less, gives me the bad news. Now I'm never going to be a writer."

"Why do you say that?" I asked.

"If someone like Preston thinks I can't write, I might as well give up. That's the last time I bother trying something I'm not cut out for."

"Did he say he thought you couldn't write?"

"Well, no, of course not."

"I see; this famous author and writing teacher doesn't tell his students what he thinks?"

"Well, no. That's not true. In fact, he's got a reputation for coming right out with his opinions to his students. He's supposed to be really tough but honest."

"But he treats you differently from everyone else?"

John began to get a little annoyed. "Well, I wouldn't think so, but how should I know? I've never met the guy."

"What do you make of the fact that Professor Preston wrote to you himself?"

"Well, I did think it was unusual. My friend Ann just got a form letter with her rejection."

"Could it mean he was impressed with some aspects of your writing and wanted to encourage you?"

"He said the story was, quote-unquote, 'promising,'" John said a little sarcastically. "But I figured he was just being nice to a dumb kid."

"So, Professor Preston doesn't mean what he says?"

"But his comments were really negative," John went on glumly. "He went through the whole story, the plot line, the characters, everything, and shot them down one by one."

I continued to reinterpret John's negative take on everything: "He must have spent several hours with your story if he gave you back such a carefully detailed critique. Don't you think?"

"Yeah, I guess he wouldn't have taken all that time and trouble if he thought it was completely worthless. He told me to apply again next year, but—"

"But he was just being nice?"

John was quiet and seemed to be thinking hard.

I went on, "Didn't you tell me that juniors aren't usually accepted into this seminar?"

"Right," John said. "Mrs. Robinson had told me not to get my hopes up, that she'd never had a junior get accepted."

"So, this wasn't really such a surprise for either of you."

"Well, actually she seemed surprised. 'I thought you would be my first junior to get accepted,' she said when I told her."

"But, she didn't mean it? Just being nice?"

John frowned.

"What did your Mrs. Robinson say when you showed her Preston's note."

"Well, I didn't show it to her. She told me to come by her office to discuss some of my other stories and applying next year, but I haven't yet."

"Because?"

John stopped talking and just the smallest hint of a smile appeared at the corners of his mouth. I went on, "Because Mrs. Robinson is being encouraging to you just to be nice?"

John nodded sheepishly. Then he asked, "Are you saying there's a pattern here?"

"What do you think?" I asked.

"You guys," he said, definitely smiling now. "You always answer a question with another question. Do they teach you that in therapist school?"

I couldn't resist: "What do *you* think?" ▲

John is down on his talents and assumes everybody else is, too. In situations that can be interpreted in many different ways, both positive and negative, he tends to go for the negative rather than seek alternative, positive explanations. When something positive happens or is said to him, he ignores it or explains it away somehow (called *negative attributions*). This, in turn, causes him to do things that reinforce his negative thinking (like missing out on the support and encouragement his teacher obviously wants to give him when he comes to her office), and the vicious cycle repeats itself.

Cognitive-behavioral therapy (CBT) is an active form of therapy. Patients are asked to monitor and record their thinking and behavior patterns. There is an emphasis on diary keeping, and "homework" is often assigned. The therapist challenges the cognitive distortions and helps patients identify automatic negative thoughts and reinterpret events more positively. There is an emphasis on the here and now, not on the past, and patients are taught to modify behaviors and ways of thinking about themselves and what happens to them (a process called *cognitive restructuring*). Many patients and families like this type of therapy because it tends to help more quickly than other types, and how it works is transparent and clearly explained. Also, it establishes concrete, structured ways to help in various situations, including emergencies.

Cognitive-behavioral therapy is the best-studied type of psychotherapy for the treatment of depression in young people, and it has been proved effective in the treatment of less severe depression.

INTERPERSONAL PSYCHOTHERAPY

Interpersonal psychotherapy (IPT) is based on the premise that depression is best understood in the context of personal connections, and that regardless of its underlying causes, depression is always inextricably intertwined with the adolescent's interpersonal relationships. IPT does not assume that relationship problems *cause* depression, but it is thought that addressing relationship problems can alleviate depressive symptoms, regardless of the individual psychological or even biological contributions to depression. Originally developed to treat depression in adults, this type of therapy has been adapted for adolescents to focus better on the relationship issues common in this age group. IPT helps the adolescent deal with problematic or unsatisfying relationships and attempts to restructure relationships to make them more fulfilling.

Like cognitive-behavioral therapy, IPT is an active type of psychotherapy and focuses on the here and now, principally on enhancing communication in the adolescent's important relationships: with parents and peers and in dating relationships. IPT tries to help the adolescent learn a more open communication style and become better at listening to others. The therapist tries to help the adolescent become aware of his need to develop adult-like expectations of himself and an increased understanding of his parents' point of view. IPT works to clarify role expectations and to address role disputes and transitions. By enhancing relationships and problem-solving skills, IPT helps strengthen the adolescent's peer and family relationships, providing an enhanced support system that he can turn to when negative things happen. It is thought that this helps the adolescent become more resilient and less likely to become depressed in the future. According to some literature, this type of therapy may be particularly suited to adolescents embedded in a cultural system that values strong family and social ties.[9]

In a study of 12- to 18-year-olds treated for depression with IPT for twelve weeks, patients reported a significant decrease in depressive symptoms and an improvement in their overall social functioning and functioning with friends and in dating relationships. They also reported improvement in their ability to think of alternative solutions to problems, to try them out, and then to use them to address difficulties.[10]

FAMILY THERAPY

There are many definitions of family therapy, but all types involve face-to-face work with multiple family members to focus on the interactions and dynamics of family relationships. This differs from interpersonal psychotherapy in a number of ways. First of all, the adolescent is no longer the single identified patient. Rather, the family as a unit is the "patient," and the goal is to help the family as a whole by working with each of its individual members equally. As such, all identified persons in the family are expected to attend the therapy sessions and work equally hard at making and sustaining positive change. In effective family therapy, this can mean a drastic increase in progress, because many people are working hard to improve the relationships, not just one. It can be a useful frame for an adolescent who is reluctant to enter therapy for fear that she will be identified as the "broken" one in need of "fixing." The family therapy approach may also be helpful when other clear sources of stress (between parents, or between siblings) are clearly affecting the adolescent. And, of course, parents who have their own history of depression may find this type of therapy particularly attractive, as it allows a more open discussion, and a deeper bonding, between themselves and their children over this common experience in a safe way.

The goal of family therapy for depressed adolescents is to decrease depressive symptoms and improve the adolescent's level of functioning by identifying and changing problems in the interactions within the family that may be responsible for initiating or exacerbating depression. As with interpersonal psychotherapy, there is less concern with the cause or causes of the depression than with current negative relationships among family members.

A depressed adolescent typically isolates herself from family members, and the irritability and disruptive behaviors that are often part of the picture of adolescent depression can poison family life. Situational stressors can cause a depressed adolescent to withdraw from family life and to rebuff parental expressions of concern that her depressive behaviors elicit. This rejection of parents' attempts to comfort and be helpful frustrates parents in turn, and they can then become angry and critical. This makes the adolescent more angry, guilty, and depressed. A vicious cycle of blame and hostility can start that becomes self-sustaining and difficult to interrupt.

Family therapy tries to help the family reestablish constructive relationships by decreasing adolescent isolation and parental criticism and bolstering family cohesion. The therapist attempts to stimulate reattachment within the family by increasing trust and desire for parental love and support in the adolescent and by helping parents reestablish themselves in their roles as empathetic caregivers.

Often the therapist will attempt to reframe depression-related behavioral problems as symptomatic problems in family relationships rather than problems that emanate only from the depressed adolescent. This may involve understanding depressive behaviors as actually fulfilling a positive function within the family. (Mom and Dad are having problems in their relationship; Johnny is acting up because he thinks a crisis will bring the family closer together.) This often has the effect of absolving blame and shifting the family's focus from "whose fault is this?" to "how do we work together to make things better?"

Family therapists encourage all family members to get their feelings out in the open in constructive ways and to improve interpersonal communications. The therapist helps the family negotiate practical family issues such as curfew, chores, and dating, balancing the need for parental authority with the adolescent's need for increasing autonomy.

Because family therapy is so wide ranging and individualized to each family situation, it has been difficult to research its effectiveness. Many studies have indicated, however, that family stresses and tensions predict relapse of depressive illnesses in adolescents. This suggests that family therapy is important when these kinds of tensions exist within the adolescent's family. Recent evidence seems to suggest that this approach can reduce depressive symptoms, even suicidal ideation, in depressed adolescents as effectively as many other therapies described in this chapter.

INSIGHT-ORIENTED PSYCHOTHERAPY

Insight-oriented psychotherapy (or *dynamic psychotherapy*) consists of individual meetings with a therapist, usually over an extended period (months or even years), in which the person in treatment discusses her past and present experiences and feelings with a goal of better self-understanding, acceptance, and personal growth. Disappointments and accomplishments, affections and enmities, fears, inspirations, passions, and worries—all are, as psychotherapists are fond of saying, "grist for the mill" of therapy. Patient and therapist will, of course, talk about such symptoms as sadness and anxiety as well, but insight-oriented psychotherapy tries to understand symptoms as signals that indicate underlying conflicts rather than as the focus of treatment in and of themselves. This more traditional type of psychotherapy emphasizes exploration of the *meaning* of symptoms and the development of self-awareness and maturity.

This type of therapy is different from most of those listed above as the therapist aims to be "nondirective." That is, psychodynamic psychotherapists never tell a patient to do anything—no homework, no assignments. Many times, therapists will even resist interpreting particular interactions, as the goal is to help patients reach their own understanding of situations without therapists muddying the waters by inserting their own opinions. The thinking behind the therapy itself, that deeper understanding on the part of the patient will naturally lead to change in behavior and attitudes, is one of the reasons that it takes such a long time, but this form of therapy is described by patients as incredibly powerful and empowering, as patients reach most of the insights seemingly on their own (though the careful, subtle guidance employed by the therapist is precisely what makes this one of the most difficult therapies to master). More mature adolescents who have good communication skills, who are capable of the introspection and self-reflection that this type of treatment requires, and who are motivated to understand themselves better are more likely to benefit from insight-oriented therapy. It also tends to be more effective for patients who can maintain a relationship, who are comfortable discussing emotions, and who are not inclined to have continual crises.

Dealing with psychological traumas and setbacks—past and present—that cause understandable feelings of sadness or anger or anxiety is a focus of insight-oriented psychotherapy, as are thinking patterns, self-attitudes, and interpersonal styles that disrupt a person's ability to be happy in relationships, effective in school or work, carefree in play, and confident about making decisions about the future. The complexity and subtlety of this kind of therapy is why psychotherapists often study and train in their profession for almost as many years as physicians do in theirs and why people are sometimes in therapy for months, even years, at a time. It is also why this kind of psychotherapy is such an intense, powerful experience and the therapeutic relationship between patient and therapist so unique.

Insight-oriented psychotherapy is often referred to as "open ended" and can continue as long as the patient continues to feel that she is benefiting from it. The goals of treatment are individual and can be quite far ranging. For these reasons, efficacy research on this type of treatment has been nearly impossible to do. That said, recent studies have attempted to compare insight-oriented psychotherapy to more modern techniques, such as cognitive-behavioral therapy. The results have been mixed. Some studies show the insight-oriented approach to be superior, some inferior, though most show it to be equivalent to CBT for the treatment of depression. It really is a matter of you and your child discussing treatment options with your child's psychiatrist and matching the type of therapy with your child's particular strengths and interests.

GROUP PSYCHOTHERAPY

Group therapy can be particularly helpful for adolescents, because they are often much more willing to talk about their feelings and difficulties to peers than to adults. Feedback and observations may have a much more powerful effect on an adolescent if coming from peers rather than from an adult therapist. In a group, young people can model and practice social skills and benefit from companionship and mutual support of others their age.

The therapist usually encourages group members to problem solve for each other and give feedback and support to one another. Group members are helped to better recognize feelings in themselves and in others, are coached on social problem solving, and are taught how to negotiate to resolve conflicts.

Group therapy is usually an adjunctive treatment to another type of psychotherapy rather than the sole treatment for depression, often to address a particular problem such as poor social skills. Substance-abuse treatment is frequently done in a group setting, where modeling of behaviors and roleplaying exercises are helpful for the adolescent to begin developing a substance-free coping and lifestyle. Group therapy helps teenagers see that others their own age have similar problems (sometimes *worse* problems) and helps them experience firsthand how peers successfully or unsuccessfully go about dealing with difficulties and setbacks. Some of the most robust evidence, ironically, relates to helping those adolescents with social anxiety—those least likely to want to participate in groups! Practicing interactions with other young persons in a nonthreatening environment tends to make these individuals more comfortable in other settings as well. Consequently, this treatment may also be good for depressed adolescents who seem to be especially asocial.

DIALECTICAL BEHAVIORAL THERAPY

In 1987, Marsha Linehan, a professor and practicing psychologist at the University of Washington, published a paper in which she outlined an adaptation of the principles of cognitive-behavioral therapy for individuals with particular problems.[11] A certain subgroup of patients, many with diagnosed mood disorders, had a difficult collection of characteristics. They seemed more irritable than sad, though they certainly had both facets; they frequently sought out, then rejected, help and authority; they sometimes had suicidal thoughts, and some responded to these thoughts with risky behaviors; they could be socially isolated; they frequently did not want to go to therapy or treatment, and had difficulty staying in therapy once started, as they rejected the idea that anything was "wrong" with them. To the attentive reader, this seems strikingly similar to our earlier descriptions of the depressed adolescent. Therefore, although this type of therapy was initially created to treat a related though separate entity (called borderline personality disorder), it will be discussed here as it can frequently be helpful in major depression in young people.

Dr. Linehan believed that cognitive-behavioral therapy had many strengths as a modality. It was concrete and easy to follow, focused on positive change, and was rapidly effective. What she did not like, however, was that some patients seemed to find it rather punitive and invalidating. For some depressed persons who are already more likely to perceive their situations and surroundings as negative, going to a therapist weekly who (kindly, but distinctly) tells you a litany of everything you are doing wrong and what you need to change can leave them feeling invalidated. Dr. Linehan noticed in her research that the rate of persons who started but prematurely terminated therapy was relatively high for CBT, and she thought she might understand why. She set out to rebalance CBT to be both validating and focused on improvement. By validating the intense struggles of the depressed person to do even the most basic of activities, while providing the skills to take on more and more challenges, a therapist can help a patient feel understood and motivated to take on the challenge of the cognitive-behavioral technique. These dialectical dilemmas are at the core of dialectical behavioral therapy (DBT) and its principles. (In a dialectic, two opposing viewpoints are resolved into a higher truth in which both are accurate—for example, "I'm doing the best I can *and* I have to change and do better.")

Like CBT, the DBT treatment itself focuses on challenging cognitions and helping the person learn skills to improve himself and his situation. It also incorporates additional domains beyond CBT, including mindfulness and distress tolerance, all aimed at helping a person accept his current circumstances without reacting emotionally. All of us have probably said things we later regretted in the heat of the moment, usually in an argument. A person struck with an irritable temperament due to depression may be even more likely to do so, setting him up for further rejection from his loved ones, deepening his sense of sadness and loneliness. DBT teaches specific concrete skills to use in just such a situation, linking the base emotional state of "I'm really mad right now and he has no right to say that to me" to the intellectual understanding of "In the greater context, I know he cares for me and I don't want to hurt this relationship." Combining the emotional and intellectual understanding of a situation results in what Linehan calls the "Wise Mind," or wise understanding, from which the correct actions may follow.

As we've discussed, DBT was initially created to treat another condition entirely. However, studies in adolescents have shown that DBT can be helpful for some of the core symptoms of depression as well, including low mood, irritability, impulsivity, and difficult interpersonal relationships. Although DBT is certainly not for every patient, it may yet find a home in treating depressed adolescents, particularly those with prominent irritability.

ACCEPTANCE AND COMMITMENT THERAPY

Acceptance and commitment therapy (ACT) is a relatively new type of treatment in the field of behavioral psychology. Although it superficially seems similar to cognitive-behavioral therapy, or other behavioral therapies, in the types of exercises it asks the patient to do, it is quite different. Almost all of the above treatments aim in some way to reduce the uncomfortable feelings and experiences accompanying depression. In CBT, this is accomplished by challenging background thoughts and behaviors, thereby controlling them; DBT takes this a step further by mitigating even the therapeutic experience itself, tempering it with understanding and acceptance. Interpersonal psychotherapy, family therapy, and group therapy all look to improve an adolescent's relationships, in one way or another, in order to improve uncomfortable interactions that worsen the depression. Insight-oriented psychotherapy seeks to resolve discomfort of which the person may not even be aware, so-called unconscious conflicts, leading the person to change. ACT is different in that its goal is specifically *not* to resolve this discomfort, but rather to allow the person to function *despite* it.

ACT bases its principles on reducing something called experiential avoidance. Many people experience uncomfortable events throughout the day. Sometimes, this is a phone call that we know we have to make even though we don't want to. Or it may be our anxiety at public speaking, or going to a party. Our natural response is usually to try to avoid these experiences. The more discomfort, the greater the avoidance. In the long run, though, avoidance actually makes us *more* uncomfortable, not less. All of the above therapies, through one method or another, aim to reduce this discomfort, allowing us to reduce the avoidance. An extreme example is in the context of CBT, in which patients are asked to undertake uncomfortable ventures. A person afraid of flying, for example, will be taken through a stepwise series of exercises aimed at lowering this fear. First, she will be asked to look at pictures of planes. Then, the therapist may take her for lunch at the airport. Next, she may (at least in the pre-TSA days) be taken onto a grounded plane and asked to sit in a seat—all the while practicing relaxation exercises until she feels more comfortable and learning to control her catastrophic thoughts ("We're going to crash!") by confronting them. Finally, she may take a short flight. ACT is different. Although the end result, flying on a plane, may be the same, the goal of the therapy would be for the patient to *accept* that flying is scary and that she will be uncomfortable, but to *commit* to getting on the flight anyway. This will reduce her avoidance of many things (the flight, her own fear), making it seem less scary and more tolerable in the long run, improving the chances of future trips.

ACT therapists do not attempt to challenge negative or scary thoughts. Rather, they encourage the patient to notice them, realize that they are just thoughts, and return to being present in the moment. This approach teaches patients to get in touch with their core self, the entity observing the thinking, and realize that their selves and their thoughts are separate things. It also emphasizes that thoughts are just that, thoughts, not facts. Rather than practicing distraction or relaxation in the face of fear, the ACT practitioner notices the thoughts and the fear and, instead of running from them, attends to them as they are in the present moment. ACT is much more meditative and present focused than the other therapies, and some adolescents find these qualities more appealing. The ACT approach does not try to "fix" the depression or negative experience, but rather encourages the person to accept it and move on, another appealing factor to some who already resent the idea that they are "broken."

In adults, ACT has shown to be effective in lowering depression scores and in improving functioning, particularly when depression is combined with other negative experiences, such as chronic pain.[12] There is increasing evidence that it can be useful in adolescent depression.[13] Although ACT is new to the field, it represents a fairly radical departure from prior approaches and may be a consideration, although few practitioners specialize in children and adolescents.

CHOOSING A THERAPY AND A THERAPIST

Some therapists are clear about the type of treatment they use. You would be able to tell by glancing at their website that they are a "CBT therapist" or a "family therapist." More frequently, however, it will take a phone call or an initial meeting to determine what specific modality a therapist employs. Many therapists are experienced in multiple treatments and will be able to adjust their therapeutic style based on their assessment of what will work best with a particular patient. A really good therapist will be able to shift back and forth as the therapy progresses, perhaps being more encouraging and directive when the adolescent is still very depressed and more passive, making the adolescent work harder, as he gets better.

Sometimes, it's not difficult to decide which psychotherapeutic technique has a good chance of being helpful for a depressed adolescent. The depressed person who tends to be self-blaming and too hard on himself and whose depression is not complicated by disruptive behaviors or substance abuse might be a good candidate for a cognitive-behavioral approach. If the adolescent relates easily to adults and usually completes the kinds of homework assignments that this treatment orientation uses, so much the better. If the depressed adolescent's irritability and disruptive behaviors have resulted in such a toxic family atmosphere that family members can hardly speak to each other without arguing, family therapy would seem like a good place to begin. Sometimes during the course of treatment, complex issues are identified that call for the more in-depth approach that insight-oriented therapy provides. An adolescent who identifies a history of sexual trauma, for example, may need longer-term psychotherapy to deal with the complex issues that such a history raises, even after the depressive symptoms have abated.

Rather than seeking out a therapist with a particular theoretical orientation or type of training, focus on finding a therapist who is experienced in the treatment of adolescents and who is good at what she does. Usually, the treating psychiatrist will be familiar with good therapists in the community, as will pediatricians, school counselors, and clergy.

In addition to getting treatment for depression symptoms, the depressed adolescent usually needs treatment for the *consequences* of having been depressed. If a hospitalization has been necessary, the return to school may be quite difficult. The young person will need to cope with the curiosity and possibly the cruelty of classmates and acquaintances, and will need help and support in formulating answers to their questions and responses to their teasing. Studies have indicated that peers often perceive the depressed adolescent as shyer and less popular than other children as well as more apt to be teased by peers. Depressed adolescents may have been outcasts and felt isolated for a while before getting treatment and will usually need help integrating back into their social situation, a situation that may have been uncomfortable for a long time.

Sometimes depressed adolescents have developed a dysfunctional peer group that they need to break away from. The youth may have developed relationships with younger, more immature children because of his poorer social skills, or with peers who are substance abusers or who engage in delinquent behaviors. The adolescent recovering from depression will need considerable therapeutic support to be able to leave these dysfunctional but nevertheless comfortable relationships and to develop relationships with healthier and more functional peers.

Adolescents also need to make peace with having a psychiatric illness and probably with taking medications, and they need help incorporating these experiences into their self-identity and coping with the stigmatization of psychiatric treatment. For all these reasons, psychotherapy is always an important component of the treatment of depression. Even if an adolescent has an excellent response to medications, she will need help dealing with these sorts of issues. All these goals can be addressed by any of the above discussed types of psychotherapy, though each will go about it in different ways.

THE PSYCHIATRIST-PSYCHOTHERAPIST: AN EXTINCT SPECIES?

You have probably noticed that throughout this chapter, we usually refer to the psychiatrist and the psychotherapist as two different individuals. Unfortunately, this has become more or less the rule rather than the exception in American psychiatry. It would, of course, be preferable for all sorts of reasons for the person prescribing medication and the person doing psychotherapy to be the same individual. But for a variety of compli-cated reasons, most adolescents with mood disorders will see a psychiatrist for medication management and a nonphysician therapist (often a social worker or psychologist) for therapy. (We discuss the various types of men-tal health professionals and their unique expertise in chapter 16.) Some of the reasons for this are the changes in medication management of mood disorders that have come about with the development of new medications: so many different pharmaceuticals are now used in psychiatry that staying skilled in their use has become increasingly time consuming. Perhaps even more significant, though, is that as more effective medications become available for more psychiatric problems, increasing numbers of people want to (and need to) see a psychiatrist for their treatment. There simply aren't enough psychiatrists to do medication management and therapy too, especially in busy clinics. Because medical school and psychiatric training take longer and cost more than the training required to become a psycho-therapist, psychiatrists are usually more expensive than other profession-als. This is particularly true for psychiatrists who have received additional training to become board certified in child and adolescent psychiatry, a field currently experiencing a national shortage. When the administrator of a busy clinic or an HMO is looking to staff a mental health program, *split treatment* (psychiatric treatment split between a psychiatrist for medica-tion management and a nonphysician therapist for psychotherapy or coun-seling) means more cost-effective treatment for patients.

The superior cost-effectiveness of split treatment allows so many more patients to receive psychiatric treatment so much more cheaply that it's difficult to envision a return to the days when psychiatrists did therapy and prescribed medications. Fortunately, there are excellent training programs for clinical social workers, psychologists, and counseling professionals that are producing superb psychotherapists. And as we have seen in this chapter, psychotherapy is becoming more specialized too. It has become nearly impossible to be both an expert therapist and an expert psychophar-macologist. For all of these reasons, two professionals rather than one will usually share the medication management and the therapy of the adoles-cent with a mood disorder.

Part III

VARIATIONS, CAUSES & CONNECTIONS

I N THIS GROUP OF CHAPTERS, we explore several related conditions and problems that frequently complicate the picture of adolescent depression. Chapter 10 addresses the complicated relationship between mood disorders and attention-deficit/hyperactivity disorder. ADHD is a common childhood diagnosis in adolescents who suffer from mood disorders. The links between these two problems are real but also complex and controversial. We explain what ADHD is (and isn't) and introduce some of the controversies surrounding its diagnosis and treatment.

Chapter 11 discusses the diagnosis of autism and how it relates to mood disorders. Since the first edition of this book, there has been a large increase in the number of children and adolescents diagnosed with autism or one of its variants (including Asperger's syndrome). Many children with these conditions at times express similar symptoms to the symptoms seen in a mood disorder, and some will have both autism and an underlying mood disorder as well. Helping persons afflicted with both of these conditions can be difficult for physicians and parents alike, and we discuss some possible approaches here.

In chapter 12, we review alcoholism and substance abuse, looking at how these problems, for most people who suffer from them, are almost inextricably interwoven with mood disorders. This topic may well be the most important of the "connections" covered in this part of the book, because the problem of substance abuse is so common and because it is the most dangerous. Numerous studies show that the combination of a mood disorder and substance abuse is perilous. Individuals with both problems are at far greater risk of harming themselves with suicidal behavior.

Next comes a review of the symptoms, classification, and treatment of eating disorders. These mysterious illnesses are seen predominantly, though not exclusively, in young women, most of whom also suffer from a mood disorder. Anorexia nervosa is one of the deadliest of all psychiatric conditions, and its successful management requires vigorous and sustained treatment of both the disordered eating behaviors and the mood disorder that so frequently fuels and sustains them.

In chapter 14, we discuss "cutting," a complication of depression that is occurring with increasing frequency and seems in many ways surprisingly similar to substance abuse and some eating disorder symptoms. It is also frequently a manifestation of a mood disorder, but as with substance abuse and eating disorders, it requires specialized treatment in its own right. This chapter also takes up the topic of suicidal behavior among adolescents.

The last chapter in this part turns away from more clinical matters and toward a more scientific one, to a topic often of intense interest to adolescents with mood disorders and their families: the genetics of mood disorders.

Attention-Deficit/Hyperactivity Disorder

No book on psychiatric problems in adolescents would be complete without a discussion of attention-deficit/hyperactivity disorder (ADHD). Depending on whom you talk to, ADHD is either an undiagnosed epidemic, with thousands of young people going untreated, or an overblown fraud that has resulted in the needless prescribing of potentially addictive pharmaceuticals to a significant percentage of children and adolescents. As is usually the case with any issue that involves human behavior, the truth is more complicated, and neither of these extreme views seems to be quite correct. In this chapter, we discuss the diagnosis and treatment of ADHD and give you some idea of how this controversy has come about. We also discuss the relationship between ADHD and mood disorders.

WHAT IS ADHD?

To understand attention-deficit/hyperactivity disorder, it's useful to examine more closely what is meant by *attention*. Psychologists have conceptualized *attention* as requiring the following separate steps and processes:

1. Becoming aware of new information in the environment (the *stimulus*)
2. Beginning to process the detected information, and filtering out competing stimuli

3. Shifting attention when appropriate to the task at hand, while resisting the shifting of attention to nonessential stimuli
4. Organizing a response to the incoming information

It is important to note that the normal attention process involves focusing on some information in the environment and actively screening out other information. If you are making a presentation to a new client at her office and hear the siren of an emergency vehicle outside, you may pay attention to the siren for a moment, but you'll then shift your attention back to the business meeting. Chances are, if another vehicle sounding its siren goes by, you won't even be consciously aware of it. In some ways, this screening out of stimuli is the more important aspect of attention.

The other important concept to understand regarding ADHD is that of *executive function*. This set of brain functions, possibly unique to humans, involves self-control and behavioral regulation, suppression of impulses, and planning and sequencing of behaviors. The executive control center of the brain allows us to think about our situation and about what might happen in the future and to plan how we can influence what happens to us for the better. Executive functions mature as a child grows into an adult. These functions seem to be carried out in the frontal lobes of the cerebral cortex, the most advanced area of the human brain. We know that this area of the brain continues developing during adolescence, which seems to provide evidence that this area is where these mature types of brain functions are carried out. In addition to problems with attention, persons with ADHD have problems with executive function. This explains their impulsivity, or inability to plan well or to delay gratification, and their tendency to overreact emotionally to stresses with angry outbursts.

A diagnosis of ADHD is considered when a child, adolescent, or adult has problems with level of attention or executive functioning that seem inconsistent with his age and expected level of maturity. The problem with making this diagnosis comes in deciding what is appropriate at any given age.

The first description of children for whom we would today make a diagnosis of ADHD was given in 1902 by British psychiatrist George Still, in a paper titled "Some Abnormal Psychical Conditions in Childhood."[1] Still described forty-three children with serious behavioral problems: aggressiveness, temper outbursts, defiance, and severe attention problems.

Many of the children had epilepsy, intellectual disabilities (formerly classified under the umbrella of "mental retardation"), or other evidence of brain damage of some kind. He suggested that these children had a "defect in moral control," meaning that they could not regulate their behavior normally. From the 1930s through the 1950s, psychiatrists emphasized the relationship between these problems and brain injuries of various types, whether actual brain trauma from accidents or damage from childhood brain infections such as what sometimes results from measles. At the same time, psychiatrists recognized that the behavioral and attention problems of these children resembled those of individuals who had suffered damage to their frontal lobes. The term *minimal brain damage* was coined to identify these cases. By the 1960s, it was recognized that many of the children and adolescents with these symptoms had no history of brain injury, so the term was changed to *minimal brain dysfunction* (MBD). More recently, the term ADHD has been used, to acknowledge that this problem may or may not be due to "brain dysfunction," and that the cause of the symptoms of ADHD is unknown.

For several decades now, the number of children and adolescents (and adults) whose problems are grouped under the ADHD umbrella has been growing significantly. Whereas the individuals given the predecessor diagnoses of ADHD were severely disturbed, often intellectually disabled, and brain-damaged children, today, adults with college degrees are being prescribed stimulant medication for ADHD because of concentration problems at work. Between 1990 and 1993, the quantity of the stimulant medication methylphenidate (Ritalin) manufactured in the United States nearly tripled, from about eighteen hundred to more than five thousand kilograms annually.[2] Are pediatricians and psychiatrists getting better at recognizing subtle cases of ADHD? Or are these medications being overprescribed? The jury remains out on this issue.

The difficulty in diagnosing this disorder is that the behaviors assessed occur along a continuum and are not abnormal in themselves: a level of attention and executive control that seems abnormal for a person of one age might be perfectly normal in someone younger. If, in the example of the business meeting given above, you interrupted your presentation by rushing over to the window every time an emergency vehicle went by, this would clearly not be age-appropriate behavior. But if a 4-year-old were to do so, no one would be surprised or would consider the child's behavior abnormal. Children are more easily bored than adults and are more easily distracted by interesting and unusual stimuli in their environment. They become more able to focus as they get older.

Age is not the only variable that affects attention and executive functioning. Just as there is a range of body height and weight that is considered normal, brain functions vary among individuals within a range that can be considered normal. At all ages, people vary in their ability to concentrate and attend. When we use more common terms such as *patience* or *maturity* to describe some of the elements of executive function, it becomes obvious that people also vary in these qualities within a wide range of "normal."

So how does one decide how impulsive is too impulsive? Or how active is hyperactive? What amount of "fidgetiness" is normal for a 7-year-old boy? And how does one objectively measure it? The psychiatrist needs to answer these kinds of questions when considering a diagnosis of ADHD.

Simply giving an individual a trial of stimulant medication to see whether it helps cannot be used as a diagnostic tool, because stimulant medications will improve behavior in healthy children as well. Stimulants *always* help with attention and concentration. This is why they are so prone to be abused.

Although the diagnosis of ADHD is difficult to make for some children, others have such severe problems with attention and executive functions that their behavior is clearly outside the range of normal functioning. There is no doubt that these children have a disorder and need help. What is the clinical picture in these children?

The two faces of the ADHD coin are that of inattention (attention deficit) and that of hyperactivity. People with this condition tend to have difficulty regulating their attention. Many people believe that ADHD describes an inability to pay attention to any single thing for a prolonged time. This isn't true. As we've said above, ADHD is an inability to direct one's attention to the task at hand regardless of outside stimuli. We have parents who come to us feeling that their child cannot possibly have ADHD. "He can play video games for hours! He's just lazy and doesn't want to do his homework." In truth, no single picture could be more indicative of ADHD than such a child. Video games are designed to constantly grab one's attention, with bright colors, loud noises, and constant action. Children with ADHD almost get pulled into the game and are able to stop scanning their environment for other stimuli. Parents will call their child's name over and over again without getting a response, not because the child is being willful, but rather because the child's entire attentional focus has been sucked into the flashing, blinking screen. Trying to attend to a less interesting task like homework is almost physically impossible for those with significant ADHD, and any other random stimulus (the family pet walking by, the phone ringing) will derail their current train of thought, so they have to start over.

The other face of ADHD is that of the hyperactive child seemingly driven by a motor. These children truly cannot sit still for any period. They seem to have more energy than any one person should. They impulsively do things without thinking about them. In psychiatric parlance, these two types of ADHD are called, respectively, the *inattentive* type and the *hyperactive/impulsive* type. Most children with ADHD have aspects of both types, but some have primarily the inattentive type. As these children tend to be more quiet and distractible, they are often overlooked by teachers. After all, they are not causing any problems but are rather passively sitting in their chair, thinking about something else. This subtype tends to affect girls more than boys and is usually diagnosed later on, usually around the third or fourth grade, when "learning to read" becomes "reading to learn." At this point, children need to use skills acquired in the first and second grades to comprehend increasingly complicated material. These skills were never laid down in children with inattentive ADHD, and their grades begin to suffer significantly.

What are the consequences of ADHD? In younger children, these problems may lead to poor grades, classroom disruptions, placement in special classes, and disciplinary suspension or even expulsion from school. Peers perceive a child with ADHD as irritating and immature (*executive functioning* is, after all, another term for what we often call *maturity*). Other children may exclude a child with ADHD from their activities, so his social skills can suffer. Peers learn quickly that it is easy to tease children who have ADHD and to set them up to get into trouble with adults. ADHD is not a benign disorder by any means, and aggressive treatment is necessary to prevent the sorts of problems these children encounter over time.

Attention-deficit/hyperactivity disorder persists into adolescence in about three-quarters of the children diagnosed with the condition. Because many of these adolescents have not acquired the basics of learning, it interferes with school performance, self-esteem, and family relationships and predisposes teenagers to high-risk behaviors. Adolescents with ADHD have worse driving habits, more accidents, and more traffic tickets. They have first intercourse at an earlier age, more sexual partners, less use of birth control, more sexually transmitted diseases, and more teen pregnancies than their peers without ADHD (all of which are likely related to increased impulsivity and a reduced sense of the consequences of their actions, or, again, immaturity).[3]

TREATMENT ISSUES

There are two main types of treatment for ADHD (as for almost any psychiatric condition): psychotherapy and medication. The "psychotherapy" for ADHD is actually more weighted toward the surrounding environment than toward the child herself. It includes parent management training (a sort of cognitive-behavioral training for parents in how to effectively manage a child with ADHD), and can also include school accommodations, such as a "decreased stimulation" environment, a high teacher-to-student ratio, and tutoring. More advanced children and adolescents can also be enrolled in study skills training. In terms of medication, the mainstay of treatment is and always has been stimulant medications, of which there are two types, *amphetamines* (table 10-1) and *methylphenidates* (table 10-2). The safety and efficacy of stimulant medications for the treatment of children and adolescents with ADHD is one of the most studied areas in the field of psychiatry. In contrast to the small amount of research on the efficacy of most other psychiatric medications in children, more than 150 randomized controlled studies have been conducted on the use of stimulant medications in children and adolescents.

These studies indicate that stimulant medications improve attention and concentration and decrease impulsive behaviors such as fidgetiness and interrupting in the classroom, and that these effects are sustained over time. Stimulant medications are unlike most of the other medications we've discussed in that they take effect almost immediately. Whereas depressed individuals must wait two to four weeks for their antidepressants to become effective, a stimulant may improve ADHD within hours.

There is much less evidence that stimulant medications help with the

Table 10-1   Stimulant Medications—Amphetamine Class

Generic Name	Brand Name
Amphetamine/dextroamphetamine	Adderall
Dextroamphetamine	Dexedrine
Lisdexamphetamine	Vyvanse

Table 10-2   Stimulant Medications—Methylphenidate Class

Generic Name	Brand Name
Methylphenidate	Ritalin, Methylin
Methylphenidate	Daytrana (topical patch)
Methylphenidate–Extended Release	Concerta

behavioral "fall-out" of ADHD. Research data indicating that medication makes a difference for problems with academic performance, peer relationships, and social skills are scarce. For these reasons, it is important to realize that medication for ADHD is only part of a comprehensive treatment plan that should include interventions in the school (such as smaller class size, increased supervision, and sometimes specialized programs to enhance social skills). Counseling and psychotherapy and sometimes family education and therapy are also extremely important to address the many types of problems afflicting children who have ADHD.

So what treatment do you pick for your child? The largest landmark study of the treatment of ADHD to date is the Multimodal Treatment Study of Children with ADHD (MTA).[4] Researchers followed almost six hundred children with ADHD who received medication, behavioral treatment, both, or no intervention (a placebo control). The children were followed for fourteen months to see how they responded. In the end, the combination of medications and therapy was the most effective. These children also ended up on lower total doses of medications than the medication-only group. Medications alone were helpful, though not as much (and at mostly higher doses). Behavioral treatment alone was no more helpful than the placebo treatment, statistically speaking. This seems to indicate that most children with ADHD should be involved in both therapy and medication management, though in a pinch, medications can help those with pure ADHD who have no sign of a mood disorder.

MOOD DISORDERS AND ADHD

Psychiatrists use the term *comorbidity* to describe two separate conditions or illnesses that frequently occur together in the same person. There is a high degree of comorbidity between ADHD and mood disorders—in some studies, as high as 75 percent.[5]

The diagnosis of both ADHD and mood disorders is difficult in young people, and the relationships between the two diagnoses are, at this point, still poorly understood. Many of the symptoms are similar (an inability to pay attention, impulsivity, irritability, disruptive behavior). The symptoms of ADHD and mood disorder can be differentiated in many youths, but some adolescents seem to have both disorders simultaneously. In one study of children already diagnosed with ADHD, 21 percent were also found to meet the diagnostic criteria for bipolar disorder by age 15. That is, they seemed to have both disorders. The children with ADHD who eventually developed bipolar symptoms had more severe symptoms and more disturbed behaviors. However, an even larger percentage of the children diagnosed with ADHD met the criteria for a diagnosis of major depression: 29 percent had major depression by age 11, and by age 15, 45 percent—nearly half—had been diagnosed with major depressive disorder.[6]

How do we understand the children whose ADHD seems to develop into a mood disorder? Did they really have ADHD symptoms in the first place, or do early-onset mood disorders mimic ADHD in their early stages? Are ADHD and early-onset mood disorder two separate illnesses that share similar symptom pictures but have different causes? Why? And what do we make of the extremely high comorbidity between ADHD and mood disorder? The answers to these questions are not yet known, and the nature of the connection between ADHD and pediatric mood disorders is unclear.

It has been suggested that the link may be genetic. In studies that look at the family members of children with ADHD, the families are found to have high rates of mood disorders. Children of parents with mood disorders have high rates of ADHD. The researchers studying the group of young people with ADHD described above investigated the prevalence of mood disorder in the family members of these children. They found that relatives of children with ADHD and bipolar disorder were five times more likely to have bipolar disorder than were family members of children with only ADHD. They also found high rates of major depression among relatives of the children with ADHD and bipolar disorder. The researchers speculate that ADHD with bipolar symptoms is a particular subtype of ADHD.[7] Or perhaps these are two separate illnesses that happen to co-occur frequently because the genes that cause them are close to one another on the chromosome and are thus usually inherited together (more on chromosomes in chapter 15). The only certainty about this mysterious connection is that much research in the area remains to be done.

The practical issues raised by comorbidity have to do with treatment. Specifically, if an adolescent has a combination of ADHD and a mood disorder, *both* will need to be treated. This makes treatment particularly difficult, as stimulant medications have been shown to worsen both the symptoms and the overall course of bipolar disorder (in adults, at least).

The combination of ADHD and bipolar disorder seems to be especially difficult to treat, and combinations of medications are often necessary. In a study of adolescents being treated for a manic episode with lithium, researchers compared treatment responses in adolescents with and without a history of childhood-onset ADHD. The adolescents with the ADHD history took significantly longer to get better during lithium treatment than did those with no history of ADHD symptoms. This appears to be further evidence that the combination of ADHD and bipolar disorder may be a subtype of illness and that it is especially challenging to treat.[8]

We know that stimulant medication can precipitate mania in patients with bipolar disorder. We know that early-onset depressions not uncommonly predict the development of mania and bipolar disorder later in adolescence. Therefore, the use of stimulant medications in depressed children must be approached with extreme caution. Many clinicians recommend avoiding stimulant medications completely in young persons with bipolar disorders.

OTHER MEDICATIONS

Although tricyclic antidepressant medications have not proved very helpful in the treatment of young people with depression, their efficacy in the treatment of ADHD is clearly proven. The newer antidepressant bupropion (Wellbutrin) has also been shown to be helpful. The problem here is the same as with stimulant medications: the possibility of precipitating mania in a predisposed adolescent.

Clonidine (Catapres, Kapvay) and guanfacine (Tenex, Intuniv), medications used to treat high blood pressure in adults, have proved helpful in ADHD. Whereas stimulant medications help with both inattention and impulsivity/hyperactivity, clonidine and guanfacine seem to be effective in reducing impulsivity/hyperactivity, though may not be as robust in treating inattention. These medications work primarily by lowering the excitement level throughout the nervous system. The human nervous system has two ways in which it can influence the body. The *sympathetic* nervous system tends to heighten awareness and excitement. It is one of the many systems responsible for the "fight or flight" response. The *parasympathetic* nervous system is primarily responsible for maintaining a calm state while the body is at rest. It is able to lower pulse, blood pressure, and breathing rate and induces a state of relaxation. These two systems are constantly in flux to maintain the body in the appropriate state for the situation. Clonidine and guanfacine seem to act by lowering the sympathetic system's ability to affect the body, effectively helping a hyperactive, impulsive individual feel more calm. As they have no stimulant effect at all, they can be useful in patients with comorbid ADHD and mood disorders. However, because they aren't all that helpful regarding pure inattention, they are rarely used in isolation and are often combined with other medications.

Recall that the most commonly prescribed antidepressants work by affecting serotonin, norepinephrine, and/or dopamine—three major chemical transmitters in the brain. The main classes are selective serotonin reuptake inhibitors (SSRIs, like Paxil and Prozac), the serotonin-norepinephrine reuptake inhibitors (SNRIs, like Effexor and Cymbalta), and dopamine-norepinephrine reuptake inhibitors (DNRIs, like Wellbutrin). In 2002, one pharmaceutical company began testing a pure norepinephrine reuptake inhibitor (NRI) for the treatment of depression. Although it seemed ineffective in treating depression, the researchers found that it was helpful in maintaining attention. Further investigations led the FDA to approve this medication, atomoxetine (Strattera), for the treatment of ADHD. It has some advantages over other treatments for this condition. Atomoxetine is not a stimulant, so the risk of it worsening a mood disorder is low. It is also not a controlled substance according to the FDA, as stimulants are, so adults with certain jobs (such as the military) are able to use it. Atomoxetine has some disadvantages too. Although it seems helpful for inattention, it has almost no effect on hyperactivity. It is more like an antidepressant than a stimulant in that it can take weeks to work. For persons who cannot take stimulants for one reason or another, however, atomoxetine has certainly carved out a niche for itself in the treatment of ADHD.

TREATMENT FOR YOUR CHILD

With all the complications delineated above, how is a parent to even begin understanding the complex treatment of a child or adolescent with a mood disorder and ADHD? How can these conditions even be told apart? As with all psychiatric illnesses, the first step is to find a qualified psychiatrist (ideally a child and adolescent psychiatrist) experienced in treating this combination of conditions. This doctor will be able to help determine which symptoms belong to which condition and develop a treatment plan unique to your child's situation. As we've said, many children need both some form of psychotherapy and medication. In cases of mild to moderate symptoms of depression and ADHD, some medications (an SNRI or a DNRI) may be able to treat both. Most persons with ADHD and a mood disorder, however, require more than one medicine to help them become the happiest, most stable, most functional people they can be. Finding the right combination can be something of a journey and is not really an endpoint so much as a continuing discussion, as both mood disorders and ADHD tend to change as the person grows and changes. That said, many highly successful people have both ADHD and a mood disorder, and the secret to their success is starting and staying in effective treatment.

Autism, Asperger's, and Related Disorders

W e've just spent some time discussing the interaction of mood disorders and another condition, ADHD. We demonstrated how the conditions can share some symptoms and may be confused for each other. Sometimes ADHD and mood disorders can be comorbid; that is, two conditions exist in the same patient simultaneously, creating unique challenges in treatment. Other conditions that can add complexity to mood disorders in adolescents are autism spectrum disorders (ASD).

Autism spectrum disorders are increasingly common. The cause of this rising prevalence is a topic of debate, even among experts. Some believe that environmental factors are making this condition more common in children. Increased screen time (video games, TV, and so on) has been suggested as a possible cause, as have food additives, wheat or lactose allergies, proximity to electrical wires (which emit subtle magnetic fields), paint additives, chemicals used in carpet and furniture manufacturing, detergents, pollution, certain infections, older paternal age, and others. One popular notion, that vaccines led to increased rates of autism, was later debunked as a scam perpetrated by competing vaccine manufacturers using falsified data. There are, however, certain genetic illnesses associated with autism, such as fragile X syndrome (so named because in people who have this syndrome, one arm of the X chromosome appears under a microscope to be thin and easily breakable).

Other experts believe that there is no real increase in the percentage of children with autism. Rather, they think pediatricians, psychiatrists, and other clinicians are paying more attention to this condition and recognizing it more and more frequently in young persons who have vague and poorly understood social difficulties. Regardless of which side of the debate you are on (and at this point, whether ASD is increasing is still a debate, with facts backing up both sides of the argument), more and more children are being diagnosed with this condition. Young persons with autism, just like all young persons, may be prone to depression and mood disorders. In this chapter, we do not try to give a complete discussion of autism, which is an incredibly complex condition. Rather, our goal here is to help parents, adolescents, and professionals better understand how a mood disorder might appear and be managed in children who, to an extent, already have some of the symptoms of depression and are by definition less able to describe their internal emotional state.

AUTISM: A HISTORY

As with so many psychiatric conditions, the history of autism is fraught with disbelief, lack of acceptance by the scientific community, misdiagnosis, and poor treatment. The term itself, *autism,* was first used by a German psychiatrist, Paul Eugene Bleuler. He was, unfortunately for the future of this disorder, also the first to describe the schizophrenic diagnoses, illnesses dealing primarily with psychosis. When Bleuler saw people who had schizophrenia who were more internally involved than externally engaged, who had retreated into themselves to the exclusion of the world around them, he labeled them autistic. The word *autism* is from the Greek word *autos*, meaning "self," with the suffix *-ismos*, which refers to a state of being. He coined the term around 1910. We now know that Bleuler was describing a particular cluster of *symptoms* without proper appreciation for fully describing the underlying *syndrome*. The term *autism* was used to characterize adults who had clear patterns of psychosis characteristic of schizophrenia as well as symptoms of internal preoccupation and internalization. When children were seen to have some of the same symptoms, even in the absence of any signs of psychosis, they were presumed to be suffering from some sort of infantile schizophrenia and were treated as such.

The first introduction of autism as a cluster of symptoms that might represent an independent condition came in the 1930s from two independent sources. The first was from Hans Asperger (for whom Asperger's syndrome was later named). An Austrian psychiatrist, Asperger used the term *autism* to describe children who showed "a lack of empathy, little ability to form friendships, one-sided conversations, intense absorption in a special interest, and clumsy movements."[1] He published a paper detailing four such cases in 1944. At about the same time, Leo Kanner, an American psychiatrist practicing at Johns Hopkins Hospital (and now widely regarded as the father of modern child psychiatry), acting independently, published a case series about eleven young persons characterized by "lacking affective contact with others; being fascinated with objects; having a desire for sameness; and being non-communicative in regard to language before 30 months of age."[2] Kanner suggested the now-defunct theory that this condition was produced by a combination of a biological predisposition and parents "lacking in genuine warmth." (We now know that parenting styles have nothing to do with the generation of autism, though parents and family members play a critical role in treatment.)

In fact, Asperger's and Kanner's descriptions seemed to diverge later in their careers. Whereas Kanner patients tended to be low functioning and have great difficulty getting on in life, some of Asperger's patients were quite successful. He described them as "little professors" (a term still used today) for their ability to pontificate wildly about their narrow focus of interest. The children Asperger described tended to be more eloquent and have more intact language than the children Kanner studied. Later in life, one of Asperger's patients became a fairly famous astrophysicist, one who went on to correct an error in Isaac Newton's original physics, an error he had noted as a child. Another of Asperger's patients was Elfriede Jelinek, an Austrian writer and Nobel laureate.

As America entered the 1950s and 1960s, a time when psychoanalytic theory held sway and most conditions were thought to be caused by life experience and internal conflicts, the idea that autistic children were the result of cold parenting was increasingly popular. The famous "refrigerator mother" theory of autism (and of schizophrenia—the two conditions were not yet fully separated) was made famous by Bruno Bettelheim in Chicago.

This theory lost influence as the science of psychiatry became more robust. Of siblings raised in the same household by the same parents, one child would have autism and another would not. Also, it was noted that children of parents who had mental illness were more likely to have autism than children whose parents did not, even if the children of parents who had mental illness were not raised by them. Finally, if two siblings were separated at birth and raised in different households and one developed autism, the other was significantly more likely to have autism than the general population. The biological side of this condition began to take hold as the causal factor, eventually eclipsing parenting styles entirely, though this took some time, until about the 1980s.

With the publication of the *DSM-III*, also in the 1980s, autism was firmly differentiated from schizophrenia, being classified as a developmental disorder rather than a mental illness. Developmental disorders are, almost by definition, biological and do not occur because of life experiences or psychological conflicts. As the century progressed, the late 1990s and early 2000s saw an increase in both the recognition and the prevalence of autism, estimated to affect 1 in 250 children (now thought to be a low estimate, but at the time a striking number).

It was at this time that other causes for autism, biological but not necessarily genetic, were explored. In 1998, a famous British medical journal, the *Lancet*, published a paper showing a link between the measles, mumps, and rubella (MMR) vaccine and an increased rate of autism in children. The author of the study, Dr. Andrew Wakefield, published a case series of twelve young people who purportedly developed symptoms of autism shortly after being vaccinated with the combined vaccine. His stance was that children should be vaccinated by three separate vaccines, and that something in either the manufacture of this combined product or the interaction of the strains themselves was to blame. This stance was problematic because the vaccine was not available as individual strains, only as the combined product.

It was later revealed that Dr. Wakefield had significant motivation to publish his (now recognized as) fraudulent paper. First, he had received more than £400,000 from lawyers involved in unrelated class action lawsuits against the vaccine manufacturer, seeking to widen their class action population and build evidence against this company. Second, Wakefield had obtained patents to manufacture his own vaccines (not surprisingly, the three separate viral strains as individual shots), which he planned to sell. The paper was finally retracted from the *Lancet*, with editorials in this journal and others citing it as "containing manipulated evidence," "fraudulent," and "the most damaging medical hoax of the last 100 years."[3]

The idea that autism is caused by external environmental influences is still a popular one. Although many of these ideas do not have firm scientific evidence, that does not make them incorrect. The human body is incomprehensibly complex, the human mind more so, and we are in all likelihood simply too scientifically naive to find definitive answers to these questions. Today, autism is seen as even more prevalent—as many as one in sixty-eight children are diagnosed with an autism spectrum disorder, with boys experiencing the condition at five times the rate of girls.

SYMPTOMS OF AUTISM

The symptoms of autism are classically divided into three main domains of function. According to the *DSM*, for the diagnosis of autism, the child must experience a failure to meet milestones in these domains before the age of 3. In about 20 percent of cases, a child who was presumably developing normally will regress, losing milestones. If this happens after age 3, however, something else is likely at play.

The first domain, and usually the most obvious to parents, is social interaction. Children who have autism simply do not bond with their parents in typical ways. These children are disinterested in their mother's and father's voices. Although they may seek out their parents to have their needs met (to be fed, for example), they couldn't care less about the human interaction that is typically such an integral part of the experience. Children who have autism fail to make consistent eye contact and do not respond to their parent's smiling face. When crying and upset, they neither seek out nor respond to parental attempts at caring and comfort. As they age, they do not play *with* other children so much as they play *beside* them. (Called *parallel play*, this is normal in younger children but tends to stop by about age 4, when typically developing children play with each other.) When children with autism do play with others, they typically use people as tools to their own ends, so that other children find them bossy and demanding. In conversation they do not so much speak *with* other people as *at* them, delivering mini-lectures on topics of interest. They frequently miss the subtle signals that their companion would like to move on to another topic or another person, and stay with the topic incessantly, refusing to cease the monologue. Children with autism rarely have friends but, unlike painfully shy children who also tend to stay alone, they have no desire for them. This pattern persists through the rest of their lives. To a greater or lesser extent, they seem to have no need of other people, aside from a certain intellectual appreciation. (We once had a patient tell us that he was engaged to be married simply because that is what people seemed to expect of him, and yes, it would probably be helpful to have someone split the responsibilities of keeping up a home.)

The second domain, the one usually most evident to the rest of the world, is language. To be diagnosed with autism, again according to the *DSM*, children must have a delay in the development of the spoken word. Some children with autism never develop the power of speech. Those who do frequently repeat what they hear, sometimes repetitively, but cannot process and internalize language in the usual way, to use it to communicate with others. Being able to repeat a favorite movie, word for word, is the kind of ability often seen as a sign of early brilliance in young children. But if they are merely repeating without internalizing the meaning of these words, this may in fact be a sign of autism. This tendency for children to repeat verbatim what they hear from others, called *echolalia*, was one of the first autistic symptoms identified by Kanner. As children with autism age, they are unable to play with language, to understand the subtleties of meaning that allow for puns, jokes, and sarcasm. This makes them the object of much teasing by their peers in school, though unusually, they don't seem to mind much (because they do not understand that they are being teased). A few people with autism, on the other hand, became fascinated by how the intonation of a word could change its entire meaning and went on to become authors, intellectually researching but never truly understanding the expressiveness of language.

The third area of function is that of fixed, repetitive interests and behaviors. Children with autism find one, usually narrow, area of focus and stick to it relentlessly. An autistic child interested in dinosaurs can out-lecture a professional paleontologist. In play, children with autism tend to be unimaginative and concrete. For example, they will not act out scenes or play with a dollhouse but might merely move the toy doll's arm up and down repetitively. They often become focused on part of a toy rather than on the whole object (repetitively spinning the wheel of a car instead of pretending to drive it, for example). Many insist on sameness and routine, playing the same game over and over again. They will insist that parents replay the same movie, or scene from a movie, endlessly. Any disruption in routine or sameness (rearranging furniture, or taking a different route to school) can result in an emotional explosion. In many children with autism, this repetitive nature also comes out in body movements, such as wringing or flapping their hands.

Some individuals on the autism spectrum turn their fixed interest into successful careers, such as the patient of Asperger who became a renowned astrophysicist. For others, the single-minded focus proves more problematic, as they avoid necessary activities to pay full attention to their particular focus, becoming upset, even enraged, when removed from it.

There are other, more subtle, signs of autism that are not part of the official diagnostic parameters in the *DSM*. Many children with autism appear to have the symptoms of ADHD, such as difficulty maintaining attention for a long period, or conversely, difficulty breaking attention from interesting objects. They may appear impulsive and have difficulty sitting still. They are frequently forgetful and cannot follow complex instructions. These shared symptoms were so common, in fact, that according to the *DSM-IV*, it was not possible to diagnose ADHD in a child with autism, because all the symptoms of ADHD were inherent in the autism diagnosis. This has changed in the *DSM-5*, because ADHD symptoms can be an important and treatable aspect of autism, and ADHD requires a diagnosis to justify treatment with the correct medications.

Many children with autism have wild and extreme temper tantrums and are poorly able to self-soothe when upset, or to accept soothing from others. Most if not all have sensory eccentricities. Broadly speaking, sensory experts divide sensory issues into *sensory seeking* or *sensory avoidant* categories, though this is usually a gross oversimplification, because many children have aspects of both. Some children will insist on eating only white foods, for example, or on eating strange and exotic foods for the textural differences. Many children with autism cannot stand the tags on the backs of T-shirts, almost as if they are painful. They may run screaming from the sound of the toilet flushing, or throw open the door to better hear an ambulance siren. Some cannot stand to be swaddled or held; for others, it seems to be the only thing that will help them calm down. Many children who are more sensory seeking use behaviors their parents see as harmful to help them regain a calm state, such as scratching themselves or banging their heads against a wall.

AUTISM VERSUS ASPERGER'S SYNDROME: THE SPECTRUM OF AUTISM

Many changes have occurred to the diagnosis of autism in the last decade. Some of the biggest were in how experts view the illness itself and how it is categorized in the *DSM*. The *DSM-IV* categorized autism as one of five disorders under the umbrella of pervasive developmental disorders (PDDs). We have discussed how mood disorders tend to appear as episodic illnesses—at times present, and at other times in remission—and how treatment with medications can make the illness entirely (or mostly) inactive. The pervasive developmental disorders are different. They are, as their name describes, *pervasive*, meaning that they are not limited to a single area of the person's functioning, such as mood or ability to pay attention. The symptoms seen in autism affect socialization, communication, and range of interests—areas that are likely to affect a person's entire sphere of life. Furthermore, PDDs are *developmental*. These disorders interfere with a child's development and are apparent early in life. This also contrasts with mood disorders, which are usually seen later, such as in adolescence, after a normal period of development.

One of the pervasive developmental disorders, Rett syndrome, has known genetic causes, and another, childhood disintegrative disorder, is controversial as to whether it exists at all. A third PDD category is "pervasive developmental disorder not otherwise specified" (PDD NOS). PDD NOS is, like mood disorder NOS, a nonspecific entity meant to capture children and adults who seem to have some features of a PDD but who do not fit cleanly into one category or another. Autism and Asperger's disorder are the remaining specific diagnoses of the five under the PDD umbrella in the *DSM-IV*. What is the difference between autism and Asperger's disorder?

The answer can be seen in the contrast between the research of Kanner and that of Asperger. Whereas Kanner worked with a group of young children who exhibited language delay (or absence), intellectual disability, and low function, Asperger had a somewhat different cohort of patients. We have already described how one revised the face of modern physics and another won a Nobel Prize. This subset of patients capture what later became known as, fittingly, Asperger's disorder. Among children, the most striking difference between autism and Asperger's is that the second group has no formal language delay (though their internalization and understanding of language still suffers in the understanding of pragmatics). People who have Asperger's disorder tend to have a normal or slightly above average IQ. Some have what are known as *splinter skills*. Anyone who has seen the movie *Rain Man* is familiar with this phenomenon. Although these persons are limited in many other ways, some of them excel in a single, narrow form of functioning. From memorizing the phone book to correcting classic theorems of Newton, splinter skills are more classically a feature of Asperger's disorder. Children who have Asperger's tend to be higher functioning than those who have autism. Though socially awkward, children with Asperger's disorder survive and sometimes excel in school. They have restricted interests, but they are often able to turn this restriction into a strength rather than a weakness. They usually exhibit a lack of social awareness or need for interaction similar to people with autism, and many people with Asperger's have sensory sensitivities and experience emotional explosiveness when routines are altered.

We've spent some time describing and delineating the different types of pervasive developmental disorders. Now we will share a secret—experts in PDDs know that the formal name of the diagnosis really doesn't matter much. Many psychiatrists have treated patients who fit every criterion for Asperger's disorder but must receive the diagnosis of autism because of a very small language delay. This is true in reverse as well—a severely "autistic" child whose symptoms were not diagnosed before the age of 3 cannot ever receive a diagnosis of autism and instead must be categorized as PDD NOS. The *DSM*, as we've said, is a research guide that has expanded to clinical circles, but it is frankly not all that useful when trying to determine the syndrome underlying a particular collection of symptoms. This was recognized by the *DSM-5* committee, and they did away with all these various categorizations and now label Asperger's syndrome, autism, and related conditions under autism spectrum disorder (ASD).

This decision was, as could be expected, controversial. Many people diagnosed with Asperger's disorder did not want to be lumped with every other form of autism, and some experts felt that it was a giant step backward in our treatment of this condition. As such, the committee instead added modifiers. So take for example a young man who in the past received the diagnosis of Asperger's disorder. Under the *DSM-5,* depending on his symptoms, this young man will be diagnosed with "autism spectrum disorder, without accompanying intellectual impairment, without accompanying language impairment, mild severity." Other modifiers include "associated with a known medical or genetic cause" and "associated with another neurodevelopmental, mental, or behavioral disorder"—which brings us to our next topic.

AUTISM AND MOOD DISORDERS

How does autism, regardless of its origin, interact with mood disorders? We've discussed the symptoms of autism: lack of interest in socialization and possibly social withdrawal; a minimal outward expression of emotionality; sleep problems; outward emotional instability, such as crying spells for seemingly no reason; finicky appetites and preferences; lack of interest in pursuits outside of a restricted interest; seeming inability to focus; and emotional reactivity and temper tantrums, which may appear as irritability. Imagine you are a psychiatrist sitting in your office. Now, imagine parents describing these symptoms in their child. You can imagine how easy it would be to think that this person might be depressed. And then, upon interviewing the child, you realize that his affect is constricted due to disinterest, not sadness. Although he may not be paying attention to you, the interviewer, he is engrossed in spinning the wheel of a toy truck or lining up his crayons in rainbow color order. He is animated while performing these tasks, though he rarely answers your questions. When he does speak, it is usually to repeat what you or his parents have said.

This boy is not depressed, he is autistic. It is uncommon, though not unheard of, to confuse the two. What is more difficult is determining if a young person already diagnosed with a pervasive developmental disorder becomes depressed. Almost by definition, children who have autism have difficulty understanding and describing their emotional world. They do not understand feelings and emotions in others and therefore have little reference point for themselves. Extensive questioning is likely to result in little meaningful information on internal symptoms. What makes this problem even more pressing is that autistic children are more likely, not less, to experience depression than the general population. According to studies, up to 24 percent of children and, surprisingly, over 50 percent of adults with autism spectrum disorders have experienced a major depressive episode.[4] Rates of depression increase along with IQ, placing those children with so-called high-functioning autism or Asperger's disorder at greater risk.[5]

There are debates on how to best approach diagnosing depression and mood disorders in this group of individuals. Many psychologists and other mental health professionals use tools to help with diagnoses in all their patients. These usually take the form of self-reports, handouts that parents and children fill out that are then "scored" by the provider. As we discuss in chapter 16, although psychological tests can be helpful, the best way to get a clear diagnosis is through a clinical interview with a trained professional experienced with the relevant population. We advise parents to be wary of providers who rely more on such reports than on face-to-face time, or who see these tools as definitive diagnostic markers (which they certainly are not). Some studies show that these tools are even less helpful when used in an autistic population, making diagnosis of a mood disorder even more troublesome.

Recall that autism is a pervasive developmental disorder. For the most part, the symptoms a child has are fairly consistent and stable. Mood disorders, on the other hand, are cyclical. The average length of a major depressive episode (untreated) is a little over seven months. When someone becomes depressed, her mood and behavior change. In adolescents, this frequently takes the form of irritability. When looking for depression in children with ASD, we look for a relatively sudden change in their behavior and mannerisms. For example, children with autism may be particularly interested in and attached to inanimate objects. A piece of string, for example, was one of our patient's constant companions. If they lose interest in this essential component of their life, we become concerned. If their emotional outbursts increase, or last longer, we begin to consider depression. In persons who can poorly describe their internal emotional experience, their external actions, and more specifically a change in their behavior patterns, signal times of distress.

APPROACHES TO TREATMENT OF THE CHILD WHO HAS AUTISM

The mainstay of treatment for autism is psychotherapeutic behavior modification. For the most part, medications are not effective in treating autism. Pharmacology can be helpful for individual symptoms, but addressing the core syndrome, the autism itself, is at this point an unknown territory. Various studies are constantly ongoing, but as of yet, there is no hard evidence that we can treat autism as we can mood disorders. There is evidence for treatments with oxytocin, the so-called love hormone, but its use is still preliminary and limited to research studies.

Even symptomatic treatments are difficult at best. Many children with autism spectrum disorders are highly ritual and routine based. If their routine changes (if they must sit in a different seat at school, for example, or if their favorite pencil is missing from their backpack), they can become almost unaccountably enraged. This feature is similar to some children with severe anxiety or obsessive-compulsive disorder, so enterprising psychiatrists began prescribing SSRI medications to try to address this anxiety. Disappointingly, a Cochrane review of nine studies found "no evidence of effect of SSRIs in children with autism spectrum disorders."[6] It seems, then, that as with so many other things, trying to work backwards from a particular symptom to the cause was ineffective. Even though these children had symptoms similar to the symptoms of anxious children, the syndrome was entirely different and not helped by the SSRI.

For children who seem to have depression and autism spectrum disorders, though, SSRIs do seem to be helpful. This is because the medicine is doing what it was designed to do: address the depression, not the symptoms of autism. In fact, from a medication standpoint, the treatment of depression does not look all that different whether the child has autism or not. We do know that children with autism are more sensitive to medication side effects, so we may start at a lower dose, but the choice of medication is not likely to be all that different. If on the other hand, the adolescent seems to have symptoms of bipolar disorder, we may make a different choice, and here we are about to contradict ourselves. In chapter 8 we spent some time discussing why antipsychotic medications are not a good first choice for mood stabilization in young people, and now we are about to describe why they may be our first choice for mood stabilization in children who have autism.

We do have some treatments that seem effective, and that are approved by the FDA, for treating a particularly troubling aspect of the autistic syndrome: aggression. When children with autism spectrum disorders become irritated, they frequently lash out, not appreciating the results of their actions. We once treated a patient whose method of getting his mother's attention was to run over and bite her arm (not because he wanted attention for attention's sake, but just because he needed something, like the phone from her purse, that only she could provide). He did not appreciate that this hurt his mother, put her at risk for infection, and so on. He had merely at some point realized that biting his mother interrupted her from whatever activity she was engaged in and forced her attention to him. Two medicines are currently approved for aggression in children with autism, both atypical antipsychotics: Risperdal (risperidone) and Abilify (aripiprazole). In children with autism, these medications are effective in reducing this type of aggression as well as the emotional outbursts that children have when frustrated. When children with autism spectrum disorders become uncomfortable, they are far more likely to act out aggressively than children who do not have autism. So, children in the midst of a mood disorder can quickly become violent—again, not with the specific intent of breaking objects or hurting people, but more out of simply not recognizing the consequences of their actions. A medication that addresses both problems (the mood disorder and the consequent aggression) would then be ideal, and these antipsychotics seem to fit this niche.

One aspect of treatment that is critical but frequently ignored is that of the parent. Multiple studies have shown that parents of children with pervasive developmental disorders have higher degrees of feeling sad, overwhelmed, and isolated than parents whose children do not have such a disorder.[7] Caring for a child with an autism spectrum disorder is a daunting task, and any treatment approach needs to take you, the parent, into consideration. Fortunately, there are many resources available for helping families, as we cover in the resources section at the back of the book. These include help groups, online communities, and practical resources such as school advocates and respite care for autistic youth. Remember what they tell you on the airline—put your own oxygen mask on first, before helping those around you. The same goes for parenting—you need to be sure to take care of yourself and your needs to be able to address your child's.

Alcohol and Drug Abuse

I n the last third of the twentieth century, young Americans achieved extraordinary levels of illicit drug use, either by historic comparisons in this country or by international comparisons with other countries.[1] As terrible as this assessment is for the health of American youth, the truth is that it has even more troubling implications for adolescents with serious depression and other mood disorders. We know from studies of adults that the combination of substance abuse and mood disorders is especially deadly: persons who have mood disorders and who also abuse alcohol or drugs have a greatly increased risk of completed suicide. Severe depression complicated by alcoholism or drug abuse has been found to be one of the most frequent diagnostic pictures in study after study on the psychiatric diagnoses of suicide victims. In a 1993 study, clinicians reviewed the medical records and interviewed the relatives of almost fourteen hundred adults who had died by suicide, in an attempt to make psychiatric diagnoses of the suicide victims. This study, which found that most of the suicide victims had suffered from a mood disorder, also found that *nearly half* (48 percent) had suffered from alcoholism or drug abuse.[2]

ADOLESCENT SUBSTANCE ABUSE

Surveys indicate that among adolescents, the number who try alcohol or drugs (substance *use*) is much higher than the number who use these substances regularly, which in turn is higher than the number who develop serious dependence and addiction problems. There are two important progressions that adolescents may move along as they develop substance-use problems. The first involves how often and how seriously they use, and the other involves which particular drugs they use.

The *stages of use* of adolescent drug use and abuse illustrate how the abused substance becomes a bigger and bigger part of the adolescent's mental life:

1. Curiosity (or pre-abuse) stage
   Does not use: opportunity for prevention
2. Experimentation stage
   Accepts alcohol or drugs from others
   May try drugs for fun and peer acceptance
   Does not usually show behavioral changes
3. Drug-seeking stage
   Seeks out a steadier supply of abused substance (either own supply
      or a peer group with easy access to substances)
   Needs more drugs to achieve the same feeling (tolerance)
   Uses more drugs, and more often, than planned
   Uses drugs more regularly to get high and to escape reality
4. Drug-preoccupation stage
   Has a significant loss of control over drug use
   Has less regard for the consequences of drug use
   Develops legal and relationship problems
5. Addiction
   Finds drugs necessary to feel *normal*
   Uses drugs daily, or even several times daily

As you will see later in the chapter, several factors determine how far along this continuum, and how quickly, an adolescent will progress. We'll jump the gun a little and tell you that depressed adolescents progress farther and faster than nondepressed adolescents.

The other type of progression is according to *substance type*, reflecting the use of increasingly "hard" drugs with increasingly severe health and legal consequences:

1. Drugs legal for adults
   Tobacco
   Alcohol
   Marijuana (in some states, under certain circumstances)
2. Less addictive illegal drugs
   Marijuana (in states where it is still illegal)
   Stimulants (ecstasy, methamphetamines, and "club drugs")
3. More addictive drugs
   Cocaine
   Narcotics

There is no doubt that tobacco and alcohol are indeed "gateway" drugs that often precede the use of illicit and increasingly dangerous substances. A glance at the results of various surveys of adolescent drug use verifies the alarming progression some adolescents make along this continuum: one review of the subject noted that adolescent cigarette smokers were 16 times more likely to use alcohol and 11.4 times more likely to use illegal drugs than nonsmoking peers. Adolescents who used alcohol were 7.5 times more likely to use marijuana and 50 times more likely to experiment with cocaine than nondrinkers. Adolescents who smoked marijuana regularly were 104 times more likely to use cocaine.[3] The farther the adolescent moves along this continuum, the farther she is likely to go. It becomes apparent that even cigarette smoking puts some young people at the beginning of a rapid trajectory of drug use that can end in physical addiction to extremely dangerous substances.

Social factors such as patterns of use among peers and the availability of particular drugs in a particular community will affect a youth's entry into and movement through this continuum. Age factors are also relevant: "huffing," the inhalation of glue and paint fumes, for example, tends to be more of a problem in younger adolescents. It is important not to regard *legal* substances as necessarily of low risk: more people die each year of tobacco-related illnesses than of any other substance-related illness. Alcohol-related illnesses and tobacco-related deaths far outnumber those due to any illegal drug. Nevertheless, increasing social impairment, legal consequences such as arrest and incarceration, and increasingly severe medical problems usually go hand in hand with the use of the "hard" drugs.

Adolescent drug abuse is a complex issue. A survey of all the substances that can be abused and the ramifications of their use for adolescents with mood disorders would require its own book. Therefore, in the following sections we cover only a few substances likely to be abused, in their order of prevalence in adolescents: (1) alcohol, because it is the most widely abused substance, except for tobacco; (2) marijuana, because it is the most widely abused *illegal* substance and can now in some areas be obtained legally; and (3) MDMA, or "ecstasy," because its rate of use by adolescents is extensive and because it has an undeserved reputation of being a "safe" high. In addition, we will discuss another substance with an alarming recent increase in use and abuse by young people: the ever-expanding category of substances collectively known as methamphetamines.

ALCOHOL ABUSE

Many medical definitions of alcoholism have been proposed over the years, and none of them involves the popular notions of what defines alcoholism: such behaviors as drinking alone or drinking before noon. Several decades of public education seem to have made most people aware that only a minority of persons with alcohol problems wind up as bleary-eyed panhandlers on downtown streets and that an alcoholic might well be able to hold down a job, pay taxes, and mow the lawn every Saturday morning. Fewer people realize, however, that an alcoholic can be someone who goes to high school and manages to maintain passing grades. As a groundbreaking article for pediatricians states, "Teenagers can and do become alcoholics."[4]

The National Council on Alcoholism and Drug Dependencies includes several factors in its definition of alcoholism: *impaired control over drinking, preoccupation with alcohol use, continued drinking in spite of adverse consequences*, and *denial*. This definition can just as easily be applied to any kind of substance abuse.

All definitions of problem drinking include a person's *loss of control* over drinking, perhaps the most important part of the definition. A teenager who drinks when alcohol is available even though he had made the decision not to is showing a loss of control over drinking. So is a young alcoholic who goes to a party intending to have one or two beers and ends up having seven or eight.

Preoccupation with alcohol means spending more and more time thinking about alcohol, about where and how to get it and how to drink without getting caught. Having availability of alcohol in mind when deciding which friends to hang out with and which parties to go to is a part of this preoccupation. Soon, alcohol is not just a part of social activities but rather the axis around which everything else revolves.

The alcoholic adolescent *continues to drink despite adverse consequences*, as alcohol begins to replace everything else as the most important thing in life and becomes the center of his world. No price is too high to pay to use it. Parental disapproval and punishment, falling grades, loss of friendships or privileges, even legal problems will not deter the alcoholic from his pursuit of alcohol.

Another important aspect of any definition of alcohol abuse (or any drug abuse) is alcoholics' *denial* of the seriousness of their problem with alcohol. The word *denial*, when used as a psychological term, means more than just a refutation or saying no. Rather, it is one of the many psychological *defense mechanisms* we all use to manage psychological conflicts and anxiety. Sigmund Freud originated the concept of defense mechanisms, and his daughter, the child therapist Anna Freud, elaborated on his ideas about them. Sigmund Freud believed that a part of the mind he called the *ego* is constantly trying to balance conflicting demands that impinge on it from within and without each individual. He called the ego's attempts to manage these conflicts *defense mechanisms* (or, more properly, *ego defense mechanisms*). Denial, formulated as an immature way to manage psychological conflict, works by simply rejecting the very existence of one "side" of the conflict. The alcoholic who wants desperately to continue drinking and does not want to think of himself as a problem drinker (and thus have to *stop* drinking) deals with these opposing sets of desires by telling himself and everyone else that he does *not* have a drinking problem. It's important to emphasize that someone in denial truly *believes* that the thing he is denying is really *not true*. The alcoholic in denial *believes* that he does *not* have a drinking problem. When the teenage alcoholic says, "I can stop anytime I want to" or "I don't drink any more than my friends do," he is not simply making excuses for continuing with a behavior he knows is a problem. Rather, the problem drinker truly believes the things he tells others about his drinking.

Although alcohol is physically addicting, and the withdrawal symptoms of abrupt cessation of heavy alcohol use are potentially fatal, a person can certainly have a drinking problem and not be *physically* addicted. Because adolescents do not have the degree of access to alcohol that adults do, true physical addiction to alcohol is less common in this age range. An important signal of physical addiction is a need to drink daily to prevent feeling "nervous" or "shaky." Persons with severe alcohol addiction also experience blackouts, episodes of memory loss that occur after a bout of heavy drinking. Blackouts may range from not remembering everything that happened at a party where the teenager became intoxicated to not remembering going to the party at all.

A person with a mood disorder is more prone to drinking than a person without a mood disorder. Individuals who have mood disorders can experience a brief reprieve from their depression in the mild euphoria induced by alcohol. Unfortunately, this experience sets them up for more problems in the future. Alcohol is in fact a depressant and can precipitate and maintain depressive episodes over the long term. In fact, some practitioners will not start an antidepressant on a person who is actively drinking because as many as one-third of those with depression who stop drinking will have a spontaneous remission of their low mood, because their depression was a pure psychological and biological consequence of their alcohol use.

MARIJUANA ABUSE

For the quarter century or so that the National Institute on Drug Abuse has been surveying drug abuse among young people in the United States, marijuana has been the most widely used illicit drug. In 2000, 89 percent of high school seniors reported that they thought they could get marijuana either "very easily" or "fairly easily." More than 75 percent of tenth-grade students and nearly 50 percent of eighth-graders reported the same thing. Obtaining marijuana has become even easier given the medical uses of marijuana for adults in certain states and the recent legal recreational use in others.

For many years, it was commonly believed that no one became physically addicted to marijuana and that it was therefore a comparatively "safe" drug to get high on. This is because cannabinoids, the active components of marijuana, are absorbed into the fat tissues during use and are slowly released when marijuana use stops, making for a sort of tapering off that often prevents withdrawal symptoms. Studies have demonstrated, however, that chronic marijuana users develop all the signs and symptoms of physical addiction. The main criteria for addiction are the development of *tolerance* to the effects of the drug and *withdrawal symptoms* when the drug use stops. In a study in which volunteers were given the same measured doses of cannabinoids daily for four weeks, the volunteers reported that the marijuana seemed to become "weaker" and that their high was becoming progressively less intense, demonstrating their development of tolerance to the drug. A number of these volunteers became irritable and hostile and developed sleep problems after the drug was stopped.[5] Other studies have confirmed that persons who use marijuana regularly and then stop completely can develop anxiety and panic, depressed mood, irritability, loss of appetite, insomnia, and physical symptoms such as changes in heart rate and blood pressure, sweating, and diarrhea.

Because these effects develop several days after stopping the drug, users can convince themselves that they are only using the drug to "self-medicate" preexisting anxiety or depressive symptoms. A regular marijuana user might say she uses it to "calm her nerves," when in fact the use is to ward off the development of withdrawal symptoms.

Marijuana abusers have the same problems with loss of control as do alcoholics, becoming increasingly preoccupied with the drug and continuing to use it despite adverse consequences. A study at the University of Colorado surveyed more than two hundred adolescents who had been admitted to a substance-abuse facility because of problems with alcohol and other drugs. This is definitely a skewed population, but nevertheless, the researchers had no trouble demonstrating the full-blown marijuana dependence syndrome: 97 percent of these adolescents had continued to use after realizing marijuana caused problems for them, and 85 percent reported that it interfered with home and school life or that they had been high in a situation where it was dangerous, such as while driving. Smaller but still significant numbers reported that they had given up other activities to get or to use marijuana and that they spent a great deal of their time getting, using, or getting over the effects of cannabis. Two-thirds of these youths reported withdrawal symptoms, and a quarter said they had used it before entering treatment in order to stop having withdrawal symptoms.[6]

There's little doubt that for these young people, marijuana was a powerful and addicting drug whose grip on them had become unbreakable. As with alcohol, some individuals appear to use marijuana "socially" and maintain control over their use, but many do not. We examine the factors that seem to help predict these differences a little later. Clearly, however, marijuana's reputation as a benign drug is undeserved.

We are fortunate authors to have colleagues willing to advise us on our writing. One such person, residing in a state in which marijuana is legal for medical purposes, believed the above discussion to be "old fashioned" and "not up to date with the current literature," to be "condemning marijuana and deriding its potential medical uses." To be perfectly clear, we are not here to weigh in on the debate as to whether marijuana is useful in medical settings or safe for recreational use. There are many drugs that have important medical or social uses, but whose inappropriate use is devastating to some individuals. Alcohol, for example, is perfectly legal for persons of a certain age. A class of medications called benzodiazepines (Valium, Xanax) work very much like alcohol and are used medically for a multitude of conditions. Pain-killing narcotics, which we discuss later, are used every day in hospitals across the country for lifesaving purposes. There is no contradiction in our minds between saying that a substance may have rational medical and even recreational use, and simultaneously saying that certain persons can develop an addiction to these same substances that harms their lives and their futures. We like to clearly point out that certain persons, especially those with a preexisting mood disorder, may be at more risk of developing addiction and need more help to break it once it has developed. Similarly, overuse of any of these substances (marijuana included) can replicate many of the symptoms of a biological mood disorder and be problematic in itself. Add to these facts the research findings showing that serious damage to the developing brains of adolescents can be caused by alcohol and marijuana and it becomes clear that the use of these substances is extremely risky for some individuals, especially if they are of a certain age.

Separate from marijuana, and pre-dating much of its legalization for medical purposes, a new crop of substances started to be seen in the United States. These were the "synthetic marijuanas," and they went by names such as spice and salvia. Unlike marijuana, these substances were being legally sold to anyone who asked for them in certain stores. People using these substances argued that they were legal and therefore must be safer than true marijuana. This argument is fundamentally flawed because of the nature of how substances gain legal or illegal status. In fact, both spice and salvia are significantly more potent than most naturally occurring marijuana. Nonmedical substances (those that do not have to go through the FDA) are "innocent until proven guilty"—that is, they are legal until they are made illegal. In essence, chemists took the cannabinoids, the active ingredients in marijuana, and chemically altered them just enough for them to be outside the definition of marijuana according to the law (thus producing a legal substance), then sold them on the street. The advent of synthetic marijuana use has been particularly problematic for the psychiatric communities, as these substances seem to be uniquely proficient at causing psychotic episodes in their users that can last for as long as the substance is in the body (which, since they are fat soluble, can be weeks). Legal status aside, we strongly encourage avoidance of all such substances, particularly in persons who may already have a preexisting psychiatric illness, which includes mood disorders.

AMPHETAMINES (CRYSTAL METH, ECSTASY, AND "CLUB DRUGS")

Amphetamines include a group of compounds (of which methamphetamine is the most abused) that are potent stimulants of the central nervous system. "Speed," "crystal meth," "ice," and "bath salts" are street names for these pharmaceuticals. They make the user feel alert, energetic, and often elated. The user experiences increased initiative, motivation, and self-confidence; enhanced concentration; and often an increase in activities and productiveness without a need for sleep. Because both physical and mental performance are enhanced, these drugs are prone to be abused by athletes, students cramming for exams, long-distance drivers, and others who desire to artificially boost their alertness and performance. The effects are brief, however, and users often experience depression and fatigue after only a few hours of amphetamine use, which may require several days of recuperation. Longer-term use or binges of heavy use over several days usually cause a crash into more severe depression, with low mood, fatigue and listlessness, and loss of interest and pleasure in activities—the gamut of symptoms of a depressive illness. Changes in appetite also occur, as well as vivid, unpleasant dreams and other sleep disturbances that can take weeks to subside completely.

The parent compound, amphetamine, is one of the stimulant medications used to treat ADHD. Diversion of these drugs from legitimate use is a source of some of the amphetamines used illicitly, but they are easily manufactured in basement laboratories from ephedrine, a related compound found in over-the-counter cold and allergy preparations, along with other fairly easily obtained chemical ingredients.

For a time in the late 1990s, a group of amphetamine derivatives started to eclipse the parent compounds in popularity, especially among young people. These substances are sometimes collectively referred to as "club drugs," or "designer drugs," and of them "ecstasy" is the most popular. The annual survey of adolescent drug use conducted by the National Institute on Drug Abuse noted a marked increase in the use of ecstasy in the late 1990s. Ecstasy is the compound MDMA (an abbreviation of its chemical name, 3, 4-methylenedioxy-methamphetamine), and a related compound is MDA (3, 4-methylenedioxy-amphetamine). Although both are illegal now, these drugs were first synthesized in the 1910s by pharmaceutical companies as possible appetite suppressants. No therapeutic use for the compounds was ever discovered, and there was little interest in them until the 1970s, when MDA (called the "love drug" for a time) began to be illegally manufactured and widely abused, prompting the Federal Drug Enforcement Administration to declare MDA and MDMA illegal substances. Underground laboratories worked to make more powerful variations of these compounds, and in the process they produced compounds that were not covered under laws against the selling, distribution, and possession of illegal substances (hence the term *designer* drugs). By 2000, nearly two hundred of these drugs had been synthesized.[7] A pill that is called "ecstasy" may, in fact, be any one of these compounds.

Although MDMA is chemically derived from amphetamine, the molecule has structural similarities to mescaline and is often classified, like LSD, as a hallucinogen. Unlike LSD, MDMA does not usually cause hallucinations, but as with other drugs in this group, users report feeling that their emotions are deeper and more meaningful and that they achieve profound self-understanding and develop new perspectives and insights about themselves and their relationships. Intense sexual arousal is often noted as well (the reason, perhaps, why MDA was called the "love drug"). The amphetamine-like euphoria and confidence the drug produces makes these experiences all the more intense and powerful. When abused, the adverse psychological effects are, as might be expected, a combination of those reported to occur with amphetamines and hallucinogens: psychotic episodes, panic, and depression.

An individual's decision to use a particular drug is determined by a balance between the perceived benefits and the perceived risks of using the drug. (This is more the case prior to the development of dependence, after which cravings take on a life of their own, and decision making is impaired.) If the perceived benefits (such as the quality of the "high" and the other pleasurable effects the drug induces) outweigh the perceived risks (adverse physical and psychological reactions; the legal consequences of drug possession or distribution), the user will decide to use. The National Institute on Drug Abuse's annual survey of patterns of drug abuse among adolescents has noted that the abuse of new drugs spreads very quickly, because it takes only a few rumors and testimonials about the "benefits" to generate interest and willingness to experiment. It usually takes much longer for evidence of serious adverse effects to accumulate and even longer for this news to be disseminated. For an illustration of this pattern, one has only to think of the decade or so during which cocaine was touted as a harmless "party drug" and widely considered nonaddictive. MDMA and its derivatives were in this "grace period" as the twenty-first century began, unfortunately abetted by uncritical media (as the spread of misinformation about cocaine was abetted). "Experiencing Ecstasy," an article published in January 2001 in the Sunday *New York Times*, reads in places like an enthusiastic endorsement of the drug and mentions little of the rapidly accumulating evidence on the dangers of MDMA.[8] Increasingly seen in the psychiatric and toxicological literature are reports of several sudden deaths in users, psychotic episodes, prolonged depressions, memory impairment, and thinking problems.

It seems that MDMA exerts its effects by potently altering the levels of serotonin in the brain. You might remember from chapter 6 that one of the groups of antidepressant medications has the effect of *boosting* serotonin levels in the brain. Serotonin seems to play a significant role in mood regulation, acting as a modulator for various brain circuits. MDMA (as well as other substances that cause a high) seems to set off a kind of serotonin "storm" that results in intense pleasurable experiences. The aftermath of this storm is an "exhaustion" of the cells that produce serotonin and, consequently, a depletion of serotonin levels in the brain. This probably accounts for the symptoms of depression that follow MDMA use. A much more worrisome aftermath of MDMA use is suggested by experimental studies in rats and monkeys. The results demonstrate that MDMA actually destroys serotonin-producing neurons in the brain. The implication of this for human users is certainly not clear yet, but we know that there is a gradual loss of neurons as individuals age, a loss that is not usually significant because of the brain's excess capacity. It has also been shown that chronic MDMA users have lower levels of serotonin than nonusers (though it cannot be definitively proved that this is due to loss of neurons). On formal cognitive testing, chronic users have significant impairment in certain types of memory and in higher cognitive functions, like executive function (see the discussion of executive function and ADHD in chapter 10).[9] If users of MDMA have depleted their "excess" serotonin neurons, killing them off by taking MDMA over a period, there is the possibility that psychiatric problems will emerge as these individuals age and progressively worsen as time goes on. Unlike mood problems brought on by alcohol use, these problems are likely to be permanent.[10]

The most recent iterations of designer drugs include "bath salts." These substances are a group of synthesized amphetamine-like compounds in the form of large crystals that superficially resemble the harmless soap-like bathing crystals, from which they derive their name. Initially developed and sold in Europe in the mid to late 2000s, they first came to the attention of the U.S. market in 2010. As with the synthetic marijuana mentioned above, these were legal compounds in the United States and so were sold over the counter in such innocuous places as gas stations and cigarette stores. In a further attempt to delay investigation of their contents, most if not all such products have clear labeling on their exteriors that they are "NOT FOR HUMAN CONSUMPTION." This warning is flippantly ignored by the person using the substance.

Around this time, poison control centers began to see an increase in patients with what seemed to be the symptoms of amphetamine intoxication (paranoia, excitability, high heart rates, panic-like symptoms, and in extreme cases, hallucinations or even heart attacks), but their toxicology tests were negative for the typical culprits, including cocaine and amphetamines. Eventually, these centers discovered the rampant use of these bath salts and since that time have put out major warnings against their use. Bath salt use was so problematic, in fact, that the United States Navy produced a warning/educational video distributed to its active service members, entitled "Bath salts: It's not a fad...It's a nightmare!" In this video, a male recruit in his early twenties opens a package containing bath salts that he has ordered from another country. After ingesting them, he attacks his friends and his girlfriend because of his disturbing hallucinations. This admittedly graphic video has as of this writing almost one million views and has developed rapid popularity among news outlets.[11] Given extreme effects of bath salts, they have successfully been made illegal in the United Kingdom and Canada and are currently illegal in forty-one states, with legislation pending in the remaining nine. Fortunately, the message that bath salts are dangerous seems to be getting through. Between 2012 and 2013, the number of teens reporting that bath salts "involve significant risk to the user" increased by 25 percent.

MOOD DISORDERS AND SUBSTANCE ABUSE

Research indicates that adolescent drug *use* appears to be more closely related to a teen's social and peer factors, whereas substance *abuse* seems to be more closely related to biological and psychological factors. This is evident from looking at the numbers of adolescents who fall into "drug *use*" versus "drug *abuse*" categories in research surveys. The National Institute on Drug Abuse's annual survey of adolescent drug use for the year 2013 indicated that about 70 percent of high school seniors had drunk alcohol and 50 percent had used an illicit drug sometime in their lives (the most common illicit drug used was by far marijuana, which was used by about 45 percent of adolescents, followed by prescription pain killers at 21 percent). Data from other surveys suggest, however, that the number of adolescents with a substance-*abuse* problem, though large enough to be of grave concern, is significantly smaller, around 10 percent.[12] In these studies, the biological and psychological factors associated with adolescent substance abuse are a family history of substance abuse (probably indicating a genetic predisposition) and a psychiatric diagnosis in the adolescent, the most common being ADHD and other behavioral problems and mood disorders. Studies also indicate that depressed adolescents are much more likely to progress from substance *use* to substance *abuse*.

Does having a mood disorder make adolescents more likely to use and abuse drugs and alcohol? Can alcoholism or drug abuse trigger the development of a mood disorder in someone who is genetically vulnerable? Do mood disorders and substance-abuse disorders have a common biochemical or genetic cause? There is some evidence to support an answer of yes to all three of these questions. Substance-abuse problems have been reported to precede the development of mood problems, to occur simultaneously, and to follow them.

Several studies support the idea that depression puts young people at risk for the development of substance abuse. In one study, 76 percent of adolescents with substance-abuse problems who had been referred to a psychiatric clinic had depression problems, and in most of these youths, the psychological problems had *preceded* the substance-abuse problems, sometimes for up to a year.[13] This supports what has been called a "self-medicating" link between substance abuse and depression: the adolescent finds that alcohol or drugs numb the psychic pain of depression, at least temporarily. After a time, however, the substance abuse takes on a life of its own because of the powerful addictive potential of these chemicals. At this point, the depression and substance abuse feed on each other. The adolescent drinks or uses drugs to get temporary relief from his feelings of depression, but since one of the after-effects of this high is a crash into worse depression, he uses again, and crashes again—and on and on the cycle spins, ever faster and more out of control.

Some studies have shown the development of alcohol and drug abuse preceding the development of mood disorders. The idea has been put forth that substance abuse somehow leads to depressive disorders. It's clear that alcohol and drug abuse adversely affect mood in the short run, especially stimulating drugs such as cocaine, amphetamines, and ecstasy. Perhaps ongoing use of drugs and alcohol can lead to more long-term problems with mood as well.

All abused substances appear to work by stimulating "reward" centers in the human brain. You have probably heard descriptions of experiments in which laboratory animals will push a lever that delivers an electrical stimulus to certain brain regions rather than push another one that delivers food to their cage, and they will continue to do so until they're practically dead from hunger. When a similar lever device is used to deliver an intravenous dose of alcohol or another drug, the substances the laboratory animals will willingly and persistently self-administer in this way are almost exactly the same ones that humans use to get intoxicated: narcotics, cocaine, and certain stimulants and tranquilizers. And these are the same substances that humans abuse and become addicted to. Some drugs, including ecstasy and cocaine, affect these brain centers quickly and powerfully; others, such as marijuana, work more slowly, but they all work in the same way: by disrupting the normal operations of the brain's "feel good" circuitry. Perhaps repeated episodes of drug use disrupt this circuitry in more profound and long-lasting ways and a mood disorder is the result. (Remember that animal studies have demonstrated that MDMA kills serotonin neurons in the brain.)

Finally, it may be that similar biological and psychological factors underlie the development of *both* mood disorders and substance-abuse disorders and that both types of problems are better thought of as two sides of the same coin.

TREATMENT ISSUES

Numerous clinical studies have shown a strong connection between adolescent substance use and adolescent mood disorders. One study followed up on a group of about seven hundred young people for approximately nine years to examine the relationship between substance use and depression. Not surprisingly, it found that depressed adolescents were more likely to use drugs and alcohol. It also found a roughly linear correlation between depression and drug use: the rate of depression problems went up in proportion to the severity of substance use. Put another way, the more severe the substance-use problem, the more likely the adolescent was to be suffering from a depressive disorder.[14]

But what about the question of whether one type of disorder *causes* the other? This question has important ramifications for treating these problems in individuals. If the self-medication hypothesis is true and depressed adolescents use alcohol and drugs in an attempt to "treat" their depressed feelings, this would suggest that successful treatment of the mood disorder should make the substance-abuse problem simply go away on its own. If the substance abuse is causing the mood disorder, then remaining abstinent from the abused substances should make the mood disorder go away. Research studies support both scenarios, which probably means that both can occur.

We think most psychiatrists who treat mood disorders have seen these two scenarios in patients, and most would agree that when a mood disorder and a substance-abuse problem occur together, they are best thought of as two problems that *both* need aggressive treatment. Either of these problems can precede and seem to trigger the other, which then takes on a life of its own and therefore requires treatment of its own as well. In our experience, patients who do not get treatment for both problems will not recover from either.

The first goal of treatment for substance abuse is to interrupt the drinking or drug use. Admission to a psychiatric hospital or other treatment facility is sometimes necessary to remove adolescents from an environment where they can still obtain and use alcohol or drugs. Family involvement is critical for treatment to be successful, by improving communication among family members and helping parents to provide guidance and set limits with the adolescent. In psychiatry there is a phenomenon called *codependence*. This is a somewhat loaded term that carries many, sometimes incorrect or exaggerated, social meanings. When psychiatrists use the term, they are usually trying to describe a simple pattern of behavior. In this pattern, one party in a relationship (in our scenario, an adolescent addicted to drugs) behaves in a dysfunctional way (misses school, for example, or commits crimes). The other person (usually the parent) inadvertently starts to support the behavior by shielding his child from the consequences of her behaviors. This usually happens with the best of intentions, that of protecting his child. What quickly transpires, however, is that the addict is increasingly insulated from the consequences of her actions, and the parent is increasingly called on to provide his protection, even if this means compromising his values. Usually this pattern becomes particularly problematic when the addict is asked to give up her addiction. Psychiatrists are constantly confronted by parents and children who want to get clean but find the process difficult and prematurely terminate the attempt. The father will sign his daughter out of rehab because it is uncomfortable or causes her suffering (even knowing that this temporary suffering is in her best interest). The mother will invite her son home from juvenile hall, knowing full well that he is likely to steal money again for drugs. This can be one of the most challenging aspects of addiction for a family to face, and it is why we always recommend that parents and loved ones pursue their own support during the treatment of the addict. This can take the form of support groups (such as Al-Anon) or even entering mental health treatment to work through their own feelings and distress. It is not usually appropriate for the same psychiatrist to treat both the child and the parent, because the psychiatrist must always have the best interest of the single identified patient in mind, which can be complicated when treating multiple members of the same family. It is becoming more and more common for psychiatry and therapy to be provided by different individuals, and in such a scenario, it may be valid for a family therapist to treat both the child and the adult, or for each to have an individual therapist as well as an individual psychiatrist.

Studies of adult alcoholics and cocaine abusers have shown that regular use of intoxicating substances alters brain functioning. Specifically, functioning is disrupted in the prefrontal cortex, an area of the brain thought to be involved in the executive functions such as self-control, delay of gratification, and inhibition of impulses (as we discuss in chapter 10). Studies of brain metabolism show that only after many *months* of sobriety do these brain areas function normally again.[15] During this time, the recovering substance abuser is still at grave risk of relapse. The treatment of substance-abuse problems must therefore be a long-term commitment. A brief "detox" admission to a hospital or several weeks of intensive outpatient treatment is not sufficient to have a long-lasting effect on substance abuse in an adolescent who has progressed beyond the experimentation stage of alcohol or drug use.

Although alcohol and drug use may stop for several months after intensive treatment, many studies have shown that abstinence does not last if the youth doesn't get maintenance treatment of some kind. According to one study of the treatment of adolescent drug abuse based on the twelve-step program of Alcoholics Anonymous, just as many adolescents who had completed a short-term treatment program relapsed by the twelve-month mark as those who hadn't even completed the program.[16] Often the adolescent needs help in developing an alcohol-free and drug-free lifestyle and in making some necessary major changes in his peer group and recreational activities, changes that the adolescent can make only with time, counseling, and support.

Some young people can move from a hospitalization or detoxification program of several days'—or weeks'—duration to outpatient care. This is often possible if the adolescent's functioning level and school and family life were not too severely affected by drug use. If drinking and drug use have reduced the adolescent's life to shambles, however, longer-term residential treatment will be necessary.

Adolescents who have dropped out of or been suspended from school, or who have developed run-away and other disruptive behaviors that make returning to live with the family tense and difficult, will probably need the structured rehabilitation of a residential or "halfway house" setting. These young people require the professional supervision and guidance, structure, and support provided in these settings to make the changes in behavioral patterns necessary to maintain their sobriety. Should this eventuality occur, it is the perfect opportunity for a parent to enter into her own treatment. Even though seeing her child destroy his life through an addiction is terribly traumatic, few things are as painful for a parent as having her child taken away from her for such a long period, especially knowing that he will likely be in psychological distress during the treatment. To brave through the experience, parents might find professional help invaluable in supporting their correct, though difficult, choices.

Adolescents who abuse alcohol and drugs to any substantial degree essentially stop the process of psychological maturation. Their emotional development is arrested at the point where they started using substances heavily. An 18-year-old who has been smoking marijuana regularly for two or three years may have the emotional maturity of a 15-year-old and will lack the more mature coping, problem-solving, and communication skills expected for her chronological age. When this adolescent gets clean, parents may be disappointed that their child seems to be immature for her age. The adolescent may find it difficult to feel comfortable with same-age peers. For all these reasons, counseling and psychotherapy, including family therapy, are often necessary and extremely beneficial for all involved. We discuss more about how to cope better with substance-abuse issues in the family in chapter 17.

Eating Disorders

Eating disorders make up a group of psychiatric syndromes that share the common element of a distortion of normal eating behaviors. Individuals with an eating disorder may eat too little or too much, but they all share a preoccupation with food, calories, and weight that comes to be all-engrossing and pathological, often with dangerous, sometimes even deadly, consequences. Ninety-five percent of persons with eating disorders develop them between the ages of 12 and 25, and 90 percent are women. Therefore, according to statistics, eating disorders are predominantly disorders of adolescent girls, and most of these individuals have mood disorders as well.

▼ Jennifer had blacked out for only a moment, it seemed, but she was still glassy-eyed and quiet when the ambulance arrived. The phys ed teacher had whisked horrified students out of the gym and called the school nurse, Mrs. Coleman, who found Jennifer's pulse to be alarmingly low and was having trouble taking her blood pressure. When Mrs. Coleman hiked up the sleeve of the girl's sweatshirt to take her blood pressure, she was taken aback by how skinny Jennifer's arm was.

"Has this girl been sick?" she asked.

"Not that I know of," replied the teacher. "At least not anything serious, I don't think. She's missed a few days here and there, but that's all."

They heard the sirens wailing up the school driveway. Good, thought Mrs. Coleman, they're here.

She looked down at Jennifer again. "Why are you wearing these heavy sweats in June?" she asked. Perhaps the girl had become overheated and fainted.

"I'm always cold," replied Jennifer listlessly.

The gymnasium doors clanged open, and three paramedics in sharply pressed blues briskly walked in. Mrs. Coleman and the teacher stood back, and Jennifer was on the gurney in seconds. One of the paramedics pumped up the blood pressure cuff that was still on the girl's arm and listened intently with her stethoscope. "Sixty-five over forty," she gasped. Another paramedic had already pricked Jennifer's finger and squeezed a drop of blood into what looked like a handheld calculator. He read the number that glowed on its little screen. "Her blood glucose is only thirty-seven, Kate." Kate looked down at Jennifer. "Are you diabetic, honey? Do you take insulin?" Jennifer shook her head weakly.

"What did you have for breakfast today, sweetie?"

"A vitamin pill."

"We're going to start an IV on you, Jennifer." In a moment, Jennifer, the gurney, and the three paramedics were moving toward the door. "Tell her parents we're taking her to Memorial. We'll need them to sign for treatment." The gymnasium doors clanged shut. As the echoes of the door's banging died away, the siren's wail started up and then faded.

Mrs. Coleman turned to the teacher. "Has this student seemed tired to you lately? Has she had trouble keeping up with the others in this class?"

"No. Jennifer's always full of energy. But this isn't really a class; it's an aerobics group for junior girls with weight problems. Participation is voluntary."

"Weight problems?" Mrs. Coleman said. "Carol, that girl does *not* have a weight problem."

"I started the group last month, and Jennifer was the first to sign up. I didn't think she looked overweight, but it's hard to tell with those baggy clothes she always wears."

Mrs. Coleman looked thoughtful for a moment, and then asked, "Do you ask these girls how much weight they want to lose when they sign up?"

"They fill out a form with their current weight and their goal weight. I remember that Jennifer left those questions blank. I just thought she was embarrassed—"

Mrs. Coleman wasn't listening anymore. She realized that this girl probably *did* have a weight problem, but not the kind of problem an aerobics class would help with. When she spoke with Jennifer's mother on the phone, she asked about the girl's eating habits.

"They're terrible. I know she's too skinny. But she won't eat with us anymore. I almost think it's better that way because every meal turned into a screaming match. We can't even talk about it around here. Her father gets so mad about it that I worry about his blood pressure getting out of control again."

"Mrs. Andrews," the nurse said slowly, "I think Jennifer might have an eating disorder." ▲

By the time pop singer Karen Carpenter died of anorexia nervosa in 1983—an event that brought eating disorders to the consciousness of most Americans for the first time—physicians had been aware of this mysterious group of psychiatric illnesses for more than two centuries. Dr. R. Morton wrote in a 1694 treatise on "consumptions" (an old word for any illness characterized by a physical wasting away) of "a nervous atrophy . . . a wasting of the body without any remarkable fever, cough, or shortness of breath" that he attributed to a "distemper'd state of the brain." In 1874, the English physician William Withey Gull coined the term *anorexia nervosa* to describe "a morbid mental state" that resulted in extreme weight loss. Gull realized that the weight loss was not due to a bodily illness like tuberculosis or an intestinal disease but was instead the result of "simple starvation."

But it was the French alienist (*alienist* is a nineteenth-century term for a psychiatrist) Charles Lasègue who first captured the essential elements of this form of the illness: a "refusal of food" that becomes "the sole object of preoccupation and conversation" such that "the circle within which revolve the ideas and sentiments of the patient becomes more narrowed." Lasègue described the disconnect between the patient's appearance and her perception of her appearance as well as her distorted assessment of her nutritional needs: "The patient, when told that she cannot live upon an amount of food that would not support a young infant, replies that it furnishes sufficient nourishment for her, adding that she is neither changed nor thinner." Lasègue also recognized the upheaval the syndrome causes in families and the frustration and powerlessness of the parents of these patients. He noted that the family "has but two methods at its service which it always exhausts—entreaties and menaces."[1]

In the 1980s, it was increasingly recognized that self-starvation is not the only serious abnormal eating syndrome. Also described were individuals, often of normal weight, who binged on huge amounts of food in a matter of hours or even minutes and then caused themselves to vomit what they had eaten. The terms *binge-purge syndrome* and *bulimia nervosa* (or simply *bulimia*) were coined to describe this condition.

More recently, descriptions have appeared in the psychiatric literature of overweight patients who binge but do not induce vomiting or use other means to compensate for their increased calorie intake, and the diagnosis *binge-eating disorder* was officially adopted in the *DSM-5*.

It has been suggested that perhaps the biggest group of persons with abnormal eating behaviors does not fit neatly into any one of these classifications; these individuals have elements of several eating disorders or shift from one clinical picture to another over time. Abnormal eating syndromes cover a wide range of problems, from those posing only minor risks to health to those that are life threatening.

As with adolescent substance abuse, the topic of eating disorders is enormous and complex. What follows, then, is a brief overview of the main symptoms of the disorders, just to introduce them and to make it easier to understand the interplay between these syndromes and the mood disorders.

ANOREXIA NERVOSA

The most dramatic and severe of the eating disorders is anorexia nervosa. People with this disorder believe they are overweight, even obese, and restrict their food intake to lose weight. They lose their objectivity about calories, weight, and appearance, and they continue to think they are overweight despite the emaciated appearance of their bodies. Their drive to lose weight takes on a life of its own, and despite their steadily decreasing weight, they continue trying to lose even more. The syndrome is, in a sense, incorrectly named, because the word *anorexia*, a medical term for "loss of appetite," does *not* characterize these individuals (except perhaps in the advanced stages of starvation, when their brain functions are abnormal in many different ways). People with anorexia do not lose their appetite but rather *fight* their hunger, and after a time, the struggle against their appetite becomes an end in itself, the focus of all their energies.

Often, the individual starts out with a desire to lose what might indeed be extra pounds, but then she cannot identify or be satisfied with a healthy goal weight. She may identify an initial goal weight of, say, 110 pounds, but after reaching this initial goal decides to get down to 105. At 105 pounds, the new goal becomes 100, then 95, and eventually the only goal is to weigh less than the day before—with no end in sight. She becomes convinced that if she starts to gain weight, she will lose control of her eating and her ability to maintain her weight and will become enormously obese. In other cases, the person realizes she is thin but nevertheless worries that some part of her body, such as her abdomen or buttocks, is "fat." Either way, eating comes to be viewed as a vice; taking needed nourishment is "giving in."

As others notice the girl's increasing thinness with alarm, eating and meals become more and more tense. As Lasègue observed in the families of his patients, "the delicacies of the table are multiplied in the hope of stimulating the appetite; but the more the solicitude increases, the more the appetite diminishes. The patient disdainfully tastes the new [foods] and after having thus shown her willingness, holds herself absolved from obligation to do more."

Individuals suffering from anorexia not only fast but also exercise excessively to lose weight. They may use laxatives and diuretics (fluid pills) to decrease calories and weight. To avoid the stares and comments of others, they dress in baggy clothing that conceals their emaciation.

Eventually, the physical consequences of starvation begin to take their toll. Menstruation stops, heart rate slows, and hands and feet become cold as the body attempts to conserve calories. Skin becomes dry, the hair may fall out, and the person complains of fatigue and is noted to be listless and lethargic. Dizzy spells and fainting occur. Eventually, sodium and potassium imbalances affect cellular functions, heart-rhythm abnormalities develop, and the girl can die from cardiac arrest.

The treatment of anorexia nervosa focuses first on refeeding the patient in order to reverse the distortions in thinking that are due to starvation.

Then, a lengthy retraining process must occur during which the patient relearns normal eating patterns and changes her feelings about herself, her weight, and her relationship with food and calories. In many cases, this eventually proves impossible to accomplish outside a carefully controlled setting. Just as many substance abusers must enter rehab to terminate their unhealthy relationship with drugs, so do many people who have anorexia require admission to a psychiatric hospital to interrupt their unhealthy relationship with food.

BULIMIA NERVOSA

The hallmark of bulimia nervosa is binge eating, during which the individual eats an enormous amount of food, often sweet high-calorie foods, over a period of an hour or so. She may eat an entire gallon of ice cream at one sitting, dozens of doughnuts, pizzas by the carton, candy by the pound, usually stopping only when physically incapable of taking in any more food. A binge is a private affair undertaken secretly and alone; the food consumption is frenzied, joyless, and obsessive, and the bulimic feels out of control, almost "out of body," while it is happening.

When she cannot force another bite, the bulimic is overcome with disgust and shame at what she has done and seeks a way to rid herself of the calorie load. The vast majority of people with bulimia do this by forcing themselves to vomit. This provides them relief from the physical discomfort brought on by the binge and also reduces their fear of gaining weight from such an enormous intake of calories. In the early stages of the disorder, individuals with bulimia usually stimulate their gag reflex by putting a finger or spoon down the throat, but later in the course of the disorder, they often become adept at vomiting at will. Those who do not manage this may actually develop a callus on the first knuckle of their finger from the repeated abrasions caused by their teeth during self-stimulation to induce vomiting. Individuals with bulimia also misuse laxatives and diuretics to get rid of calories and water weight.

The binge is often an unplanned and impulsive response to some uncomfortable emotional state. Like those with anorexia nervosa, these girls and young women are abnormally preoccupied with their weight and body image and, outside their binges, are often strictly controlling their diet and avoiding high-calorie foods.

Individuals with bulimia nervosa are usually impulsive in other areas of their lives, and they often have a history of substance abuse, self-mutilation, and suicide attempts. Many people with anorexia also have bulimic behaviors, and approximately 40 percent of them have a more prolonged bulimic phase in the course of their illness or recovery.[2]

Most individuals with bulimia are of normal weight or are slightly overweight. Physical complications of bulimia nervosa are mostly related to the purging behaviors discussed above, including vomiting. These purging practices are dangerous. They can cause severe dehydration or imbalances in the body's natural electrolytes that can lead to cardiac arrhythmias or seizures. The stomach acid repeatedly forced up the throat can cause blistering and, over the long term, cancer.

Binge-eating disorder describes the behaviors of people who binge but do not purge, use laxatives, or engage in other behaviors to get rid of the extra calories. Their binges have exactly the same qualities as those of a bulimic—they can be impulsive or, conversely, highly ritualized. The person feels physically unable to stop and can eat well over her daily allotment of calories in one sitting. We once treated a patient who would consume three family-sized buckets of fried chicken in a single episode—he would begin crying halfway through but was still unable to stop the bingeing episode. As might be expected, many people with binge-eating disorder are overweight.

The treatment of bulimia nervosa includes helping patients identify the precipitating factors of a binge, addressing their distorted body image and abnormal attitudes toward food, and teaching them healthy eating habits and coping patterns other than binge eating during periods of emotional distress. As with anorexia, persons with bulimia have a great fear of food and can be highly resistant to entering treatment. Though many are of normal body weight (as opposed to people with anorexia), they fear that giving up their abnormal behaviors (primarily the purging) will result in their ballooning up to an enormous weight. Forcing a patient to refrain from vomiting after even a normal-sized meal can result in a seemingly calm, rational patient flying into a violent rage. As may be expected, treatment of bulimia is similarly difficult to treatment of anorexia and may require an inpatient psychiatric stay.

UNDERSTANDING EATING DISORDERS

Like substance-abuse problems, eating disorders are best understood as complex self-reinforcing *behaviors* that entrap vulnerable individuals. The challenge to understanding eating disorders in this way is that of understanding how self-starvation and bingeing and purging can possibly be self-reinforcing, that is, why patients, on some level at least, are *attracted* to these behaviors in the same way substance abusers are attracted to alcohol and drug use. It helps to first identify the vulnerabilities that are the setup for these behaviors.

Social and cultural factors are very important. Eating disorders are seen almost exclusively in industrialized countries where food shortage is not significant. Western culture's glorification of thinness in females is also a significant factor. One need only glance through any magazine marketed to teenagers to see the idealized feminine physique: willowy thin supermodels or buxom but toned and wiry beach beauties—often photographed and touched up in such a way as to make them look even thinner than they are in real life. Surveys show that up to 70 percent of young women in Northern Europe and the United States feel they are overweight even when they are thin or normal in weight. Most girls simply do not have the genetic endowment needed to look like the women they constantly see depicted in magazines, on billboards, and in films and television programs. Adolescent boys feel some of the same pressures, but the emphasis is on being muscular rather than thin. This is one of the reasons eating disorders are thought to be so much rarer in males (and perhaps why steroid abuse is almost exclusively a problem of young men).

There is also something of a class consciousness attached to thinness, exemplified by the old saying that "a woman can never be too rich or too thin." In contrast to cultures in which food is scarce and plumpness is valued, where food is plentiful, slimness and the avoidance of obesity are valued and associated with wealth. Being overweight is associated with laziness, poor self-control, and self-indulgence; thinness is associated with good health and self-discipline. Young people constantly see and hear that thin is good and fat is bad, and they incorporate these ideals into their view of what sort of body type is attractive and desirable.

While some young people are relatively unaffected by this barrage of messages about weight and appearance, those with serious self-esteem problems can take these messages to heart in a very serious way. Adolescence is a time of difficult transitions and worries about identity and fitting in. Fears about sexual maturation crop up for younger adolescents, and older ones may equate entering adulthood with being abandoned and isolated. The adolescent fears losing control of her life in several important ways and may feel ineffective and helpless to influence the outcome of these developmental processes. At this point, some adolescents become preoccupied with food and weight control to distract themselves from these frightening issues.

When they restrict their food intake and experience weight loss, these young women experience a surge of competence, self-confidence, and control. Complimentary and congratulatory comments from others on successfully losing weight further reinforce weight loss as an admirable goal. Fasting and food preoccupation become a "safe place" where the girl feels in control and knows that her efforts will pay off in predictable and measurable ways. The girl with anorexia begins to take pride in her ability to adhere to stricter, narrower, and more abnormal diets and to restrict further and further. Thinness, fasting, and exercise come to be seen as virtues and eating as a vice. The adolescent becomes intoxicated by her success at losing weight and by reaching ever more ambitious weight-loss goals.

Experiments to study the psychological effects of starvation, in which healthy volunteers have gone on extremely restricted diets, have shown that constantly hungry people begin to think about food constantly, talk about food constantly, and even have dreams about food. As her food intake decreases, the girl with anorexia experiences ever stronger, and now physiologically induced, food cravings. She finds that she must work even harder to keep the weight off. She develops increasingly irrational fears about what would happen if she were to begin to eat normally, imagining that her body would balloon to immensely obese proportions if she were to stop restricting. More fasting leads to more craving and hunger, which leads to more food preoccupation, more fear of losing control—and this leads to more fasting. A vicious circle has developed: the young woman with anorexia has become intensely fearful of eating, and fasting is the only way she knows of to deal with her anxiety. There is no escape.

Eventually, malnutrition begins to affect brain functioning. At this point, the individual becomes physically incapable of making good decisions about eating or realizing how dangerous a situation she is in. This is why, at very low weights, hospitalization is necessary to accomplish refeeding.

Individuals with bulimia follow a comparable course. They are affected by the same sociocultural factors regarding thinness and also start out worried about their weight. They often go on diets that are unreasonable and overly strict, and their initial binges are the result of impulsive and out-of-control eating to quickly alleviate their hunger pangs. Alternatively, the binge may have developed as a means of dealing with depression, loneliness, and anxiety. In either case, binge eating becomes the coping mechanism and simultaneously the cause of shame, guilt, and disgust. The bulimic starts purging to rid herself of the physical discomfort and calories that result from the binge, but this behavior (and perhaps the weight gain that results from it as well) causes more shame and guilt, precipitating more binge eating, and another vicious cycle begins.

In the treatment of eating disorders, normal eating behaviors and healthy attitudes toward food and body need to be retaught to the patient. She must also learn new ways of coping with uncomfortable feelings and address self-image and self-esteem issues. For many of these individuals, there is also an underlying mood disorder that fuels the maladaptive coping mechanisms and that requires treatment in its own right.

MOOD DISORDERS AND EATING DISORDERS

Many people with eating disorders have mood disorders as well, usually depression. One clinical study of American high school girls with eating disorders found that more than 80 percent of them suffered from a depressive disorder, mostly major depressive disorder.[3] Another study found that dysthymic disorder was more closely associated with eating disorders than major depression.[4] But whatever the details, the pattern is clear: the combination of an eating disorder and a mood disorder occurs too often to be explained away as simply coincidental. The cause or causes for this correlation are hotly debated. There is some evidence that genetic factors are at play. A study of twin girls with anorexia nervosa found evidence that genetic risk factors are important for the development of the eating disorder and "substantially contribute to the observed comorbidity between anorexia nervosa and major depression."[5] Perhaps personality traits such as obsessiveness or a tendency to be shy and introverted have a genetic basis, and perhaps these traits interact with social cues to set up the adolescent female for anorectic behaviors. We know that a person's degree of impulsivity has some genetic basis and that a tendency to be impulsive is frequently seen in individuals with bulimia.

The bad feelings that arise from a mood disorder may precipitate eating disorder behaviors and sustain them over time. An Italian study of patients with bulimia found that many of them had a *prodrome*, or preliminary phase, to their eating disorder characterized by low self-esteem, depressed mood, loss of interest and pleasure in activities, and irritability—all symptoms of depression.[6]

The relationship between eating disorders and mood disorders is likely one of complex interactions that differ from one individual to another. The optimal treatment of the combination is quite clear, however: when they occur together, *both* problems require treatment. As with the combination of substance abuse and mood disorders, treating one problem does not usually make the other go away.

Several double-blind placebo-controlled studies have shown that patients with bulimia can reduce the frequency of their binges when they are prescribed antidepressant medications as part of an overall treatment plan that includes psychotherapy and therapy aimed at the eating disorder behaviors.[7] Studies on antidepressant treatment of patients with anorexia nervosa at first appeared to be less impressive, but more recent studies suggest a reason to be optimistic. It seems that antidepressants have little effect when the patient with anorexia is still significantly underweight, perhaps explaining the results of studies on still-malnourished hospitalized patients that have not shown antidepressants to be of much benefit. When fluoxetine (Prozac) was given to patients who had been discharged from the hospital at normal weight, however, the medication had a significantly beneficial effect on relapse rates. Perhaps biochemical abnormalities in the brains of malnourished, underweight patients prevent antidepressant medications from working properly, and only when weight has returned to normal can medication be effective.[8]

The treatment of severe eating disorders is complex and requires a team of experts. Severely malnourished patients are best served in psychiatric hospitals that have a special eating disorders unit and a treatment team that is experienced in the therapy of such disorders. In addition to treating the abnormal eating behaviors, all the treatment options for addressing the mood disorder that usually accompanies an eating disorder are required. A psychiatrist with experience in treating eating disorders, mood disorders, and children and adolescents is optimal, though it may be difficult to find someone with this level of expertise, as the only specialty of the three eligible for separate certification by a governing board is that of child and adolescent psychiatry. Additional members of the treatment team should include experienced psychotherapists, family therapists, and nutritionists, all of whom are necessary to treat these complex and very dangerous illnesses.

"Cutting" and Other Self-Harming Behaviors

We have described in the last two chapters two types of self-harming behaviors that frequently complicate mood disorders: substance abuse and eating disorders. As Drs. Paul McHugh and Phillip Slavney point out in their book *The Perspectives of Psychiatry*, a disorder is something people *have* whereas a behavior is something people *do*.[1] This distinction is important when developing a treatment plan for a psychiatric problem. Treating a disorder is often easier than stopping a behavior. In this chapter, we talk about a group of behaviors often seen in people with mood disorders, behaviors in which individuals intentionally injure themselves. "Cutting" behaviors and other forms of self-mutilation, as well as the ultimate self-harming behavior, suicide, fit into this category.

SELF-MUTILATION

This account from Jill (14 years old) appeared in the *New York Times:*

I was in the bathroom going completely crazy, just bawling my eyes out, and I think my mom was wallpapering—there was a wallpaper cutter there. I had so much anxiety, I couldn't concentrate on anything until I somehow let that out, and not being able to let it out in words, I took the razor and started cutting my leg and I got excited about seeing my blood. It felt good to see the blood coming out, like that was my other pain leaving me too. It felt right and it felt good for me to let it out that way.[2]

Self-mutilation is deliberate *nonsuicidal self-injury* (NSSI), usually by cutting or burning the body. By definition, it is self-injury that does not involve the desire to end one's life; the self-injury is, rather, an end in itself. This behavior inspires horror and disgust and seems utterly irrational to others, but it is increasingly common. Even suicide is, in a sense, easier to understand as possibly arising out of a desire to end suffering or out of a profound hopelessness and despair. The intentional self-infliction of pain and disfigurement, on the other hand, is incomprehensible, at least at first glance. Unfortunately, self-mutilation is not rare, and it has been estimated that "cutters" and other individuals who repeatedly harm themselves number in the millions—this behavior occurs in about a thousand persons per hundred thousand population per year.[3] Among young persons being treated for other psychiatric conditions, the prevalence can be as high as one in five.[4] Like substance abuse and eating disorders, self-inflicted injury is a complex behavior with no single "cause." Rather, it is best understood by examining the variety of factors that are involved in its development. Self-mutilation occurs in vulnerable individuals, is precipitated by emotional distress of various types, and is then sustained by additional and usually different factors.

In this section, we discuss what has been called *repetitive*, or *episodic, self-mutilation*. Elsewhere in this book, we describe other forms of self-harm, such as the repetitive head-banging occurring in severely developmentally disabled persons and the self-mutilation in response to hallucinations or delusional ideas in individuals with psychotic illnesses. Repetitive self-mutilation, on the other hand, occurs in nonpsychotic individuals who cannot resist impulses to harm themselves physically.

Again, it's important to stress that this is not suicidal behavior, that is, individuals are not acting out of a desire to end their life. Rather, they report that the behavior gives them rapid, though short-lived, relief from a variety of uncomfortable emotional states such as depression, anxiety, and anger. They describe how, while they are engaging in the self-harming behavior, they go into a trancelike state (called *dissociation*) and do not experience pain from their actions. Usually the individuals feel guilty and ashamed afterward and attempt to conceal what they have done. This pattern shares many behavioral elements with eating disorders, especially bulimic behaviors, and in fact, many patients with repetitive self-mutilation behaviors have eating disorders too.

Secondary effects of the behaviors help sustain them. As with eating disorders, it's quite a challenge to understand how self-mutilation can make a person feel *better* in any way and what feelings draw people to hurt themselves again and again. As with eating binges, episodes of self-mutilation seem to start out with a building sense of inner tension or distress that gradually increases to a point where it is unendurable. Patients report that injuring themselves provides an instant relief of this unbearable tension. They compare the relief they experience to lancing a boil, popping the lid off a pressure cooker, or bursting a balloon. The injury focuses frustration and emotional pain in the harmful act, and some patients report a sense of regaining control of their mental state by their self-injury. This sense of relief may last for hours, and the person often goes into a deep sleep afterward. Sometimes the act is highly ritualized, including a careful laying out of the cutting instruments and the materials to bandage the wound afterward.

The range of self-injuring behaviors is broad. Some individuals make only superficial skin scratches with their fingernails or pick at skin blemishes. At the other end of the continuum are those who collect razor blades, surgical gauze, and antiseptics and make careful incisions, which they then cleanse and bandage. Burning with lit cigarettes or heated metal objects is another common method of self-harm. For some people, self-mutilation seems to be a brief, time-limited behavioral syndrome, playing out over weeks or months. Only a minority of persons who repeatedly injure themselves go on to develop a sort of addiction to the behavior that can go on for years. Many of these individuals have mood disorders, but we still don't know how many mood disorder patients repetitively self-injure themselves or how many self-injuring individuals have a mood disorder. As with eating disorders, the individuals who self-mutilate appear to be predominantly female. The most important personality vulnerability factor seems to be impulsiveness. One study of women with self-mutilating behaviors found that about half of them had a history of or later developed an eating disorder, and about one-fifth had a history of alcohol or drug abuse, compulsive stealing, or shoplifting.[5]

The ability of the self-mutilating behavior to shock and horrify others, especially family members, is another proposed explanation for how such behaviors develop. Rendering family members (and therapists) gasping and helpless, as these behaviors do, can be a potent and dramatic way to act out anger and replace fear and depression with feelings of power and control.

The number of persons with this problem is growing, and it's fairly clear that young females are especially at risk. Articles and books in the lay press that describe and discuss "cutters" have appeared with increasing frequency.[6] The practice of self-mutilation has been glorified through the vast availability of information on the Internet. Sites like YouTube and Instagram carry sometimes graphic depictions of self-injury.[7] The same kinds of social factors that influence the development of eating disorders may be at work to increase the numbers of young women who are drawn to "cutting" behaviors. In 1992, *People* magazine published excerpts from a biography of Princess Diana that revealed not only her eating disorder behaviors but her repeated episodes of cutting herself as well. Film idol (and teenage heartthrob) Johnny Depp displayed scars on his forearm and told *Details* magazine in 1993 that he cut himself with a knife to mark special times in his life.[8] Just as the glorification of thinness and the societal pervasiveness of dieting lead increasing numbers to attempt to lose weight and trap a few of them into eating disorder behaviors, the glamorizing and romanticizing of self-injury in the famous may be leading more and more to try cutting. The increasing prevalence and acceptance of such body modification behaviors as tattooing, piercing, and scarification (producing tissue injury to develop decorative scars) among young people may also be a factor, reducing the barriers to trying cutting by making painful and visible assaults on the body more acceptable.

The treatment of self-mutilation resembles that of eating disorders: the individual must be persuaded to give up a behavior that, however perverse, is powerfully addictive. Treating underlying depression is, of course, always necessary. Therapy to identify other sources of uncomfortable emotional states and to help the individual learn alternative ways of coping with them is extremely important. Treating repetitive self-mutilation is complex and requires intensive, long-term multidisciplinary therapy, preferably by specialists in the treatment of these problems.

A specific technique for treating patients who engage in repetitive self-mutilation is a form of cognitive therapy called *dialectical behavioral therapy* (DBT). We discussed DBT in chapter 9 as a form of therapy that may be helpful for many young people with depression. DBT focuses on emotional regulation and distress tolerance, on learning to cope with negative feelings without acting irresponsibly to end them. DBT has now been validated to help with many different forms of negative experiences, but it was specifically created to help patients with chronic suicidal or nonsuicidal self-injury, particularly those with borderline personality disorder.[9] Dr. Marsha Linehan, the founder of this technique, later admitted that she was a former cutter herself and that this influenced her development of DBT: "I developed a therapy that provides the things I needed for so many years and never got."[10] DBT focuses on helping the patient identify and interrupt the thinking and emotional processes that lead up to an episode of self-mutilation (or other poorly adaptive behaviors, such as aggression) and consists of weekly individual psychotherapy and group therapy sessions. There is a strong emphasis on learning how to tolerate distressing emotional states, on learning to better regulate emotions, and especially on changing behavior patterns to eliminate self-harm. For adolescents who have repetitive problems with self-mutilation, seeking out a therapist who is trained and experienced in DBT is an essential part of the treatment process. DBT has also been shown to help in multiple domains beyond self-injury, including generally tolerating distress and reducing emotional reactivity. As you can imagine, in many ways it is tailor-made for the tribulations of adolescence. In fact, a modified form of DBT specifically for adolescents includes their parents in the treatment, which can greatly reduce strife in this relationship. This form of DBT externalizes the dialectical debate. Whereas classic DBT focuses on the internal mental processes of a single person, DBT for adolescents works on bringing together the sometimes opposing viewpoints of parent and child.

In the introduction to an issue of a psychiatric research periodical devoted to the topic of self-mutilation, the scientific editor, a well-known psychiatrist, stated, "The typical clinician treating a patient who self-mutilates is often left feeling a combination of helpless, horrified, guilty, furious, betrayed, disgusted and sad."[11] As in treating other destructive but addictive behaviors, the intense and specialized treatment required for self-injury behaviors is often difficult and time consuming; recovery can be frustrat-ingly slow. Fortunately, more and more research on the causes and corre-lates of this syndrome is being done, and the number of therapists who are skilled in its treatment is increasing.

ADOLESCENT SUICIDE

In the chapters in this part of the book, we have been discuss-ing complex behaviors that often complicate mood disorders but that are shaped and precipitated by many factors and influences—behaviors that do not have any simple cause. Suicidal behavior also falls into this category.

We discuss the danger signals of an impending suicide and talk about suicide prevention later in this book (chapter 18). Here, we want to discuss adolescent suicide a bit more abstractly and address some misconceptions about suicide in this age group.

The rates of suicide among adolescents rose steadily in the United States during the second half of the twentieth century. In 1956, the completed sui-cide rate among 15- to 19-year-olds was just over 2 per 100,000 individu-als per year, a number that turned out to be the lowest of the century. By the mid-1980s, this number had increased nearly five-fold, to about 11 per 100,000 per year. Most strikingly, boys almost entirely accounted for this dramatic increase in the number of adolescent suicides, with the suicide rate for males in this age range approaching 20 per 100,000 per year in 1988. The rate has declined slightly since then, likely due to increased education and a larger awareness of adolescent depression itself. The adolescent sui-cide rate hit a low of 10 per 100,000 in 2000, though since then it has crept back up slightly to 12 per 100,000 in 2013. During this time, suicide rates for young women stayed about the same, so this fluctuation is again almost entirely due to increased rates among young men.[12]

The number of adolescents who make *suicide attempts* is far larger than the number who actually kill themselves. For every adolescent who com-mits suicide, more than a hundred others have made an attempt. Most of these attempts do not result in any injuries, and many are medically incon-sequential, such as taking a handful of aspirin tablets or making superficial scratches on the wrists. Studies have indicated that only about 2 to 3 percent of adolescents who have made a suicide attempt seek medical treatment.

Studies also show that twice as many adolescent girls than adolescent boys make a suicide attempt, but more than five times more boys than girls actually kill themselves. Boys who attempt suicide do so by more lethal means. In fact, of all suicide attempts resulting in death, half involve a gun and a quarter involve suffocation (which includes hanging). These two methods are those most commonly attempted by boys. It has been suggested that those who *attempt* suicide and those who "succeed" in killing themselves are two different (though overlapping) groups. But a review of the research studies on individuals who make suicide attempts and on those who die from completed suicide reveals that, aside from the differences in sex ratio, the characteristics of the two groups don't appear so terribly different clinically. Also, most adolescents who actually kill themselves have previously made a suicide attempt. It appears that both groups usually suffer from psychiatric problems, most commonly mood disorders.

For many years, mental health experts held on to what might be called the "Romeo and Juliet" theory of adolescent suicide, the idea that adolescence is a time of stress and that any individual exposed to an intolerable amount of psychological stress is at risk for suicide. The theory was a natural outgrowth of the early Sturm und Drang ideas about adolescence that we discussed in chapter 2: that all adolescents are volatile, impulsive, and raging with emotions, and those who attempt suicide are, like Romeo and Juliet, simply more volatile and impulsive and under greater environmental stress. This is clearly not the case. The majority of adolescent suicide victims suffered from a mood disorder. Environmental stressors seem to play some role in the behavior, but the underlying psychiatric illness appears to be the most important factor. For this reason, suicide prevention programs aimed at adolescents are beginning to shift away from "stress management" models to programs that educate adolescents and their families on how to recognize mood disorder symptoms and on the importance of treatment.

One model for understanding and preventing adolescent suicide, increasingly accepted in psychiatry, is that developed by David Shaffer and his colleagues at Columbia University in New York (figure 14-1). This multifactorial model proposes that suicidal thinking originates in an adolescent because of an underlying psychiatric disorder, but it smolders under the surface until more active consideration of suicide is precipitated by some stressful event; at that point, actual suicidal behavior is either facilitated or inhibited by a combination of mostly external factors.

Numerous studies have found that almost all adolescents who commit suicide suffer from depression, forming the basis for the proposed first step of this model: development of an underlying psychiatric disorder. Studies of adolescent suicides indicate that the most common underlying disorders are mood disorders. In boys, a combination of a mood disorder and a substance-abuse problem is especially dangerous. In a study of 6,483 adolescents aged 13 to 18, 12 percent had considered suicide, and 4 percent had attempted. Twenty-four percent of those who had attempted suicide abused alcohol, and 35 percent abused other drugs. Seventy-five percent of those who had attempted suicide also suffered from a mood disorder. More than 50 percent of this last group had shown signs of the disorder that were severe enough for them to already be in mental health treatment prior to their suicide attempt.[13]

The suicide attempt is precipitated in these vulnerable individuals by what Shaffer calls a *stress event*, an event such as being in trouble with the police or at school, the breakup of a relationship, or simply a recent distressing or humiliating experience. Often the stress event can be understood in relation to the underlying disorder: the stress event leads to an acute emotional crisis, with the development of extreme anxiety, dread, and hopelessness; a sense of inner tension and agitation builds, and the adolescent feels compelled to "do something."

At this point, external factors either facilitate or inhibit suicidal behavior. A strong religious belief about the sinfulness of suicide would be an inhibitory factor, whereas living in a culture where suicide is seen as an acceptable solution to problems (as was formerly the case in Japan) would be facilitating. The availability of a supportive, trusted influence such as a family member, a close friend, or a therapist to help soothe and decompress the situation would be an inhibitory factor. Studies suggest that feelings of connectedness to family are protective against suicide. Being or feeling isolated and unable to reach out for comfort or support, on the other hand, appears to facilitate suicidal behavior. This factor has been cited as important in understanding the much higher rate of suicidal behavior among adolescents who experience questions and conflicts over same-sex romantic at-

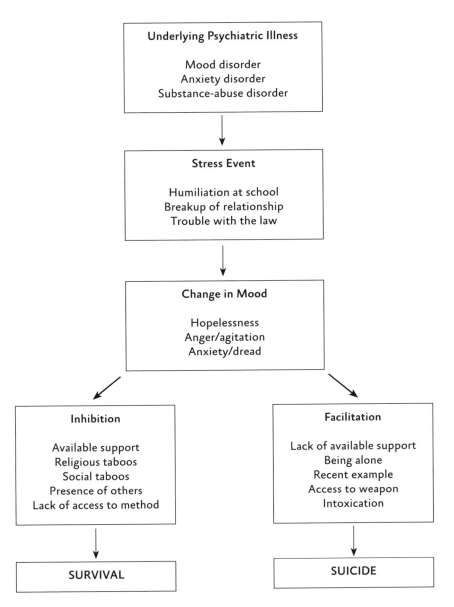

Figure 13-1 A model of adolescent suicide
Source: Described in David Shaffer and Leslie Craft, "Methods of Adolescent Suicide Prevention," *Journal of Clinical Psychiatry* 60, suppl. 2 (1999): 70–74.

traction and who feel unable to discuss this issue with family, friends, or the other usual sources of support.[14]

Another facilitating factor is the recent suicide of someone known to the adolescent or even someone simply living in the same community, serving as a model for suicidal behavior. The issue of *suicide contagion* has received attention: adolescent suicides often occur in clusters, and the suicide of one adolescent may lead to a series of suicide attempts by others. In February 1990, a physician notified the Centers for Disease Control (CDC; now the Centers for Disease Control and Prevention), the federal agency that investigates epidemics and the spread of illnesses, that two adolescent boys had committed suicide in Santa Fe County, New Mexico, within four days of each other. The New Mexico Department of Health investigated and found that the number of persons under the age of 20 who had been evaluated for a suicide attempt or suicidal thinking had *tripled* that month, a finding interpreted as strongly suggesting that one suicide can lead others to make an attempt. The study also found that the rate of suicide attempts had been consistently lower during June, July, and August for the preceding three years, giving support to the idea that school problems can be a precipitating factor for suicidal behavior.[15] A more recent Canadian study found even higher numbers, that adolescents were four and a half times as likely to attempt suicide after a schoolmate had done the same.[16]

Media coverage of an adolescent suicide that seeks to comfort a community may have the unwanted effect of promoting the clustering of suicides. Portrayals of a poignant family and community tragedy, with emotional descriptions of grieving friends and family and of moving eulogies given at well-attended funerals, have the effect of presenting suicide in a positive way and making it more acceptable. In 1994, the CDC issued media guidelines for reporting on suicide and listed several aspects of media coverage that may promote suicide contagion, including presenting simplistic explanations for suicide or presenting suicide as an understandable way of coping with personal problems ("John had recently broken up with his girlfriend"). Focusing on the victim's accomplishments and positive characteristics is also discouraged, as it may make suicide more attractive to vulnerable adolescents who feel that those around them do not appreciate them.

Other suicide facilitators include opportunity and access factors, such as being alone at home and the availability of a highly lethal suicide method, such as access to a gun. It is quite clear that the presence of a firearm in the home greatly increases the risk of suicide. One study showed that the presence of *any* firearm increased adolescent suicide risk, and whether the weapon was a handgun or a long gun, kept loaded or unloaded, locked up or not, made no difference.[17]

Perhaps the ultimate facilitating factor is intoxication of some type. Not only does a substance-abuse diagnosis greatly increase the risk of suicide, but most persons who kill themselves have alcohol in their bloodstream when they do so.

Public health efforts at suicide prevention in adolescents are increasingly focusing on the start of the process that leads to suicide: identifying the psychiatric disorder and getting the adolescent into treatment. Although hotlines and crisis services have been popular efforts, there is little research evidence to suggest they have much effect on suicide rates in a community. Efforts to educate high school students and parents about the self-identification of depression and referral for treatment also show no clear effect. Actually screening students for symptoms of depression and suicidal thinking and making further evaluation and treatment available to students who screen positive for symptoms may be the most effective means of reducing suicide rates in the community. According to a study by the CDC in 2009, 16 percent of all children in grades nine through twelve have seriously considered suicide, and almost 10 percent report attempting suicide within the past year.[18]

Suicide is still the third leading cause of death for those aged 15 to 24 years old. That said, recent data indicate that reduction in adolescent suicide coincided with the introduction of more effective SSRI antidepressant medications, and some have suggested that improved treatment of serious depression in adolescents may be an important factor in this welcome trend. Many factors are at work, however, and much research into the causes of and solutions to suicidal thoughts and behaviors remains to be done before the startling epidemic of adolescent suicide over the last fifty years or so can be truly under control.

The Genetics of Mood Disorders

A s has long been recognized, mood disorders cluster within families. Dr. Emil Kraepelin, who more or less invented the modern concept of mood disorders, wrote in his landmark textbook of psychiatry about one family in which "of the ten children of the same parents who were both probably manic-depressive by predisposition, no fewer than seven fell ill the same way; of the five descendants of the second generation, four have already fallen ill."[1]

For many years, research on the genetics of mood disorders was hampered by foggy diagnostic criteria and a lack of laboratory methods to identify genes. But this is changing. Not only have psychiatrists become more skilled in the diagnosis of mood disorders, but the biochemical methods available to locate and identify genes on the human chromosomes have become tremendously more sophisticated. These developments will, sooner or later, lead to a better understanding of the genetic mechanisms of mood disorders, which will in turn lead to better diagnosis and treatment of these illnesses.

GENES, CHROMOSOMES, AND DNA

A brief discussion of the principles of *genetics*, the scientific study of the inheritance of biological attributes, is necessary before turning to a discussion of the heredity of mood disorders.

The patterns and rules of inheritance in living things were first described by Gregor Mendel, an Austrian monk who, over many years, performed elegantly planned and executed experiments with plants, mostly garden peas, in his monastery garden. Prior to Mendel's work in the latter half of the nineteenth century, it was thought that the traits of one parent were simply blended with those of the other parent in their offspring, who thus had traits that were intermediate between those of the two parents. Mendel discovered that this was not always or even usually true. He found, for example, that crossing a pea plant that produced tall plants with a pea plant that produced short ones (which he did by transferring pollen from one plant to the other) did not give rise to seeds that produced medium plants—that is, an intermediate form. Instead, Mendel discovered that *all* the seeds formed from this cross gave rise to tall plants (figure 15-1A). When he then crossed the offspring plants and planted the next generation of seed, exactly *three-quarters* of them produced tall plants and *one-quarter* produced short plants (figure 15-1B). There were no intermediate forms and no blending of traits. The offspring received either a "tall" inheritance or a "short" one—there were no "in-betweens." Mendel concluded that each parent contributed something that determined plant size, and these "somethings" were distributed to the next generation, determining plant size in that generation. These "somethings" are now called *genes*, the units of inheritance.

We now understand that genes are sets of instructions for building proteins. All plants and animals are constructed (in part) and operate by means of proteins. Myosin (muscle protein), hemoglobin (the oxygen-carrying protein of red blood cells), and collagen (the structural protein of skin and cartilage) are just a few examples. Even the nonprotein structural materials of the body, such as the calcium salts in our bones, depend on proteins. Proteins called enzymes direct the manufacture of bone from calcium salts by expediting certain chemical reactions. Many hormones are proteins (insulin, for example), and those that are not (such as testosterone and cortisol) are manufactured by protein enzymes. In earlier chapters, we discussed some members of the protein family that are of enormous interest to those studying mood disorders: G proteins and the receptors for neurotransmitters. All proteins are built according to specifications contained in genes.

For many years, it was believed that genes were proteins also, that genetic information was somehow encoded in protein molecules. But by the

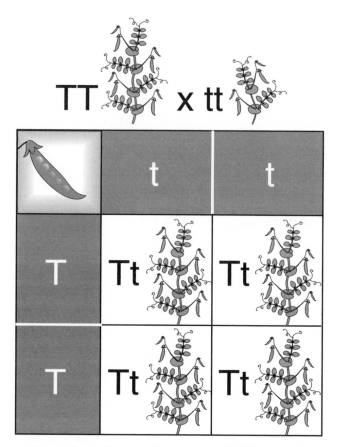

Figure 15-1 *Above*: Mendel's cross between a tall (*TT*) and a short (*tt*) pea plant. Each offspring (seed) receives two tallness genes, one from each parent plant. The seeds from this cross grew all tall plants because all received the *tall* gene (*T*), which dominates over the *short* gene (*t*). *Next page*: When the next generation of plants is crossed, one-fourth of them receive no *tall* gene (*T*) and therefore grow short plants.

mid-1940s, experiments with bacteria had proved that a far simpler family of biochemical compounds, called *nucleic acids*, contained the genetic information. In 1953, James Watson and Francis Crick published a paper in the British scientific journal *Nature* describing the structure of the most important of these compounds, deoxyribonucleic acid (DNA). With this discovery, the modern age of genetics had begun.

DNA molecules are long spiral chains, their links consisting of four simpler compounds called nucleotides. The four types of DNA nucleotides,

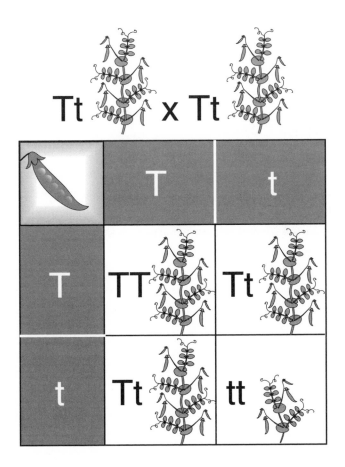

containing adenine, cytosine, guanine, and thymine (usually abbreviated as A, C, G, and T), are the elements of an elegantly simple code used to write out instructions for the manufacture of proteins. Just as you can write out a Morse code version of *Hamlet* using only dots and dashes, you can write out instructions for building hemoglobin, myosin, collagen, or any other protein using A's, C's, G's, and T's. That's what DNA does. You can think of the physical structure of a gene as the section of a DNA molecule that codes for one protein.

When the DNA molecule is doing its work in the cell, it is unraveled and stretched out and surrounded by a whole retinue of ultramicroscopic attendants busily reading the coded instructions and making proteins. When it's time for the cell to divide, another set of attendants carefully coil the DNA molecule into a compact cylinder and surround it with protective proteins to form the threadlike structures you probably looked at under the microscope in high school biology: the chromosomes.

GENETIC DISEASES

Sometimes the pathways from a certain gene to a certain protein to a certain trait or disease are easy to follow (although, in medicine, as we'll see, the understanding of these paths has usually been approached from the other direction: disease to protein to gene). Sickle-cell anemia is one disease for which the pathway from gene to disease is easy to follow. If you looked at the blood of a person with sickle-cell anemia under the microscope, instead of seeing the normal saucer-shaped red blood cells, you'd see abnormal crescent-shaped (sickle-shaped) cells. When scientists had the biochemical methods to look at the components of blood cells, they discovered that people with sickle-cell anemia had an abnormally shaped hemoglobin molecule, which tended to form abnormal chains within the cell, stretching the normally disk-shaped cells into the characteristic sickle shape seen under the microscope.

Because hemoglobin is easily purified, it was one of the first proteins whose structure was completely described (a feat that earned Cambridge University biochemist Max Ferdinand Perutz the Nobel Prize in 1962). Sickle-cell hemoglobin (hemoglobin S) was found to differ from normal hemoglobin by only a few atoms, the equivalent of a single substitution of one nucleotide for another in the gene of the DNA molecule. Because of a number of biochemical factors that made the hemoglobin gene especially accessible and easy to work with, scientists could pinpoint its location early on in the search for genes that caused human diseases. We now know that at one particular spot on the DNA molecule of persons who have sickle-cell anemia, there is an A instead of a T in the set of instructions. An abnormal hemoglobin molecule results from the reading of these incorrect instructions. The abnormal hemoglobin causes the abnormally shaped red blood cells, which block blood vessels and result in the symptoms of the disease. The pathway from abnormal gene to abnormal protein to abnormal cells to symptoms was completely described.

Genes have been identified and located for several other human diseases whose inheritance patterns indicate that they are single-gene illnesses. In some cases, this has been possible even though the identity or function of the protein that the abnormal gene codes for is unknown. Huntington's disease (or Huntington's chorea), the degenerative brain disease that afflicted folk-singer Woody Guthrie and his family, is one example. We know that the affected gene, the HTT gene, produces a protein called *huntingtin*, but we don't know what precisely the function of this protein is in the brain.

Scientists searching for "disease genes" now often use *linkage studies* to locate and identify genes. These studies take advantage of the fact that genes located close to one another on the same chromosome tend to stay together when the chromosomes undergo the process that apportions them into egg or sperm cells. In linkage studies, geneticists use gene maps that show the location of marker genes. First, DNA tests are performed on a blood sample of persons with the condition being investigated as well as on unaffected family members. Scientists then perform sophisticated mathematical analyses of the presence or absence of marker genes in affected and unaffected subjects to find an association between the condition and marker genes. If an association is found, the known location of the markers pinpoints the location of the gene for the condition. This method has been highly successful in locating the genes for several other single-gene diseases, including cystic fibrosis and Duchenne muscular dystrophy.

Studies have indicated that depressive disorders and bipolar mood disorders are probably related genetically at least some of the time. Serious depression is two to ten times more likely to occur among relatives of persons with bipolar disorder than in families of persons who don't have the illness. When we examine the family tree of persons with major depressive disorder, however, the data are not quite as clear; more persons with bipolar disorder than would be expected are found in some studies but not in others. This has been interpreted as indicating that when major depressive disorder shows up in families with bipolar disorder, the depressive illness is genetically similar to bipolar disorder, but that depressive illness in the absence of bipolar disorder in the family has more varied causes and may or may not share the same genes as bipolar disorder.

When several genes might be involved in an illness, the problem of gene identification becomes tremendously more complicated. And if the illness takes several forms or is difficult to diagnose, the task becomes monumental. Unfortunately, all of this applies to mood disorders. Most scientists looking for genetic causes of mood disorders agree that these are not one-gene illnesses like sickle-cell anemia or Huntington's disease. Mood disorders are caused, in all probability, by several different genes, perhaps as many as a dozen or so. The illnesses take many different forms and are sometimes difficult to diagnose.

In the late 1980s, several reports appeared that purported to link a mood disorder, specifically bipolar disorder, to specific regions of chromosomes. The most significant report was of an Amish family that seemed to carry a gene for bipolar disorder on one end of chromosome 11 (human cells have twenty-two pairs of chromosomes, numbered 1 through 22, and a pair of sex chromosomes). In this study, the researchers thought they had overcome at least one of the usual hurdles to finding a "bipolar gene." This particular family pedigree seemed to indicate Mendelian (that is, single-gene) inheritance at work. Even if several possible genes could cause bipolar disorder, this particular family seemed to pass on the disorder through only one gene. Mathematical analysis of previously identified DNA markers pointed to chromosome 11, and the statistical significance of the findings appeared solid. Zeroing in on a mood disorder gene seemed within reach.

These results were called into question within months, however, when another team of scientists took a look at the mathematical analysis. But it was the issue of diagnosis that ultimately scuttled this ambitious study. Several of the individuals who had been classified as unaffected when the data were originally collected developed symptoms of bipolar disorder later on. When the new numbers were crunched, the results fell apart completely.[2]

Linkage studies have pointed to several different locations on different chromosomes as possible sites for "mood disorder genes," but results are still preliminary. The most promising candidates currently are genes involved in creating a certain type of channel in the neuron. When a neuron gets a signal to release neurotransmitters (for example, serotonin or norepinephrine), the mechanism by which this occurs is quite complicated. It's not as simple as the electrical impulse directly shooting forth the chemicals. In fact, the impulse causes channels in the neuron to open and allow the entrance of calcium ions. As the concentration of calcium in the neuron increases, other chemical changes occur, leading to the release of neurotransmitters. In certain genome-wide studies, a particular gene, CACNA1C, has been closely associated with the development of bipolar disorder. Functionally, this makes sense—lithium, one of the oldest and best-studied medications used to control this condition, lowers the influx of calcium, essentially making the neurons less excitable. Although it would be silly to think that this one gene is responsible for all of bipolar disorder (in studies, most persons with the genetic mutation do not develop bipolar disorder), it is certainly reasonable to say that scientists may very well have found a strong risk factor for developing the condition.

Looking for genes involved in major depressive disorder has been even more challenging, because this disorder can be more difficult to diagnose. A 2014 review article examining "the nine published genome-wide association studies" for major depressive disorder found, in the authors' words, no significant genetic associations, a conclusion echoed in many of the papers and reviews of the field.[3] Studies of *childhood-onset* major depressive disorder, however, have demonstrated that this form of the illness is especially likely to run in families, suggesting that studies of the childhood-onset illness will prove the most useful for studying genes for major depression.

People who develop mood disorder symptoms most likely have inherited *several* genes that predispose them to these illnesses. There is even some thought that these are relatively common genes that many people carry without ever developing a mood disorder. Perhaps a certain number of genetic "hits" are necessary to make a person vulnerable to developing mood disorder symptoms, and perhaps certain environmental conditions are needed as well. Furthermore, genetics don't seem to tell the entire story of bipolar disorder.

Monozygotic twins are those sets of siblings who have exactly the same genetic information. Almost immediately after the mother's egg is fertilized (forming the *zygote*), it splits in half, forming two zygotes from the original one (*mono-*). Two separate eggs that happened to be fertilized at the same time result in *dizygotic twins*, that is, twins originally from two (*di-*) zygotes. Even in monozygotic twins, if one twin develops bipolar disorder, the second twin has only about a 70 percent chance of developing the condition—leaving 30 percent up to other factors, likely the environment. These findings and factors make the search for mood disorder genes all the more daunting.

WHAT WE KNOW

Until we identify specific genes and discover what proteins these genes code for, we can talk about the inheritance of mood disorders in only a general way. What we can say is that the children of persons with mood disorders have an increased risk of developing a mood disorder. Assigning a number to that risk is tough, owing to some of the same problems that have made the search for mood disorder genes so difficult, especially problems of diagnosis. But the risk appears to be several times that of the general population, around 10 percent, for those with a family history of the disease.

The risks in bipolar disorder can be quantified more precisely. The chance that a child whose parent has bipolar disorder will also develop bipolar disorder parallels the numbers above for mood disorders in general: the risk is about 10 percent, several times the risk for the general population. However, children of persons with bipolar disorder are also at a higher risk for unipolar (depression only) illness, and when you add this risk in, the percentages go up into the high twenties. This means that the children of persons with bipolar disorder have about a one in four chance of developing some kind of mood disorder and about a one in ten chance of developing bipolar disorder.[4]

Persons with mood disorders need to be alert to signs and symptoms of mood disorders in their children and get them into treatment if these signs appear. Although we may be uncertain about the details of the inheritance of these illnesses, we are not at all uncertain about the importance of early diagnosis and treatment.

THE SEARCH CONTINUES

Several factors make scientists optimistic about eventually discovering genes for mood disorders. In 1999, scientists of the Human Genome Project and Celera Genomics announced the "first draft" of the full sequence of human chromosomal DNA. Specifically, the pattern of A's, C's, G's, and T's in human DNA had been worked out. Based on this work, scientists can now perform multiple types of chemical analyses on an individual DNA strand to look for small or previously unknown mutations. Researchers can now look for single nucleotide polymorphisms (called SNPs, pronounced "snips"), changes in a single genetic base pair, across the entire genome.

But the number of identified genetic markers used in the linkage studies that *will* determine gene locations continues to rise. These markers, like signposts along the length of the chromosome, designate particular locations in the DNA molecule: the more genetic signposts there are, the easier it will be to find a particular gene. More precise diagnoses will also help, as will the study of larger family pedigrees and the development of technological advances—both biochemical methods and more powerful computers and software to do the mathematical analyses.

Even when genes are identified and tests developed that can look for these genes in individuals, predictions about who will develop symptoms will probably still be imprecise. Several genes are likely involved and genetics is unlikely to be the whole story. Environmental factors are probably operating to determine who will and will not be affected: psychological and perhaps physical stresses and traumas may be important. Some evidence suggests that viruses play a role in the development of some psychiatric disorders. So even when a gene or genes are identified and can be tested for, finding that a person has a mood disorder gene will probably mean that she has a much higher chance of developing symptoms than someone who does not have the gene, but that developing them is not a certainty—the risk is not 100 percent. This will raise many difficult questions about who should and should not be tested and who is entitled to know the test results (siblings? spouse? employers? insurance companies?).[5]

But finding the genes responsible for mood disorders may lead to new treatment approaches that will benefit everyone with these illnesses. Gene identification, and identification of the function of these genes or their gene products, will undoubtedly shed light on the biochemical basis of mood disorders. It may then be possible to design medications or other treatments based on knowledge about the causes of symptoms at the cellular or biochemical level—rather than stumbling on treatments by accident, as has been the case so far. This science is called *pharmacogenomics*. It is already widely used in the treatment of cancer and certain other conditions and is just beginning to be examined for use in psychiatry. Genetics research is one of the most challenging but also the most promising areas of investigation of mood disorders and could truly revolutionize the treatment of these illnesses.

Part IV

GETTING BETTER & STAYING WELL

K EEP IN MIND THAT DEPRESSION and other mood disorders of adolescence are not "cured" by any of the treatments discussed in part II of this book. We are getting better and better at treating these problems, but talk of cures is still years, perhaps even decades, in the future. In the meantime, however, many things can be done to promote good mental health. Millions of individuals who have been diagnosed with mood disorders are living happy, healthy, and productive lives. Unfortunately, many are not. These chapters are intended to help you and your adolescent maximize the chances of staying in the first category and out of the second.

But if you're looking for a simple list of do's and don'ts, we're afraid you will be disappointed. Instead, in chapter 16, we lay out some general principles that underlie the sorts of advice and recommendations usually given to patients in the doctor's office or clinic. We hope that after reading this chapter, you'll have a better understanding of why some of the do's and don'ts that you hear from the doctor and therapist are so important. We also address what the terms "doctor" and "therapist" actually mean and describe in detail the various types of mental health professionals so that you can make more informed decisions when seeking treatment for yourself or your child.

Adolescent depression doesn't just affect the teenager. Inevitably, family members are affected in countless ways, both directly and indirectly, and chapter 17 addresses this aspect of the illness. We go over what family members can do—and just as important, what family members cannot and should not try to do—to help their loved one who has a mood disorder.

In chapter 18, we've collected together some principles for dealing with emergencies and highlighted the types of emergency situations that, in our experience, patients and their families often fail to prepare for. It's so tempting to put off thinking about and planning for things that we hope won't happen; we emphasize in this chapter how important it is not to give in to this temptation and how easy it is to be prepared for emergencies.

Finally, we provide a short chapter that looks into the future and explores some of the exciting possibilities that may help us to better understand mood disorders. With this knowledge, it should be possible to improve the diagnosis and treatment of these illnesses, and perhaps one day, we might be able to cure them.

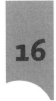

16

Strategies for Successful Treatment

This chapter presents some principles of good treatment for mood disorders in adolescents. In depression and bipolar disorder, perhaps as in no other kind of medical problem, treatment must be carefully tailored to each patient's needs. In part III of this book, we discussed how complex treatment can be when a person has complicating problems such as substance abuse or an eating disorder along with a depressive disorder. But even when these complications are not in the picture, the best treatment approach to adolescent depression is often a matter of much dispute. Experts frequently disagree on what should be considered standard treatments for these illnesses, which often makes treating patients more of an art than a science.

The prescription of medications for the treatment of adolescents with mood disorders is frequently off label (see chapter 5), and new medications are being touted all the time as useful for treating mood disorders years before they are approved, or even evaluated, by the FDA. How should parents make decisions about medication, about choosing a therapist, about hospitalizing their child? How can parents know whether their child is receiving the best possible treatment?

Because these illnesses are so complex and poorly understood, and because the treatment for each individual must be so, well, individualized, we cannot say which medication should always be tried first or tell you at what point a different or an additional pharmaceutical should be tried. We can lay out some principles that underlie successful treatment and that will usually, though perhaps only slowly, put your child on the road to recovery.

DIAGNOSIS, DIAGNOSIS, DIAGNOSIS

You've probably heard the old saw that the three most important factors in the real estate business are location, location, location. A similar saying would be well heeded by all mental health professionals: the three most important factors in the development of a treatment plan in medicine are diagnosis, diagnosis, diagnosis.

Occasionally, we speak to a parent who is interested in getting a consultation about her adolescent's problems and who tells us something like, "Our son has been diagnosed with major depressive disorder, ADHD, obsessive-compulsive disorder, generalized anxiety, separation anxiety, and a learning disorder, and his therapist is wondering if he's not developing a personality disorder, too. We want to be sure he's getting the proper treatment for all his diagnoses so that doesn't happen." Not infrequently, the adolescent is on a different medication for *each* of his "diagnoses" and is experiencing so many side effects that any kind of normal functioning is impossible.

This problem of accumulating diagnoses in psychiatry seems to us to be a direct result of the checklist method of the *DSM*, which lists different symptoms of various disorders and asks for several from this column and a few from that one to meet diagnostic criteria. It's easy to go through these various diagnostic checklists and, before you know it, compile a collection of "diagnoses" on the patient's chart. But this is not what the diagnostic process is all about. Rather, the job of the diagnostician is to put together *all* the information about symptoms, family history, medical history, and the findings on examining the patient in order to formulate a coherent diagnostic impression that pulls together the entire story—in *one* diagnosis if possible.

The overlap of the symptoms of bipolar disorder and ADHD is a good example of how this kind of diagnostic confusion can develop. Some of the symptoms of ADHD, such as impulsivity, impatience, disorganized thinking, and poor concentration, are also seen in adolescents with bipolar disorder. These are distressing symptoms that deserve attention, but more important, they deserve the right kind of attention. If they are an expression of the mood changes of bipolar disorder, then medication for ADHD won't help. (In fact, the medications used to treat ADHD, stimulants and antidepressants, may make things worse.) Adolescents with depression are especially vulnerable to irritable mood states that lead to behavioral problems, which might suggest an additional diagnosis of conduct disorder, oppositional defiant disorder, or again, bipolar disorder. We want to persuade you that giving these young people additional *diagnoses* often doesn't clarify their situation; it just confuses the picture. This is a central tenet that is critical to, but often forgotten in, the diagnostic process. If a child is diagnosed at age 7 with ADHD, but later on it is discovered that he had the symptom of inattention only because of a developing depression, some clinicians will diagnose him with ADHD and depression, rather than re-evaluating the picture in light of new evidence and removing prior diagnoses.

In the field of medicine, such errors of continuation without critical examination are called "chart viruses." These include statements, recorded in the diagnostic record, that may or may not continue to be true. In hospitals, these diagnoses lay indolent and spread throughout the hospital record, only becoming virulent when they seem most applicable. For example, a person asked while in the hospital how her headaches are doing, even though she hasn't had a headache for twenty years, may be experiencing the results of a chart virus. These chart viruses can infect the field of psychiatry as well—not through bad intentions, but rather through the reluctance to doubt previous clinicians' diagnostic acumen without becoming familiar with a case in depth.

When we see a patient, particularly a young one, who seems to have too many diagnoses, we wonder how much information gathering and critical thinking went into the diagnostic process. The same applies when there seem to be too many medications. Does the patient really have several different disorders that need treatment with different medications—an antidepressant for depression, a tranquilizer for anxiety, a mood stabilizer for "mood swings," and so on? Or have too many medications accumulated to treat various symptoms of one underlying disorder?

Making a diagnosis is the process of attempting to identify the one process that can explain all the patient's symptoms. There is a scientific principle called *Occam's razor,* named after the medieval theologian-philosopher who developed it, William of Occam (or Ockham). This principle states that the simplest explanation for a phenomenon is always preferable to a more complex one and is more likely to be correct. Obviously, a patient may have two or three or four different disorders that require different treatment approaches. But if all the symptoms can be understood as expressions of *one* disorder, treating that one will likely alleviate all the symptoms. Even when there are clearly several problems, formulating the relationship between them often makes the treatment plan priorities clear. For example, an adolescent may have a depressive disorder that is "fueling" eating disorder behaviors and precipitating alcohol abuse. These three problems all need attention, but unless the depression that is driving the behavioral problems is aggressively treated, treatment aimed solely at behavioral problems will not be very effective. We have seen many young people go through extensive (and expensive) substance-abuse rehabilitation programs only to relapse as soon as they leave the program, because a mood disorder underlying the substance-abuse problem was never identified and properly treated.

Such mistaken thinking can run the other way as well. An adolescent with recurrent substance-abuse issues and problems with stealing, who sometimes feels morose when the result of his actions run into him (for example, failing a test from partying the night before), may appear depressed at that time. This does not mean that he has a major depressive disorder and that a simple medication will cure all his problems. At the risk of sounding redundant, taking the time and energy to determine the true diagnosis and to develop a well-rounded and thought-out treatment plan is critical to success.

Another diagnostic pitfall is putting too much emphasis on psychological testing and rating scales. We occasionally see parents who have been told their child has a particular psychiatric diagnosis solely on the basis of psychological testing (meaning paper-and-pencil testing) or even of a score on some rating scale administered by someone. Frequently, parents think this is the definitive diagnostic procedure.

Sometimes parents insist that psychological testing be administered to their child as part of the assessment. Rating scales and psychological testing are helpful tools for the diagnostic process, but they are not sufficient in themselves to make a psychiatric diagnosis and are rarely the final answer to the diagnostic process. Many people think that a psychological test is like an x-ray: by means of trick questions and other mysterious methods, a psychological test will reveal what's "really" there, just as an x-ray can reveal a break in a bone that is otherwise undetectable. This is nonsense. In fact, the opposite may be true. One of us once treated a very bright child who, unfortunately, leaned toward the lazy side. He quickly found a particular quirk of many psychological tests, that those who do more poorly are asked fewer questions. He found that by intentionally flubbing examinations, the testing would be over sooner. The subpar results of his testing clearly did not match up with his clinical picture according to the psychiatrist, and so the test was quickly declared invalid for this child—in this instance, the acumen of the physician was far more important than any testing. Most psychological tests simply compare the way an individual answers standardized test questions with the way groups of others have answered the same questions, then assume that the individual being tested resembles the group whose answer patterns are closest to his answers. Psychological tests are useful for helping to identify personality styles quickly, but they don't do a good job of making diagnoses of psychiatric disorders. A depression rating scale might show that someone is depressed, and might even be able to say whether he is mildly or severely depressed, but it won't do a good job of determining whether he is suffering from major depressive disorder, bipolar depression, dysthymic disorder, or more minor temporary depression. And when a person is depressed, psychological tests aren't even that good at what they usually do best—revealing personality style—as the depression will alter the profile of answers. If the individual being tested isn't very honest in completing questions, the results will be practically meaningless.

This is not to say that psychological testing is never useful. It is accurate and precise in grading people on the mental abilities that we call intelligence. The same goes for tests of memory, some types of problem-solving abilities, and other types of mental functioning (again, this is true only as long as the person is answering honestly and putting forth her best effort). Paper-and-pencil tests are also helpful in screening large groups of people for the possibility that they might have some psychiatric disorder, identifying those who need a more in-depth evaluation for a particular problem (in psychiatry, these kinds of tests are globally known as *screeners*, because they screen for potential problems and hint at further evaluation but make no attempt at actual diagnosis). Various rating scales are useful in assessing changes in the severity of a disorder's symptoms over time. An individual who is suffering from depression might fill out a depression rating scale at each visit to the doctor or therapist, who can then make a more accurate assessment of progress, or lack of it, by following how the scores change over time.

The decision to give an adolescent an antidepressant cannot be made on the basis of a depression questionnaire. The diagnosis of attention-deficit/hyperactivity disorder cannot be made on the basis of a score on a screening test for ADHD. A battery of psychological tests is rarely necessary for the accurate diagnosis of mood disorders; a thorough psychiatric assessment is sufficient (and, as we make clear in the next section, necessary). Like any other laboratory test, a psychological test can answer a specific question that comes up during a psychiatric assessment (How intelligent is this person? How introverted is this person compared with most people?). But putting an individual through a battery of tests to "see what shows up" is not good practice.

One last warning about the diagnostic process. In a popular book for parents about mood disorders in young people, we read something to the effect that parents should be wary of a doctor who "takes too long to make a diagnosis." We are going to tell you the exact opposite: beware of a doctor or therapist who seems too eager to make a diagnosis, especially multiple diagnoses, too quickly. Adolescent mood disorders are often complex, subtle, and difficult to diagnose, especially if the adolescent has come to treatment reluctantly or has trouble describing how she feels. If there are complicating factors like substance abuse or behavioral problems, it may take several visits over a period of weeks or even months to get the best sense of how the various problems relate to each other and what the best treatment approach should be. Quick, confident diagnoses may feel satisfying—like an answer to the question "What is wrong with my child?"—but frequently lead to sloppy, ineffective treatments.

CHOOSING THE TREATMENT TEAM

We hope we have convinced you by now that adolescent-onset depressive disorders are serious illnesses that require serious treatment by specialists. The foregoing section should make it clear that the diagnostic process is vital in starting treatment on the right track. For that reason, a full evaluation by a board-certified psychiatrist experienced with adolescent mood disorders, or even better, by one specifically board certified in child and adolescent psychiatry, should be part of the treatment process as early as possible. There are places for many different types of professionals in the treatment of depression, but the point of entry should be with an individual who has the most training and experience in the treatment of psychiatric illnesses: a psychiatrist. Sometimes this is impossible, as busy psychiatric clinics will insist on initial appointments with a therapist, but the psychiatrist should still be involved as soon as possible.

Psychiatrists have attended medical school, where they have learned about the structure and biological functioning of the human body (anatomy and physiology); the biological chemistry of the body and the principles of treatment with medication (pharmacology and therapeutics); the methods for examining bodily and mental functioning by physical examination, mental status examination, laboratory tests, and medical imaging (x-rays, MRI scans [magnetic resonance imaging], and other methods); as well as the principles of treating medical and surgical diseases. After medical school, psychiatrists train in the specialty of psychiatry for four or more years, applying what they have learned in medical school about diagnosis and treatment of disease to the evaluation and treatment of psychiatric problems of all types. They also learn a set of therapeutic skills that are somewhat different from those of their colleagues in other medical specialties: the principles of psychotherapy. By studying the works of behavioral scientists—Freud, Erikson, and others—psychiatrists learn about the theories of psychology, and by counseling and doing therapy with patients, they learn the practice of psychotherapy. At the conclusion of their training, most psychiatrists apply for certification by the American Board of Psychiatry and Neurology. They undergo two full days of examination, including written tests and a review of cases on video. These exams are created by experienced psychiatrists who have themselves passed the tests. The examiners have a vested interest in making the tests challenging, for by certifying the performance of the test takers, they are welcoming them to the public as representatives of their own profession. Applicants who pass these rigorous examinations are said to be *board certified* in general psychiatry. This board certification is somewhat equivalent to obtaining a black belt in martial arts. Though it seems like the final point of mastery to the uninitiated, it is really only the beginning of the psychiatrist's practice and opens the door for further specialization. An old saying is this: "The path to black belt is about the creation of technique. The path beyond black belt is about learning to implement technique effectively."

Part of the requirements for general psychiatry training is that, at some point, trainees must spend two months working with children and adolescents. The form this work takes, however, can be highly variable. In the training program at Johns Hopkins Medical School, senior trainees work on child inpatient units for that time, receiving a good overview of the most intense forms of treatment. At other programs, however, first-year trainees (called interns) may only have to observe a clinical session once a week, leading to a thin experience. Alternatively, they may work in a college counseling center or somewhere similar, which certainly doesn't help them later when their patient is a 12-year-old. For psychiatrists interested in treating younger patients, a separate training follows their general psychiatry residency. Called a *fellowship*, it entails two additional years of working exclusively with children and adolescents. Psychiatrists who enter this realm of work train with a variety of experts in the diagnosis and management of conditions in young people, and in various settings. After completion of this work, the trainees are eligible for board certification in child and adolescent psychiatry, an additional full day of testing and examination.

One thing that many people don't know is that no authority requires psychiatrists to receive board certification for treating young people (and there are psychiatrists who decide simply that they'd like to add younger people to their patient list, without having any sort of experience in the matter). In fact, any licensed physician could in theory open a psychiatry practice with no experience at all. Therefore, it is up to you, as an educated consumer, to ask any potential providers about their training and board certification. You can also go to the American Board of Psychiatry and Neurology website (abpn.org) and look up the current status of any physician you are considering seeing.

Psychiatrist clearly signifies a specific type of training. The term *psychotherapist* more appropriately describes what someone does, rather than how the person was trained. The term describes anyone who does counseling and psychotherapy, regardless of professional education and training experiences. This can include psychiatrists as well as a number of other professionals. At times this number can seem daunting, and more professionals are becoming involved all the time. Just as physicians typically place letters after their names, such as MD (for medical doctor) or DO (for doctor of osteopathy), most if not all psychotherapists will have some letters after their names that tell you something about their educational and professional background.

A *psychologist* has a doctoral degree in the science of human behavior: psychology. Psychologists usually place PhD (doctor of philosophy) or PsyD (doctor of psychology) after their names. The field of psychology covers the whole range of mental life and functioning: language development, how visual images are represented in the brain, the neural basis of learning, crowd behaviors, and the accurate measurement of intelligence—these are only a few of the areas within this immense and fascinating field. Psychologists may focus on understanding normal human—or animal—behaviors through research (experimental psychology); on the dynamics of groups of individuals (organizational psychology); or on the treatment of psychological problems (clinical psychology). *Clinical psychology* is the subspecialty of the field involved in the treatment of emotional problems. Clinical psychologists usually have a four-year college or university degree plus several more years of education toward their final degree. Clinical psychologists have focused on theories of human behavior as they relate to the development of psychological problems, have learned various methods of psychological assessment (such as giving and scoring intelligence tests, personality assessments, and other tests of mental functioning), and have learned about psychological disorders and psychological treatments: counseling and psychotherapy. Doctoral-level psychologists must go on to complete a year of postgraduate training (called an *internship* or sometimes a *residency*), in which they gain practical experience in assessing patients and doing therapy. There is no national accrediting body for clinical psychologists, but most states require psychologists to be licensed in order to see patients. Typical licensure requirements include passing a written and sometimes an oral examination and having completed a degree and an internship in a program approved by the American Psychological Association.

After psychologists achieve their doctorate degree, they may go by the title "doctor," but this is not the same as being a medical doctor—most psychologists have no training in the practice of medicine. Although some states have given psychologists permission to prescribe certain psychoactive medications, we shudder to think of anyone taking a prescription written by a professional who has no training in how it might affect her physical body, or interact with other medications she may be taking. Many mental health professionals see the medications we prescribe as benign; they underappreciate how significant the effects of medications can be. A colleague of ours was asked if it might be possible to put together a training on the effects of medications for prescribing psychologists, so that they might begin to appreciate the medications' more general effects on their patients. He replied "There already is one. It is four years long and called medical school." We firmly agree.

Many, perhaps even most, psychotherapists have a degree in social work, a field that emphasizes the interactions of individuals with their various social groups: their family, community, and culture. A *clinical social worker* specializes in helping individuals, couples, or families with emotional or relationship problems by means of counseling and psychotherapy. Most clinical social workers have a master of social work degree (MSW), though some have a doctoral-level degree (DSW or PhD). Many social workers instead list their licensure after their names. An LGSW is a licensed graduate social worker. After additional training and supervision, a social worker may apply for licensure as a licensed certified social worker, or LCSW. After yet more training and experience, licensed certified social workers may apply for an added modification so that they are recognized as an LCSW-C (in which the last C stands for "clinical," the subspecialty of social work focused on direct mental health treatment of patients, much like clinical psychology). Social workers may apply for membership in the Academy of Certified Social Workers of the National Association of Social Workers after submitting professional references and passing a written examination if they have a master's degree in social work from an approved program and two years of supervised social work experience. The letters ACSW in a social worker's title indicate this membership. A more advanced certification is the diplomate in clinical social work, requiring additional years of experience and a more advanced examination. These social workers use the designation DCSW to indicate this certification. The American Board of Examiners in Clinical Social Work is another organization that issues a certification in advanced practice to social workers who have a master's degree in clinical social work from an approved college or university program, have practiced in the field for five years and seen clients under supervision for a certain number of hours, and have had colleagues and supervisors attest to their competency. Clinical social workers with this certification add the designation BCD after their name.

Some psychiatrists decide to limit their practice to psychotherapy and become primarily psychotherapists, though this is becoming increasingly rare. Individuals with degrees in nursing may also work as psychotherapists. Often they have taken advanced training in therapy to do so. Their names typically end in RN (registered nurse, an associate degree), BSN (bachelor of science in nursing, a college degree), or MSN (master of science in nursing). All these providers must practice under a licensed physician. Nurse practitioners (NPs) and doctors of nursing practice (DNP) are in many states able to practice independently. These professionals, in contrast to psychologists, have training in the physical body and in the medications they prescribe.

Some psychotherapists have a degree in counseling and have trained specifically in this field. *Counseling* differs from psychotherapy in its emphasis on giving advice and guidance rather than treating disorders. School counselors often have this kind of training background. A more advanced degree in counseling allows counselors to put LCPC (licensed clinical professional counselor) after their names. Alternatively, a counselor with a college degree may choose instead to get licensure as a marriage and family therapist (MFT). These therapists, as their title indicates, typically focus more on couples and family therapy than on individual therapy, so they are not as likely to work individually with children. Though there is certainly a lot of overlap between counseling and psychotherapy, counseling can be thought of as helping psychologically healthy individuals to improve and enhance their functioning and coping skills, and psychotherapy as treating individuals with psychological problems, helping them return to normal functioning. Clergy may get training in pastoral counseling and even pursue advanced training in psychotherapy. Pastoral counselors usually emphasize spiritual growth, of course, and the religious and ethical principles of their particular faith will guide their work with clients. The National

Board of Certified Counselors offers various certifications in counseling to individuals with diverse educational backgrounds.

Of all these professionals, the one with the most training and experience in the treatment of persons with illnesses is the psychiatrist. It's difficult to think of a reason that parents who suspect serious depression in their child shouldn't *begin* the evaluation with a psychiatric consultation, but this isn't always possible. Many busy mental health clinics practice an alternative structure in which a patient meets with a therapist or counselor first, before seeing the psychiatrist later. Typically this is because of the relatively small number of psychiatrists and is not ideal. This shortage of psychiatrists is a problem especially in child and adolescent psychiatric clinics. As of 2013, there were only about eight thousand board-certified child and adolescent psychiatrists in the country, about one for every ten thousand children. This severe deficiency of child and adolescent psychiatrists is a well-recognized phenomenon. We are obviously aware that not everyone will be able to find a board-certified child and adolescent psychiatrist in his area, but if possible, it really is the best option. If you are faced with a situation in which a child and adolescent psychiatrist is unavailable, be certain to question the psychiatrists you consider for your child about their training and experience with this age group. Far from being insulted, any qualified psychiatrist will be delighted to inform you, and impressed that you care enough and know enough to ask.

As with choosing any other physician, choosing a psychiatrist must usually start with a review of your medical insurance plan. Psychiatry is considered a specialty referral, and depending on your coverage, some phone calls and investigation will be necessary and will save a lot of headaches later. If your family is enrolled in a health maintenance organization (HMO), your child will be able to see only a psychiatrist approved by the plan and usually only with the referral of your child's primary care physician. If your family is covered by a preferred provider organization (PPO), the primary care referral may or may not be necessary, and you may be able to go outside the organization's list of approved doctors for psychiatric care at a lower reimbursement rate (you will be required to pay for a higher percentage of the fee).

HMOs and PPOs frequently outsource their mental health services. This usually involves contracting with a particular mental health practice or other provider group. Sometimes this group provides all treatment services; sometimes it provides certain services and manages others, contacting other providers and approving treatment with them upon receipt of written treatment plans. (Chapter 18 goes into more detail on these insurance issues.)

More and more psychiatrists, especially child psychiatrists, are opting not to participate in insurance plans because of all the paperwork and other kinds of extra work involved in dealing with managed care organizations. These practitioners require their fees be paid in full at the time of each visit; patients must then submit receipts to their insurance plan and deal with the reimbursement issues themselves. Unfortunately for individuals needing care, the best practitioners often fall into this category, making for some difficult financial decisions. Many psychiatrists will operate on a sliding scale, so it is always worth calling to inquire.

Once you know what your options are from an insurance standpoint, you can narrow your decision making. Pediatricians usually have a consultative relationship with a psychiatrist, or with a psychiatric practice, to whom they are confident referring their patients. This is perhaps the best referral source. If you live in a community where there is a university with a medical school, the medical school will have a department of psychiatry and usually a practice affiliated with the faculty. These clinics can often be the best resources available, but because of their value, they typically fill up quickly.

Some psychiatrists choose to provide a full range of services, including psychotherapy. Many do not, so it may be necessary to assemble a treatment team including both a psychiatrist and a separate psychotherapist. Choosing a psychotherapist will involve a similar process. It may be easier, in fact, because psychiatrists almost invariably have working relationships with several psychotherapists to whom they refer their patients. Because the fees of nonphysicians are usually lower than psychiatrists' fees, paying a psychotherapist out-of-pocket may be a bit more feasible. But remember that psychotherapy sessions are often weekly for many months, so the total outlay may be substantial. Given the devastating effects of untreated depression on the lives of adolescents, however, this is clearly a good investment.

Another factor to keep in mind when going through this selection process is that the management of mood disorders is a long-term proposition. One of the most important requirements for successful treatment is a *long-term* relationship with the treatment professionals. We cannot emphasize this point strongly enough. One of your goals in selecting a professional is to find someone who will be providing care for *years* to come.

Do not be afraid to get a second opinion about treatment. When your child doesn't seem to be benefiting from treatment, getting another clinician to take a fresh look at the diagnosis and treatment plan can be very helpful. The treating physician will not, or at least *should* not, object to a request for a second opinion. In fact, a physician often welcomes the opportunity to get some help and advice in managing a difficult case. Many university medical centers provide consultation services and often have mood disorder experts on the staff. The consultant will be able to help most if he can review as many treatment records as possible, so some advance work on your part, collecting records in preparation for a consultation, is well worth the effort. The consultant's report usually has a "have you thought of . . ." tone and will often raise questions rather than answer them, but this approach is usually the most helpful for the clinician who already knows the patient well and who will thus be able to incorporate new ideas into the treatment plan.

Beware, however, of the temptation to get too many opinions in a tough case. It is *not* useful to radically alter a treatment approach every month or so based on yet another consultant's recommendation; a parade of experts can result in more confusion than clarity.

The treatment of mood disorders must often adjust to the clinical situation: medications are started and stopped, added and taken away; therapy may need to be more intense and frequent at times, but the patient may be able to take a "vacation" when things are going well. Especially for adolescents, who often have trouble expressing their feelings and who sometimes are just plain oppositional, having a psychiatrist and a psychotherapist who know them well is a tremendous asset in their treatment.

Keep a treatment record for your child. This can be in chart form, as in figure 16-1, or it can simply be a diary. Record what medications your child has taken, including dates of starting and stopping, doses of medications, and blood levels (if they have been ordered). List any side effects or problems your child has had with the medications and also the treatment response.

This sort of list is extremely useful in many different situations: if there is a change in doctors, if you request a second opinion, or if treatment seems to have stalled for some reason and a detailed review of all treatments and responses is needed to see what hasn't yet been tried. Many parents assume that the physician is keeping a detailed history of each patient's prescriptions. The reality is that they probably are not. The information is available, but it may be embedded deeply within the individual progress notes and treatment records. Keeping your own succinct "cheat sheet" can be one of the most important contributions you make toward your child's improvement.

ELIMINATING PATHOLOGICAL INFLUENCES: MOOD HYGIENE

The word *pathological* is derived from the Greek word for "disease," and by *pathological influences,* we mean factors in the patient's environment that make illness symptoms worse or more difficult to treat. Just as an adolescent with diabetes must make lifestyle changes (including dietary changes, such as what to eat and the timing of meals) as a part of controlling blood sugar, so an adolescent with a mood disorder must make lifestyle changes to have the best control of mood symptoms. Sometimes this means a minor adjustment, sometimes a major overhaul, but this is *not* an optional part of the recovery process.

What is meant by *mood hygiene*? Simply put, it refers to practices and habits that promote good control of mood symptoms in persons with mood disorders. *Hygiene* is a word that we probably don't use as much as we should in medicine—and we certainly don't use it as much as we used to. Hygeia was the Greek goddess of health, the daughter (or in some versions of the story, the wife) of Aesculapius, the god of medicine (figure 16-2).

Hygiene, or *hygienics*, is the science of the establishment and maintenance of health (as opposed to the treatment of disease) and concerns itself with conditions and practices that are conducive to health. The hygienic conditions and practices we think of today are usually related to cleanliness, but the word has a much broader meaning. Johns Hopkins University's School of Hygiene and Public Health (founded in 1916; now the Bloomberg School of Public Health), University of London's School of Hygiene and Tropical Diseases (1924), and other such institutions were founded to study methods for the prevention of disease and for promoting and improving the

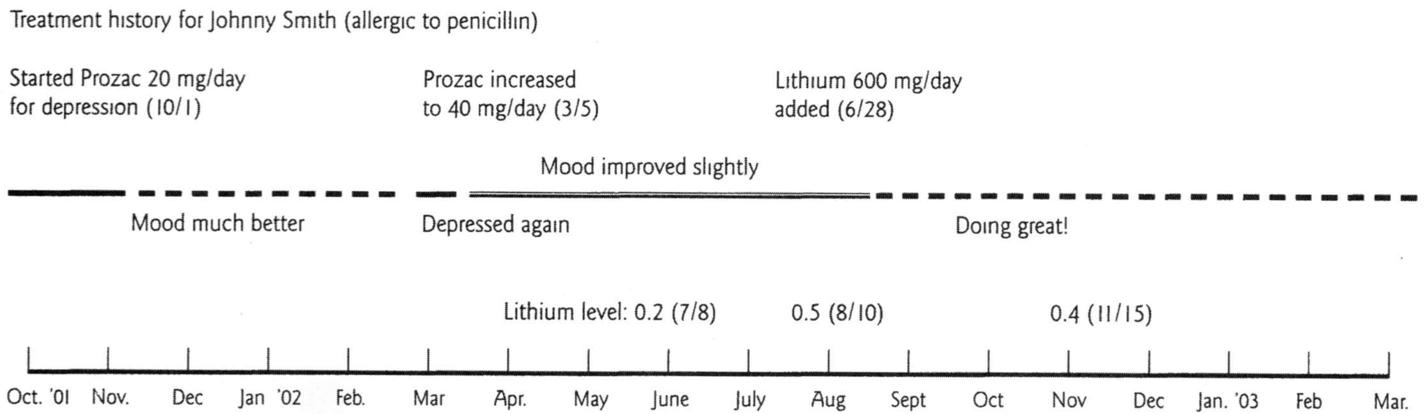

Treatment history for Johnny Smith (allergic to penicillin)

Started Prozac 20 mg/day for depression (10/1)

Prozac increased to 40 mg/day (3/5)

Lithium 600 mg/day added (6/28)

Mood improved slightly

Mood much better

Depressed again

Doing great!

Lithium level: 0.2 (7/8)   0.5 (8/10)   0.4 (11/15)

Oct. '01 Nov. Dec Jan '02 Feb. Mar Apr. May June July Aug Sept Oct Nov Dec Jan. '03 Feb Mar.

Figure 16-1 A sample treatment record. This sort of chart is extremely helpful in recording medication response, especially when a mood disorder is difficult to treat and multiple medications have been tried.

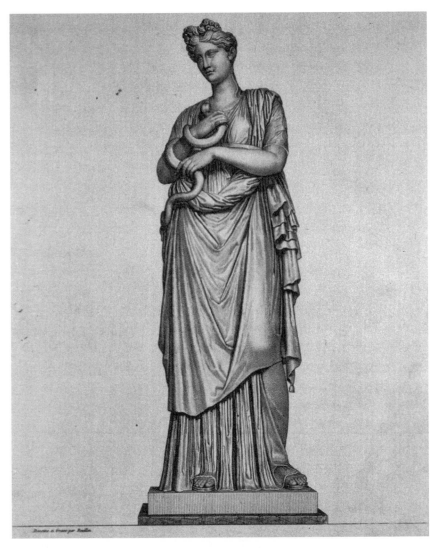

Figure 16-2 Hygeia. *Source*: Courtesy of the National Library of Medicine.

health of whole communities. Pre-dating these was the Mental Hygiene Association, founded in 1909 by former asylum inmate Clifford Beers (who probably had bipolar disorder) and now called the Mental Health Association; its purpose is to promote emotional health and well-being and to advocate for better and more available treatment for psychiatric illnesses.

Several areas of research on mood disorders, especially bipolar disorder, show just how important preventive measures can be for improving symptom control in these illnesses. Things like stress management and lifestyle regularity make a big difference.

One of the most astute students of the study of mood disorders, German psychiatrist Emil Kraepelin, noticed in his patients with mood disorders that early in the course of illness, their mood episodes often came on after a stressful event in their lives. In the final edition of his textbook of psychiatry (which was almost ten times longer than his first edition), published early in the twentieth century, Kraepelin noted: "In especial, the attacks begin not infrequently after the illness or death of near relatives . . . Among other circumstances there are occasionally mentioned quarrels with neighbors or relatives, disputes with lovers . . . excitement about infidelity, financial difficulties . . . We must regard all alleged injuries as possible sparks for the discharge of individual attacks."

Kraepelin was quick to point out that these events were triggers, not causes, and that "the real cause of the malady must be sought in permanent internal changes which . . . are innate." Kraepelin noticed, however, that later in the course of the illness, attacks occurred "wholly without external influences," and he proposed that at this later stage, "external influence[s] . . . must not be regarded as a necessary presupposition for the appearance of an attack."[1]

Research has shown that severe depressive episodes in many young persons are preceded by the death of someone close to them or by some other loss or difficulty. One study found a significant association between adolescent depression and repeated episodes of loss or significant separation during childhood. The most interesting finding of the study was the lack of an association between depression and only one episode of serious loss. *Multiple* events were necessary to trigger depression.[2] Studies on adults with bipolar disorder have shown that the initial and early mood disorder episodes are often related to psychological stresses, but that after several episodes, the illness can take on a life of its own, and episodes are more likely to arise spontaneously.

These sorts of findings are quoted to support the idea of a *kindling* phenomenon in mood disorders: a match held to a pile of wood may start a small flame that quickly dies out; but if the process is repeated often enough, a fire is kindled, and no more matches are needed. In a similar way, repeated episodes of psychological stresses, especially loss, set off a chain of events in vulnerable individuals (perhaps individuals who have inherited a genetic vulnerability to mood disorders) and an episode of depression results.

An interesting parallel in animals can be demonstrated by repeatedly giving animals small doses of stimulants, such as cocaine. Over time, animals become *more* rather than less sensitive to the stimulant, and repeatedly giving the same small dose causes *increasing* amounts of behavioral stimulation in the animal. A close examination of the brain cells of these animals, with and without the prolonged stimulant treatment, reveals that a certain gene that was not previously active has been turned on by the repeated stimulant exposure. This same gene can be made to turn on by stressing the animals (by depriving them of water, for example). This work with animals, showing that electrical and chemical stimulation as well as stress can bring about long-term changes in behavior (possibly through alterations in gene function), is thought by many experts to be highly relevant to the study of mood disorders.[3] The observation that anticonvulsant medications, which have "anti-kindling" effects, are highly effective in treating bipolar disorder is one piece of evidence cited in support of this line of thinking.

Several direct observations on patients indicate that kindling may occur in individuals with mood disorders. First, patients sometimes have more environmentally triggered mood episodes early in the course of their illness and more spontaneously occurring episodes later. Second, they sometimes have an acceleration in their illness as they age, with episodes occurring more and more frequently as time goes on. And third, mood episodes make patients more sensitive to stress than they might otherwise be and more likely to relapse. In a study of fifty-two adult patients with bipolar disorder followed up for two years, those who relapsed during the time of the study were much more likely to have experienced some stressful event. In this group of patients, those with a greater number of prior mood episodes were *more* sensitive to these stresses: they were more likely to relapse under stress, and they relapsed more quickly.[4] The worsening of depressive illnesses as individuals age has been demonstrated in many studies.

Given the observations that (1) psychological stress can make a person with bipolar disorder more vulnerable to having a mood episode, and that (2) as the person has more and more episodes, the symptoms can be triggered by smaller and smaller amounts of stress and adversity, then (1) *preventing* relapses of depressive episodes is extremely important, and

(2) individuals with mood disorders need to work hard to minimize situations of emotional stress in their lives.

After the development of antidepressant medications made the medical treatment of severe depression widely available in the 1960s, the question quickly arose of how long antidepressant medications should be prescribed. Although we do not have enough information yet to answer this question definitively, the information we do have supports long-term treatment.

Studies in adults clearly indicate that an antidepressant medication that has been effective for an individual with a serious depression should be continued for at least twelve months. We tell patients and parents of patients that anyone who has had a serious depression that has responded to treatment with an antidepressant medication shouldn't even consider discontinuing the medication for at least a year. For some individuals, this becomes difficult. Taking a daily pill, which may have minor but annoying side effects, to prevent a depression they do not feel, seems less and less important. For other individuals, however, it is a blessing. They recognize that they had been more depressed and more severely depressed than they had ever realized while in the grip of their illness. These are the individuals who had never really known what a normal mood was like before starting on medication. Not infrequently, these patients come to their appointment at the twelve-month mark ready to plead with us to let them *continue* taking antidepressant medication. They never need to plead. We are only too happy to let individuals who have been helped by antidepressant medication take it for as long as they wish. We are convinced by our personal experiences of treating many patients with mood disorders that every relapse of depression increases the chances of the illness becoming more difficult to treat. Research data clearly indicate that early-onset depression is a more severe illness. Some guidelines for the treatment of adults with depression recommend that individuals with the onset of severe depression before the age of 20 take medication indefinitely because of the higher probability of relapses.[5] Instead of asking, "Why should I continue taking antidepressant medication?" people who have had serious depression should probably ask, "Why *shouldn't* I continue taking antidepressant medication?" Individuals who have a family history of either bipolar disorder or recurrent major depressive disorder are especially well advised to take this long view.

For individuals with bipolar disorder, the evidence for the necessity of long-term treatment with medication is much more compelling. True bipolar disorder is clearly a relapsing illness that must be treated continuously and indefinitely to prevent the development of episodes. This piece of evidence re-affirms how essential it is to reach—and get—a correct diagnosis. Many irritable adolescents receive a misdiagnosis of bipolar disorder, which sets them on a path of taking medications for years of their lives that they may not have needed in the first place.

ADDRESSING SUBSTANCE ABUSE

The surest recipe for treatment failure in mood disorders is the continued use of intoxicating substances. For many reasons, adolescents with mood disorders must not drink alcohol and must certainly not use marijuana or other drugs.

The first is that alcohol and many drugs have direct toxic effects on the brain. In the chapter on substance abuse, we mentioned that drugs such as ecstasy have been shown to kill neurons. We know that chronic alcoholics develop memory problems and the wide-ranging decline in all mental abilities that psychiatrists call dementia. These damaging effects are more significant in the developing brain (neurons and their interconnections are still growing and developing in an adolescent's brain). Substance abuse in young people is thought to interfere with the brain's developmental process and may disrupt brain development in permanent ways that, currently, we can only guess at.

By altering the chemical functioning of the brain, substance abuse has effects on mood as well. Persons who abuse alcohol and individuals who are crashing from binges of cocaine or amphetamines can go through profound depressive episodes that seem to be directly related to the chemical effect of the intoxicating substances. It's thought that the high of getting intoxicated from alcohol or anything else results from a massive stimulation of the pleasure centers of the brain. These centers become exhausted and depleted of their chemical messengers because of this massive overstimulation, and this depletion is what is thought to result in the depressive crash and other mood changes that occur after intoxication. Thus, for individuals undergoing treatment for mood disorders, getting intoxicated interferes with the therapeutic process to relieve depression or to stabilize mood. A simple way of thinking about this is that getting intoxicated depletes the chemicals that antidepressants are trying to boost. We tell patients that drinking or getting high when under treatment for depression is like punching holes in a bucket that you are trying to fill with water—continued substance abuse makes treatment for a mood disorder pretty pointless.

We believe that abuse of marijuana is the most harmful in this regard, because it is the most insidious. Because marijuana is slowly absorbed into the fat cells of the body and slowly released between episodes of "getting high," crashes into depression and obvious withdrawal symptoms are less apparent. It's as if the usual time line for these phenomena gets so stretched out as to become almost undetectable. We've seen many persons with depression in all age ranges who refused to stop using marijuana because they were convinced that marijuana had no effect on their mood, or that it even helped their depression—and whose depressions never quite went into remission.

A striking lesson in how marijuana use can be a powerful obstacle to treatment of depression comes through in the story of a young adult one of us was treating for severe depression. We'll call him Joe.

▼ Joe's severe depressions only partially responded to aggressive treatment with medications. A combination of quite a few medications was the only approach that kept him out of the hospital, and he was nearly nonfunctional in his family life and was unable to work. Joe insisted that marijuana was the only thing that helped him feel better for a few hours, and he absolutely refused to give it up.

One day, I stepped into the clinic's waiting area to ask Joe to come back to the interviewing room for his medication appointment, but I didn't see him among the patients waiting for their appointments. There was a young man with a neck brace who looked familiar, but it seemed that Joe must have stepped out to the restroom. When I turned to the receptionist and asked if she knew where Joe had gone, the young man with the neck brace stood up. It was Joe, looking so bright-eyed, relaxed, and energetic that he was unrecognizable.

It turned out that Joe had been in a swimming accident that had injured him badly enough to put him in a rehabilitation hospital for nearly three months—long enough for the marijuana to get out of his system completely. His depression steadily improved over this period, and by the time he got out, most of his medications had been discontinued, and he was taking only a single antidepressant. We had both learned an important lesson about the connection between depression and substance abuse the hard way (though it had certainly been a lot harder on Joe).   ▲

Substance abuse is, in a way, a means of coping with adversity by retreating into getting high. As we explained in chapter 12, substance abuse also has the effect of crowding out other activities like school and family life. Another activity it crowds out is emotional maturation. Learning how not to get caught takes the place of learning how to trust and be trusted. Learning how to find and secure a steady supply of alcohol or drugs takes the place of learning how to make and keep healthy relationships with peers. Planning for the next high takes the place of planning for the next five years. Every mental health professional who has worked with adolescents can tell you that young people who are substance abusers seem to stop maturing emotionally at the age they started using. A 19-year-old who is able to stop using alcohol or drugs may have the emotional development of a 13-year-old, if that's when he started using. Catching up from this "maturity deficit" can take several years and a lot of therapy.

The most difficult issue parents face when their child is abusing substances is knowing how much intervention on behalf of the adolescent is helpful and how much is *enabling*. The concept of enabling a substance abuser has developed out of the treatment literature on alcohol abuse and refers to helpful actions on the part of family members that turn out to sustain rather than stop the substance abuse. The classic example is the wife of an alcoholic who calls her husband's boss to report that her husband is "sick" and won't be in to work, when he is actually hung over from his latest alcoholic binge. Rather than helping her husband, she is actually enabling him to escape the consequences of his alcoholism—consequences that could force him to face his problem and decide to get treatment. Parents must decide how much interceding on their child's behalf with school authorities, other family members, and even the police is helpful and how much is enabling their child to remain a substance abuser. Because adolescents have a difficult time appreciating the long-term consequences of their actions, this is an even tougher problem. At what point is "tough love" too tough? There are no easy answers. In his powerful account of his daughter's struggle with alcoholism, Senator George McGovern writes, "The trouble with waiting for people to 'hit bottom' is that they may do so only after they have destroyed their lives or the lives of others."[6] (More on this dilemma in the next chapter.)

ADOPTING A LIFESTYLE THAT PROMOTES MENTAL HEALTH

Just as physical stress is to be avoided by persons with certain physical problems, psychological stresses need to be identified and addressed by individuals who suffer from mood disorders. Although most of us have little control of when and how stress and conflict come into our lives, we sometimes have *some* control, and we can learn how to better manage the stress and conflict we can't avoid—and here we will put in another plug for counseling and therapy. Serious, *vigorous* attention to any ongoing sources of significant stress is critical in the management of mood disorders. It's no accident that family therapy is so often recommended as an adjunct treatment in adolescent mood disorders. Numerous clinical studies show that ongoing family conflict is a major risk factor for relapse of depressive disorders in adolescents.[7] Relationship difficulties, too much advanced coursework at school, an overly ambitious schedule of extracurricular activities—all these things can make for too many demands, too much stress, and can be risk factors for relapse of the mood disorder.

Adolescence is a time of developing lifestyle habits that will last a lifetime. Putting things off until the last moment invariably raises stress levels. Eliminating procrastination as a way of dealing with things goes a long way toward eliminating a lot of stresses. A growing body of research supports the notion that external regulators like regular sleep and activity schedules help with mood stability. *Establishing and sticking to a personal schedule* is essential. Establishing regular times for going to bed and getting up in the morning—seven days a week, if possible—is highly recommended. Adolescents need more sleep than adults, not less. For many 12 to 18 year olds, nine to ten hours every night is optimal (though rarely possible). Research on sleep shows that many other lifestyle factors contribute to or detract from good sleep. Adolescents might consider cutting caffeinated beverages out of their diet completely, or at least making a habit of not drinking caffeine-containing soft drinks or coffee or tea after noon. Heavy meals late in the day should be avoided. Regular exercise has been shown to benefit sleep and has many other benefits besides, on blood pressure, for example. These factors are even more important for adolescents with mood disorders because of possible medication side effects on appetite and energy level. Several medications increase appetite and can be mildly sedating at first. Attention paid to healthy diet and exercise habits will go a long way toward improving energy level and avoiding unwanted weight gain. Consultation with a nutritionist can be helpful, and developing an exercise program through the physical education department at school is often an option.

It is impossible in these few paragraphs to distill this process of taking stock of personal conflicts and stresses and to detail the kind of individual attention it takes to deal with them. There's no list of helpful hints or do's and don'ts that we can give you here. Rather, we are recommending *serious examination* and *fundamental change.* This change may involve something as minor as cutting back on participation on a team or as major as changing schools. Adolescents face many important decisions: decisions about selecting a high school and a college, after-school jobs and career paths, and for older adolescents, moving away from home and sometimes even getting married. These decisions need to be considered even more thoughtfully and carefully for those with a mood disorder. Counseling and psychotherapy are an invaluable help in sorting through options and making these decisions.

The Role of the Family

When a child is miserable, parents want to make things better. Small children aren't very hard to cheer up. They will delight in a little toy surprise, a trip to a fast-food restaurant, helping mom or dad in the kitchen or with washing the car. But when an adolescent is seriously depressed, no amount of cheering up can help. Worse, when the symptoms of depression take the form of oppositional behavior and irritability, parents may discover that their child has become a hostile stranger who seems intent on tearing the family apart. Parents may be frightened and angered to discover that their son or daughter is drinking, using drugs, or engaging in other dangerous behavior. It's easy to be so paralyzed by fear and anger that ordinary decisions become overwhelming.

As in any illness, the role of the family includes support, understanding, and encouragement of the person who is ill, and the role of the parent includes nurturing, protecting, and supervising. The first step in being able to provide this kind of support is understanding some important facts about the illness. It's also vital to get the help and support *you* need to be there and be strong for your child.

RECOGNIZING SYMPTOMS

Never forget that someone with a mood disorder does not have control of his mood state. People who do not suffer from a mood disorder sometimes expect the person who does to be able to exert the same control over his emotions and behavior that they themselves are capable of. When we sense that we are letting our emotions get the better of us and we want to exert some control over them, we tell ourselves things like "snap out of it," "get a hold of yourself," or "pull yourself together." We are taught that self-control is a sign of maturity and self-discipline. We are indoctrinated to think of people who don't control their emotions well as being immature, lazy, self-indulgent, or foolish. But you can only exert self-control if the control mechanisms are working properly, and in someone with a mood disorder, they are not.

People with mood disorders cannot "snap out of it," as much as they would like to (and understand that they *desperately* want to do so). Telling a depressed adolescent something like "pull yourself together" is simply cruel; in fact, it may reinforce the feelings of worthlessness, guilt, and failure already present as symptoms of the illness.

The first challenge facing family members is to change the way they look at behaviors that might be symptoms of the illness—behaviors like not wanting to get out of bed, being irritable and short tempered, or being "hyper" and reckless or overly critical and pessimistic. Our first reaction to these sorts of behaviors and attitudes is to see them as laziness or meanness or immaturity and to be critical of them. In a person with a mood disorder, this almost always makes things worse: criticism reinforces the depressed adolescent's feelings of worthlessness and failure, and it alienates and angers the hypomanic or manic individual.

Keep in mind, however, that these behaviors are symptoms primarily when individuals are in the midst of an episode of a mood disorder. Our response to some of these same behaviors in adolescents who are not experiencing an episode should not necessarily be the same as when they are. We have both treated patients who are perfectly well (what we would term *euthymic*) but claim to suddenly develop a deep depression if and only if they are asked to participate in things they would rather not do; they then return to euthymia after the stressor is relieved. One of us even treated a patient who eventually admitted that there was an upside to being depressed. As she put it, "My boyfriend is only nice to me when I'm depressed," meaning that he took care of her and did not expect her to act or function independently. Just as an accurate diagnosis is essential in putting together an effective medical and psychiatric treatment plan, it is also critical in creating a "family" treatment plan that helps you best address behaviors that may—or may not—be symptoms of an underlying illness.

This is a hard, but critical, lesson to learn: don't always take behaviors and statements at face value. Learn to ask yourself, before you react, "Could this be a symptom?" Little children frequently say "I hate you" when they are angry at their parents, but parents know that this is just the anger of the moment talking and that these are not their child's true feelings. Irritable, depressed adolescents will say "I hate you" too, but this is the illness talking, an illness that has hijacked their emotions. The depressed adolescent might also say, "It's hopeless. I don't want your help." Again, this is the *illness* and not your child rejecting your concern.

GETTING INVOLVED IN TREATMENT

Frequently, parents don't know what role to take in their child's treatment, and sometimes the seemingly contradictory messages given by therapists and psychiatrists can be confusing. Be interested in your child's life, but not nosy. Be assertive and set limits, but do not be overly controlling. Be sensitive to changes in your child's behavior, but don't jump to conclusions. Inform the therapist of all you observe about your child, but don't expect the same in return. Respect your child's privacy, unless you're afraid for her safety! In many ways, negotiating the role of the parent in treatment is similar to negotiating the role of the spouse in a relationship, and it requires the same amount of careful consideration, and possibly continual adjustment. Although we go through some general guidelines here (and into some specifics especially around the delicate nature of confidentiality), your role as parent is best understood through a continued discussion with both your child and your child's therapist.

Different therapeutic modalities will require different levels of involvement. In discussing medication effects, parents and child will be expected to report on everything and anything they've observed that may be helpful or a side effect. Cognitive-behavioral therapy is similar in that parents can participate in the treatment, both in the office and at home, when their children are trying to use the skills they've learned. In psychodynamic treatment, on the other hand, parents may learn to expect a closed door with very little, if any, information at all. Different phases of treatment will also require different levels of involvement. During standard outpatient therapy during a relatively stable time, parents may be able to take a small step back. Should an emergency develop or a hospitalization be required, however, parents sometimes have to take time off from work due to the necessary level of involvement.

Every individual's health care information is protected from unauthorized access by a law entitled HIPAA (the Health Insurance Portability and Accountability Act of 1996). In short, this law makes the identifiable health information of each individual his or her own property. There are exceptions to this, of course. For the purposes of this discussion, the health information of children is the property of their parents or legal guardians. Certain states have made exceptions to this rule in regards to reproductive and psychological health, but generally, parents have the legal obligation and the right to consent to or deny psychiatric treatment and medications for their children under the age of 18. The details of said treatment, however, are a little murkier. Parents have a right to ask questions and get answers about their child's treatment, particularly medications. The intimate details of individual therapy sessions, however, are expected to be confidential between the therapist and patient, provided that there is no risk to the child's health or safety. If, for example, a patient stated that she was planning on committing suicide, the clinician would legally have no choice but to tell the parents. However, should the parents ask, "Is Sally still dating Tommy? She won't tell me," the clinician will usually decline to answer or, in the best-case scenario, encourage that sort of a discussion with all parties in the room. Most clinicians lay out these delicate ground rules about privacy issues at the beginning of treatment.

On the other hand, after age 18, the patient is the only person who has the right to his own treatment information and records, a change that can feel both abrupt and shocking to parents. Psychiatrists experienced at dealing with these matters will always make parents aware of this change well before the child's adulthood (years before, preferably) and will attempt to negotiate the terms of this adulthood with the child. Unfortunately, this change can come at exactly the time when parents are most curious about the activities of their children, who may even have moved to college or elsewhere. The therapist cannot answer simple questions from parents, such as "Did Mark come to his appointment today?" Doing so would be considered a breach of ethics, unless the patient has explicitly signed a legal document giving the clinician permission to discuss his treatment with his parents.

Fortunately, many therapists are savvy enough to directly involve parents in the treatment of their children. Many clinicians will see parent and child together, at least initially. As the child ages, more and more time is spent with him alone, although the parent is usually brought in toward either the beginning or the end of the session for more information and discussion. Some clinicians will also give parents their own time to discuss their child's life; however, even these individual sessions must follow the confidentiality rules described above. Remember, your child is the patient. He should be given all (well, most) of the same rights you would expect from your own treatment provider. Just as you would probably not appreciate your therapist telling your child all about your own session, so would your child appreciate some degree of confidentiality in his. Your own individual meetings with his therapist should not be seen as your chance to "see into his mind," or to find out all the little details about his life that he wants to keep private. Quite the opposite! These are chances to discuss any changes you have observed and how you should best handle them.

Even though you are expected to respect your child's privacy in therapy, you are also expected to participate in the treatment as far as it affects your relationship with your child and your interactions. Your child's treatment isn't exactly like seeing another type of physician. You should not expect to drop them off at the door and pick them up in an hour. Also, don't ask the therapist or psychiatrist to confront your adolescent about behaviors you've observed if you can't be there to back up your observations. We find that separate conversations with the patient and the parents about these sorts of issues often become "yes, he did—no, I didn't" sessions that are simply not helpful for anyone. Going along with your child to doctor's appointments and sharing your observations and concerns during the visit *in your child's presence* eliminates miscommunication and ensures that everyone—therapist, parents, and patient—is operating with the same set of information. This can at times be uncomfortable, but that is exactly what therapy is for—making room for difficult discussions and issues so that they can be resolved productively.

Above all, parents should resist the impulse to bring the therapist to "their side." Conversations in which parents plead, "You can't tell her I know about this, but…" or "Don't tell her but…" can make ongoing therapeutic work difficult, to say the least. In general, children are very sensitive to perceived slights, and any feelings that their therapist and their parents are conspiring against them can ruin any further work that might have been done.

Parents sometimes err on the side of not being involved enough in their child's treatment, however, for fear of being a "tattle-tale"; they assume the clinician will notice the same things they've noticed about changes in moods or behaviors. One of the most valuable ways in which a family member can help in treatment is to provide a clear, undistorted view of the situation to the clinical team treating the adolescent. In our experience, family members are frequently the first to pick up on subtle changes in behaviors and attitudes that signal the beginnings of a relapse. We don't know how many times we have seen a patient in the clinic or even in the emergency room who has reassured us that she was feeling fine, whose behavior and mood seemed normal, whom we sent on her way, making a note in the chart that she was doing well, only to receive a panicked phone call from a parent or other relative a few hours later. "Didn't she tell you that she's lost ten pounds?" "…hasn't slept in three nights?" "…got suspended from school?" Contrary to popular belief, psychiatrists cannot read minds! Communicate your concerns openly, sincerely, and supportively—almost anything that might otherwise seem intrusive can be forgiven. Your goal is to have your child trust you when she feels most vulnerable and fragile. She is already dealing with feelings of deep shame, failure, and loss of control related to having a psychiatric illness. Be supportive, and yes, be constructively critical when criticism is warranted, but above all, be open, honest, and sincere.

Don't ask the psychiatrist or therapist to make parental decisions, and don't abdicate parental authority to the treatment team. The professionals are there to make recommendations and suggestions but not to make family decisions. Saying something like "you can't go to Tampa on spring break because the doctor said you can't" gives the adolescent the message that the parent has ceded authority to the professionals or, even worse, is incompetent to make decisions. It may cut off debate and argument in the short run but will inevitably backfire, actually encouraging defiant behavior. Remember that one of the goals of family therapy is to clarify roles and *your* parental authority. Adolescents need to know and to feel that their parents are in charge in the home. Your psychiatrist will back this up. When our patients ask us if something is OK to do, we always say that they will have to discuss it with their parents. In psychiatry, there's a phenomenon called *splitting*. It's something that every parent will be familiar with. The most common situation is that a child will ask one parent for something (say, staying out past curfew) and, if she doesn't get the answer she wants, ask the other parent. A more wily adolescent may start playing one side against the other or using other tools to manipulate the situation. "Mom said I could stay out late as long as you don't need the car," or "Dad's so strict! It drives me crazy. He won't even let me stay a half hour later! Can you believe that? Of course you can. You're cool, not like dad." For parents, our advice is always to be on the same page.

The exact same thing can happen in treatment. Parents will ask us if it's OK, from a mood disorders standpoint, to change their child's curfew, or to go on a trip. In the absence of a true psychiatric emergency, our reply is almost always, "What do *you* think?"

SAFETY ISSUES

Never forget that mood disorders can occasionally precipitate truly dangerous behavior. The dark specter of suicidal violence haunts those with serious depression, and rageful irritability can lead to frightening assaultive behavior. Violence is often a difficult subject to deal with, because the idea is deeply embedded in us from an early age that violence is primitive and uncivilized, a kind of failure or breakdown in character. Of course we recognize that the person in the grip of psychiatric illness is not violent because of some personal failing, and perhaps because of this, people sometimes hesitate to admit the need for a proper response to a situation that is getting out of control—when there is some threat of violence from the adolescent, toward himself or others.

Although family members cannot and should not be expected to take the place of psychiatric professionals in evaluating suicide risk, it is important to have some familiarity with the issue. As we've mentioned, young people who are starting to have suicidal thoughts are often intensely ashamed of them. They often hint about "feeling desperate," about not being able to "go on," but may not verbalize actual self-destructive thoughts. It's important not to ignore these statements but to clarify them. Don't be afraid to ask, "Are you having thoughts of hurting yourself?" People are usually relieved to be able to talk about these feelings and get them out in the open where they can be dealt with. But they may need permission and support to do so.

Remember that the period of recovery from a depressive episode can be a time of especially high risk for suicidal behavior. People who have been immobilized by depression sometimes develop a higher risk for hurting themselves as they begin to get better and their energy level and ability to act improve. Also, patients having mixed symptoms—depressed mood and agitated, restless, hyperactive behavior—may be at higher risk of self-harm. In fact, there is some evidence that mixed, or dysphoric, mania is the most dangerous mood state in this regard.[1]

Another factor that increases the risk of suicide is substance abuse, especially alcohol abuse. Alcohol not only worsens mood, it lowers inhibitions. People do things when drunk that they wouldn't do otherwise. Increased use of alcohol increases the risk of suicidal behaviors and is definitely a very worrisome development that needs to be confronted and dealt with.

The development of serious suicidal risk calls for action. Have an emergency plan and be prepared to use it. Involve your child and, if possible, the therapist or psychiatrist in developing this plan so that everyone is on the same page and there are no surprises. Don't hesitate to invoke involuntary commitment procedures if you are really worried and your child is not cooperating with the need for evaluation.

A less frequent but nevertheless real risk of violence is the violence toward others that can occur in mood disorders. Friends and family members should not hesitate to call for police help if they feel threatened. "What will the neighbors think?" should not be a concern when anyone's safety is at risk. If the situation is becoming dangerous, don't call the psychiatrist's office or the local emergency room—dial 911. Police officers are accustomed to dealing with psychiatrically ill individuals. They know safe physical restraint techniques, and they will be familiar with psychiatric emergency services in the community. In our experience, police officers will have the same goals you do in the situation: transporting your child quickly and safely to the appropriate health care facility so that he can receive proper treatment.

ARRANGING HOSPITALIZATION AND INVOLUNTARY TREATMENT

Every community has laws and procedures to safeguard individuals who are unable to care for themselves. Laws allowing the removal of children from the care of parents who are abusing them are the most obvious example. Another set of laws allows the treatment of individuals for psychiatric illnesses against their will in certain circumstances. One of the most difficult things parents might be called on to do for their child with a mood disorder is to sign for hospitalization over the child's protest or to initiate involuntary treatment or commitment.

The laws governing the admission of minors to psychiatric facilities and the involuntary commitment laws for adults are usually state laws, so they vary from one state to another; in addition to these state-by-state variations, local procedures can differ from community to community. This means that we can't provide a step-by-step procedure here, only general principles—but in our experience, it's not the procedures that confuse people but the general principles, so we think a brief discussion of this matter is worthwhile.

There are generally two types of admissions to the hospital: voluntary and involuntary. In nonemergency situations, parents must *consent* to the hospitalization. This gives them the legal right to voluntarily admit their child to the hospital. Part of the consent is also the right to refuse to consent—that is, to decline an admission. In some states, minors of a certain age are given the right to consent to or to refuse their own psychiatric treatment independent of their parents' wishes. Other states do not consider the wishes of the minor, relying solely on the parents' judgment. A third option exercised in some areas is to ask the minor to *assent* to this decision. This means that the minor agrees with her parents' decision to have her admitted. Minors cannot admit themselves if the parents do not first consent. Similarly, minors can refuse to assent (that is, they can *dissent*), in which case a judicial process of some kind is typically initiated to protect the rights of the minor. This process is similar to that for minors admitted involuntarily to the hospital. It is to prevent a parent from dealing with a troublesome child by simply signing her into a psychiatric hospital. Thus, the admission of a minor to a psychiatric hospital, though sometimes technically a "voluntary" procedure, might involve a judicial hearing similar to those held in the case of involuntary commitments (sometimes this is true even if the adolescent is willing to be in the hospital).

Law and legal procedures governing the provision of psychiatric treatment (or any kind of medical treatment, for that matter) against a person's stated wishes are based on the knowledge that, first, an individual whose judgment is immature and unformed cannot make sound decisions about medical treatment, and second, an adult whose judgment is clouded by the symptoms of an illness often does not make the same decisions about treatment that he would make if his judgment were not impaired. The delirious motor vehicle accident victim who has suffered massive blood loss may moan, "I want to go home," as he loses consciousness on the stretcher, but the ER team will ignore such a statement and proceed to do what they have to do to save the person's life. It is presumed that if the person were alert and thinking clearly and understood the implications of "going home," he would not make such a request. No one would ask a screaming toddler for written permission for a needed blood test. Similar principles underlie psychiatric commitment law: treatment is given to persons against their will if immature or clouded judgment prevents them from making good decisions about their treatment. Minors fall into this category. Depressed older adolescents may feel so hopeless that they think treatment has no chance of helping. Thinking processes in mania can be so disorganized and scattered that seeking out and cooperating with treatment is not possible. In either case, there are mechanisms to get needed treatment for persons whose immaturity or psychiatric symptoms blind them to the need for it.

Fortunately, these laws also have safeguards built in to prevent confinement in a psychiatric hospital for the wrong reasons. Decades ago, it was easy to invoke commitment law, often requiring only the signature of a relative or family physician to hospitalize a person for weeks or months, even years. People were hospitalized for all kinds of bogus reasons, and serious abuses of individual rights occurred. Laws became much stricter in the 1960s and 1970s to prevent these abuses. The main change was the addition of *dangerousness* as a commitment criterion. Unless an individual's behavior is truly dangerous to self (usually meaning suicidal behavior) or others, the person cannot be committed for involuntary psychiatric treatment. In the case of minors, the need for and appropriateness of the level of treatment are the sorts of criteria used.

Requests or petitions for psychiatric hospitalization do not necessarily mean that the person who is alleged to be psychiatrically ill will be hospitalized. Parents cannot simply sign a child into a facility; only a doctor can admit someone to a hospital. A parent's request for admission or involuntary commitment usually allows the young person to be transported to an emergency room, where a physician will make a decision about hospitalization. The child may be released if she does not meet legal criteria for admission or commitment.

Involuntary commitment is a serious legal procedure in which an individual is confined against his will and temporarily loses some rights of self-determination. For this reason, the law and the courts take involuntary psychiatric treatment very seriously, and many safeguards against abuses are built into the procedures. The person requesting an involuntary commitment must usually appear at the local courthouse or police station to give information and, in some jurisdictions, must make a sworn statement before a judge or magistrate. Parents will be asked for specific and detailed information about their child's behaviors. This is often frustrating for those trying to get help for their loved one. They may feel that being asked a lot of questions is uncaring, or that someone is questioning their judgment or their motives. It's important to remember that in the days when individuals could be confined to psychiatric hospitals simply because a relative or a doctor "thought it was best" for them, significant abuses of civil rights resulted. With serious attention on the part of the issuing magistrate or judge to documenting the facts and a close questioning of the need for psychiatric admission for minors and involuntary treatment of adults, we know the system is working.

Some form of judicial review (a *commitment hearing*) occurs at some point in the process (usually a few days after hospitalization), at which a judge or hearing officer determines that the admission procedure was done properly and legally. Although this is a legal proceeding, it is not a big courtroom scene. Usually a conference room in the hospital is used, only a few people are present, and the proceedings are kept confidential (not a matter of public record). The patient is allowed legal representation—in fact, an attorney will be appointed if the patient does not have one. As noted above, in some jurisdictions, even when both parents and child agree to hospitalization, a similar hearing occurs to safeguard the rights of the minor.

Involuntary commitment for psychiatric treatment does not usually affect people's other legal rights. This is changing, though, and certain states now forbid the possession of firearms to anyone who has had an involuntary hospitalization (sometimes for a limited time, such as five years, and sometimes for life). This change may have rather serious implications for anyone interested in a police or military career and is worth investigating. Other rights, such as wills or other legal instruments the committed person has executed, are not invalidated, and patients do not become legally "incompetent" in other areas. Hospitalization and treatment are the only issues that are addressed in commitment hearings.

We are aware that the topic we're discussing here is frightening. It might seem that a person's liberty and the right of self-determination can be taken away all too easily. At the risk of sounding glib, however, we want to reassure readers that involuntary commitment of an individual is *not* a quick and easy procedure. On the contrary, in our experience, most people are surprised at how difficult it is to invoke these laws, how many safeguards are built into the procedures, and how seriously the strict interpretation of the laws is taken by everyone involved. These laws have been carefully written in the interest of helping, not simply confining, people with severe psychiatric illnesses. In our experience, they are effective at doing just that.

GETTING THE SUPPORT *YOU* NEED

It is important that family members recognize their own need for support, encouragement, and understanding in dealing with adolescent mood disorders. Mental health professionals go home every day and leave behind their work of dealing with psychiatric illnesses, an option that most parents and other family members do not have. Dealing with a seriously depressed adolescent day after day and living with a frequently irritable, cranky teenager can be frustrating and exhausting. The changes and unpredictability of the moods of someone with a mood disorder intrude into home life and can be the source of severe stress in family relationships, straining them to the breaking point.

Perhaps the most difficult challenge is that posed by an adolescent with a mood disorder who is consistently resistant to getting treatment. The most astonishing learning experience for medical students and interns is encountering their first patient who repeatedly refuses to continue with a treatment that will keep him well and that is often the only way to avoid hospitalization. As a resident, one of us had the experience of reading the chart of an adult patient with bipolar disorder who had been admitted to the hospital dozens of times after stopping lithium, and wondering why on earth a person would make such a foolish decision again and again. In perspective, three capsules of lithium a day seemed a small inconvenience compared with spending what added up to several years of this patient's life in a psychiatric hospital. We have since learned that making peace with having this illness and staying in treatment are much more difficult than healthy people realize. Sticking with treatment is especially rough for individuals who must start taking medications at an age when none of their peers have to bother with such things—when the only people they know who take medication are "old people" and "sick people." It's very difficult for a young, physically healthy person who's feeling well to take medication every day. The idea of the medication controlling one's moods and mental processes is also daunting.

But the harder lesson for parents is learning that no one can *force* an individual, even one's own child, to take responsibility for treatment. Unless the individual makes the commitment to do so, no amount of love and support, sympathy and understanding, cajoling or even threatening can make someone take this step. Even parents who understand this at some level may feel guilty, inadequate, and angry at times when dealing with this situation. These are normal feelings. Parents should not be ashamed of these feelings of frustration and anger but should get help with them instead.

But even when the adolescent does take responsibility and is trying to stay well, relapses can occur. Family members might wonder what *they* did wrong. *Did I put too much pressure on her? Could I have been more supportive? Should I have been tougher and set firmer limits? Why didn't I notice the symptoms coming on sooner and get her to the doctor?* A hundred questions, a thousand "if only's." Another round of guilt, frustration, and anger.

On the other side of this issue is another question: How much understanding and support for the adolescent with a mood disorder might be *too* much? What is protective and what is overprotective? Should you call your child's coach with excuses for why she isn't at practice? Should you pay off credit card debts from hypomanic spending sprees caused by dropping out of treatment? When an irritable outburst ruins a family occasion, should the teenager be grounded for her behavior? We've already discussed the concept of enabling a substance abuser to continue abusing by shielding him from the consequences of his problem. The same dynamic can operate even when substance abuse is not at issue. What actions constitute helping a sick person, and what actions are helping a person to be sick?

These are thorny questions and complex issues. To say that they have no easy answers sounds pat and rather feeble, but it is frustratingly true. Punishing the teen for symptoms like irritability and low energy and motivation isn't fair, but not holding the teenager accountable for *any* of her actions isn't helping her either. Clearly, putting the adolescent too much in charge of her treatment is not right, but letting her have no say in treatment decisions isn't right either. Parents need a forum to process their decisions and strategies; by walking through their successes and failures with experienced peers or a professional, they can learn from others. You will need and deserve a lot of support and encouragement for the tough work of helping with these illnesses—just for hanging in there, every day, day after day.

For all these reasons, it's vital that family members seek out support groups and organizations and consider getting counseling or therapy for themselves to deal with the stresses caused by these illnesses. Like many chronic illnesses, mood disorders afflict one but affect many in the family. It's important that *all* those affected get the help, support, and encouragement they need. At the end of this book we have included names and contact information for some reputable organizations that can provide further information and support. Some of these are for parents by parents, and others are led by mental health professionals. Of course, the best way to ensure that you are getting precisely the individualized support you need may be to find your own therapist. This is not the same as seeing your child's therapist regularly, or even taking your child to family therapy. This is about you, sitting alone with your therapist, talking about your concerns. It may seem like an extreme step to consider, but we can say from experience that all parents we have ever engaged with who have taken this step have later told us that it was possibly the single greatest turning point in their family's recovery from their child's mood disorder.

Planning for Emergencies

The decisions we are forced to make in a crisis situation are frequently not the decisions we would make under other, calmer circumstances. When an emergency arises for which we are unprepared, we are usually forced to make up our response as we go along. One of the best ways to prepare for an emergency is to have a crisis plan ready to go.

In speaking to many readers of the first edition of this book, we learned that some skipped this chapter because "My son was depressed but never suicidal," or "Well, we didn't think we'd need a plan and wanted to get through the book." We caution readers that the best strategy regarding an emergency plan is that "it is better to have one and not need it, then to need one and not have it." Although some people may find even the specter of an emergency stressful and the planning process anywhere from overly laborious to anxiety provoking, take home this message—at the very least, bring up the topic with your child's therapist or psychiatrist. They have put together many, many safety plans in their time and can give you a better and more individualized opinion of what may be best for your family. What follows are some general guidelines that we always consider when having these discussions with families.

Because so many highly effective treatments are available for a mood disorder, we sometimes forget that these disorders are potentially fatal illnesses. And in dealing with a disease that has the potential to become life threatening, the last thing you want is an improvised response to an emergency situation. One of us once faced just such a situation.

▼   The frustration in the nurse's voice was apparent as she spoke into the emergency room phone.

"I hear you, Mrs. Winters," Susan said, "but the magistrate won't approve a petition for involuntary treatment because you think she needs treatment. I need more information before we can—"

Suddenly, Susan put down the phone. "I can't believe it. She hung up on me!" She looked down at her note pad and then turned to me. "Does the name Anne Winters mean anything to you? That was her mom. She wanted someone to come out to their house and bring Anne into the emergency room. She said the girl might be suicidal."

"The name doesn't ring any bells with me," I replied. "Let's try the computer to see if she's ever had any treatment here before; maybe we've got some records. Then we can try calling Mrs. Winters back." As Susan stepped over to the emergency room's computer terminal, I glanced at my watch. It was almost noon, and I had a lunchtime lecture to give. "Susan, I have to go and give my lecture to the medical students. If we have a chart on Anne, can you order it from medical records? I'll be back a little after one, and we can see what we're dealing with and get back with Mrs. Winters."

It was just minutes past one when my beeper went off, with a message to call the emergency room.

"Frank, this is Susan. Mrs. Winters and her daughter are here in the ER. Well, that's not exactly true. Mrs. Winters is here, but Anne won't get out of the car. Do you think you can come down?"

I hadn't done any parking-lot therapy for a while, and as I walked past the "Authorized Personnel Only Please" sign that marked the door to the emergency room, I wondered what I would find. Susan was waiting for me. "I went out and persuaded the girl to come in. They're in room five. Anne has secretly been making cuts on her wrist for several days, so I think she'll need to be admitted. I'll call and see if we have any beds on the adolescent unit."

"How old is the girl? Has she been here before? Were you able to get some records?" I asked.

"She's sixteen, and she was seen about two years ago in the emergency room. We should have the record soon, but the computer information shows that the discharge diagnosis from the ER was major depressive disorder."

"Well, that's some help. Let me go see them."

As soon as I opened the door to the interview room, I could see that (as usual) Susan had sized up the situation pretty accurately. Anne was a tall girl dressed in baggy denim pants that looked to be at least four sizes too big, held up by bright yellow suspenders. She had on a gray sweatshirt with sleeves so long that her hands were invisible. A few brownish smears on one of the sleeves must have been what clued Susan in to asking the girl about hurting herself. She was slumped in a chair in the corner of the room, staring at the floor. Mrs. Winters was smartly dressed in a business suit, which made me think she had been at work before all this started. She didn't wait for me to ask a question to get started.

"The principal called me from school this morning and said Anne had told one of her friends she wanted to die. She's been staying with her father and me since spring break last week and is supposed to be going back to her mother and stepfather this evening. I could tell something was wrong with Anne, but her father's been gone on business for the past several days and I thought we'd talk to her together when he got back. This is a total shock to me. The school counselor suggested I call the doctor Anne was seeing, but when I did, I found out she's retired from practice. Then Anne tells me she hasn't taken her antidepressant for a month—I didn't even know she was on medication!"

Anne answered my questions with only angry glares, so I took Mrs. Winters to another office and let Susan try to sort out what had happened at school with the girl. It took a while to get Mrs. Winters calmed down, and even longer to get the whole story.

Anne's father had shared joint custody of the girl with his ex-wife since they had divorced about three years previously. He had married the present Mrs. Winters a year later. This Mrs. Winters knew nothing about Anne's mood disorder. She had gotten Anne to agree to come to the ER only by threatening to call the police, and she'd been worried the girl would jump out of the car the whole way downtown.

A phone call to Anne's father revealed that the girl had begun psychiatric treatment following the ER visit two years previously. She had started psychotherapy and some medication and after a few months had recovered well from her symptoms. She was no longer in therapy but was supposed to be seeing the psychiatrist every month. I recognized the name of the psychiatrist as a colleague who had retired about three months earlier. I knew for a fact that she had sent letters announcing her retirement several months before she quit her practice group.

It turned out that when Anne ran out of medication, Mr. Winters had persuaded her pediatrician to continue it "until we can make other arrangements." That had been months ago, and Anne still didn't have a psychiatrist.

I heard a knock on the door. Susan peeked in. "Doctor, can I see you for a moment?" "Excuse me," I said and stepped outside. Susan was holding the PPO and HMO list that was posted on the ER bulletin board. "Mr. Winters's medical insurance changed in April, and the new plan doesn't pay here. If Anne needs to be admitted, she'll have to go to Harris Memorial."

As Susan filled in more details of Anne's history and suicidal thinking, it became clear that the girl would indeed need to be in the hospital. "Great," I grumbled. "Her step-mom had a terrible time getting her here. I don't think we should let Mrs. Winters transport the girl. Can you have the secretary call patient transportation, and I'll call—"

Susan's frown stopped me. "Our transportation won't take patients to a hospital outside our system," she said. "We'll need to call an ambulance."

"That will cost them several hundred dollars," I said. "We can't use our people for a three-mile ride?" Susan gave me her best "I don't make the rules, I just follow them" look and said nothing. I took a deep breath and prepared to go in to tell the Winters that it would probably be several more hours before Anne could be admitted to a hospital. ▲

People usually enjoy making plans—vacation plans, wedding plans, retirement plans. Planning for a psychiatric emergency is much less enjoyable, but if you have a family member with a mood disorder, it is, unfortunately, much more important. Unlike with vacation plans, you won't be disappointed if you don't need to use your emergency plans. But if you do need them, odds are you'll be very glad you made them.

It seems that Mr. Winters was operating under the assumption that his daughter's mood disorder was an easily treated problem that didn't require a specialist. As we've emphasized already, adolescent-onset mood disorders can be difficult to treat, and vigilance to signs of relapse is vital. Mr. Winters made a big mistake switching Anne's care to a busy pediatrician so soon after she had received her diagnosis and started treatment. It also seems that no one was monitoring her medications to be certain that she had a good supply and was taking them regularly, which is unfortunately common. Although many parents want to give their children autonomy over their medications, this is typically easier said than done. It is common for parents to reach the end of the month, time for a new refill, and find the bottle half full with medicine. Clearly, something went wrong. This would be a matter to discuss further with the adolescent or, if it is more appropriate, with his psychiatrist so a more detailed plan can be put in place (for example, taking a pill every night right before brushing one's teeth, and keeping the medicine next to the toothbrush, or setting a reminder on a cell phone). Similarly, many adolescents cannot, or will not, take responsibility for filling their own prescriptions, particularly at a local pharmacy, where they may be recognized by friends. All of these details can be discussed and worked out with the adolescent, preferably in the presence of the psychiatrist.

In the example above, Mr. Winters and his new wife had obviously not had a discussion about Anne's mood disorder and what the step-mom should do if symptoms flared up. Mrs. Winters didn't know what to do or whom to call when Anne refused to come to the ER. Last but not least, the Winters were unfamiliar with their medical insurance plan requirements, so Anne wound up being taken to a hospital where their insurance would not approve hospitalization.

How long would it have taken to avoid all these mistakes? An hour or two? Maybe three? Obviously, this would have been time well spent.

KNOW WHOM TO CALL FOR HELP

Every young person with a mood disorder should be under the care of a child psychiatrist who is familiar with the patient's symptoms and course of illness. This means getting established with a new physician when your family moves to a new community or when any other event (such as the retirement of your child's psychiatrist) leaves your child "uncovered." Changes in insurance plans sometimes force a change in psychiatrist too. Don't put off making an appointment to get your child established as a patient in a new community or with a new practice. Because of increasingly long wait times, it can sometimes take a month or more to get in the office to see someone. It is always better to make an appointment and then cancel if something comes up than to wait for a crisis to prompt an urgent visit. Also, because it can sometimes take months for records to be transferred from one office to another, ask the old office for a copy of your child's records or a letter of introduction that you can take to the new doctor at the first appointment. At the very least, such a letter should include your child's diagnosis and medication or medications.

Be sure to inform your pediatrician or family doctor about your child's treatment for a mood disorder, including diagnosis and any medications your child is taking. Keep a list of these medications on you as well to give to medical staff in case your child is taken to an emergency room or admitted to a hospital for *any* reason.

In choosing a new psychiatrist, there are many practical realities to consider. In addition to asking about the factors we've already mentioned (board certification, experience with adolescent age patients, and so on), don't hesitate to ask how the practice is covered after office hours. Also ask how easy it is to get a routine office appointment. Are appointment times set aside so that patients can get an appointment in a day or two for emergencies? Every psychiatrist or mental health clinic should have some means of seeing patients within twenty-four hours in cases of true emergency. Be sure you know how to contact the psychiatrist or the office at any time of the day or night and what arrangements are in place to handle emergencies. Does the psychiatrist see her own emergency patients, or does everyone in the practice rotate emergency on-call duty? The on-call system, though not ideal, is the standard in many communities, meaning your child may well see a doctor other than his regular one if there is an acute emergency. Are you prepared for such an arrangement, so that your child will be under the care of a psychiatrist who comes highly recommended? Less commonly, some psychiatrists make it clear that they do not have after-hours coverage and that any crisis is expected to be dealt with in the emergency room. If this is the protocol for your psychiatrist, ask which emergency room she recommends, whether the hospital has child psychiatrists available, and what other services are available there.

Which hospital or hospitals does the psychiatrist or the practice have a relationship with? Is it the hospital you prefer? The hospital where your insurance covers inpatient psychiatric treatment? Some psychiatrists do not do inpatient work at all; that is, they do not secure admitting privileges to a hospital but refer patients who need hospitalization to colleagues who do. This is especially true of child psychiatrists. This means a loss in continuity of care and sometimes lost time while a new psychiatrist gets to know the patient. Ask about whether the psychiatrist cares for her patients in the hospital and, if not, to whom she refers her hospitalized patients.

If the answers to these questions are not satisfactory, consider your options. Many psychiatrists are well aware of their own limitations and are more than happy to have a frank discussion about other providers who may be a better fit for your family's needs. Alternatively, ask your family doctor, family members, and friends for recommendations. Call the local chapter of Mental Health America, the Depression and Bipolar Support Alliance, or another advocacy group for a referral. (These groups are listed in the resources, following chapter 19.) Sometimes, your options are limited by medical insurance coverage—which brings us to another important aspect of being prepared.

INSURANCE ISSUES

Be familiar with the details of your medical insurance coverage of psychiatric illness. Unfortunately, most plans do not treat psychiatric illnesses in the same way they treat nonpsychiatric illnesses. For example, for psychiatric illnesses, plans frequently have different and stricter limits on hospitalization coverage, number of outpatient appointments they will pay for, and the percentage or amounts that patients must pay out-of-pocket for certain services (*copayments*). These practices have been minimized to a degree by the 1996 Mental Health Parity Act, the Mental Health Parity and Addiction Equity Act of 2008, and the Patient Protection and Affordable Care Act of 2010. Nonetheless, many people who are working to obtain mental health care for the first time are shocked by the red tape involved, so it pays to contact your insurance provider now to find out the exact details of your coverage.

This does not have to be a confrontational exchange. Many insurance companies have dedicated care coordinators who are invested in maintaining the health and well-being of their company's beneficiaries (thereby financially avoiding the more expensive emergency and hospitalization expenses). Care coordinators can explain exactly what is and is not covered and even how to find providers in your area. Some will contact provider offices on your behalf.

Some of the questions to ask include whether there is a "cap" on psychiatric services. This might be a limit on days of hospitalization or on number of outpatient appointments per year, or it might be a dollar-amount limit to coverage. If your insurance company denies coverage for a hospitalization or for several days of hospitalization, what procedures must you follow to appeal the decision?

Hospital stays of all types are getting shorter, and psychiatric hospitalization is no exception. Hospitalization is reserved almost exclusively for life-threatening emergencies now, and patients are discharged as soon as possible. As a rule, patients are no longer hospitalized on a psychiatric unit or in a psychiatric hospital for weeks or months (an exception might be the inpatient treatment of a very malnourished patient with an eating disorder, and even these stays are becoming briefer). Does the psychiatrist have access to a *partial hospitalization* program? (Sometimes also referred to as a *day hospital*.) This alternative to traditional hospital treatment provides hospital-like monitoring and treatment during the day (or sometimes for only part of the day) but allows patients to return home in the evening and spend the night there. It is a useful treatment option for mood disorders because it offers a way to provide daily monitoring of mood symptoms and treatment response without the disruption to personal and family life that staying in a hospital causes. This can also be a useful transitional step between an acute inpatient hospitalization and returning to the outpatient world. Some insurers cover a partial hospitalization (even insist on it), but others do not. Know where your insurance company and your psychiatrist stand on partial hospitalization.

Everyone these days seems to be talking about *managed care*. If you are a member of an HMO, you are part of the managed care picture. (In a *health maintenance organization*, members pay a monthly fee to receive their medical care from the organization.) But even if you are not in an HMO, aspects of managed care practice probably affect you in one way or another, no matter what kind of insurance you have.

Managed care means that the organization that is financially responsible for your child's medical care (your medical insurance company or HMO, for example) supervises or manages how much medical care your child receives. This is accomplished in a variety of ways, some that may be visible to you, some not. The main purpose of this management is to minimize the use of more expensive types of medical care, usually meaning hospitalization and treatment by specialists. In an HMO, the patient may have to be referred by a primary physician to any specialists (including a psychiatrist) in order to be covered. Lab tests may be covered only if the primary physician approves of them (this can make getting the blood tests needed to monitor therapy with lithium and some other psychiatric drugs inconvenient).

A newer alternative to the HMO is the ACO, or accountable care organization. Unlike the HMO, the ACO is held accountable (hence the name) for both the quality of care it provides to patients and their overall health. This mitigates somewhat the greatest criticism of the HMO, which some felt was designed solely to save money no matter how it affected the health of its members.

Before a person can be admitted to a psychiatric hospital, the physician often needs to get approval for hospitalization from the individual's insurance company, a process called *pre-admission review*. This consists of phoning an insurance company representative (usually a nurse or social worker) and giving the details of the clinical situation that justify a hospital stay. If this reviewer does not think a hospitalization is justified by the facts the physician relates, a doctor-to-doctor review is usually arranged. This pre-admission review can be a lengthy process, involving multiple phone calls to and from insurance company representatives and clinical staff. After the patient is admitted to a hospital, the treating doctor may be called every few days by someone from the insurance company asking why the patient still needs to be in the hospital, a function called *utilization review*. If this reviewer (usually a nurse) thinks your child should be discharged, your child's doctor (and you) will be told that coverage will be denied after a certain date and that you will be financially responsible for any additional inpatient treatment. (A variety of appeals procedures usually kick in at this point if your child's doctor disagrees.) Once limited to inpatient treatment, managed care now monitors outpatient treatment as well, and psychiatrists are being asked to fill out forms specifying a treatment plan and requesting a certain number of office visits. All these hassles are the reasons many psychiatrists who can afford to do so do not participate in insurance plans.

If the insurance plan includes coverage for pharmacy charges, you may not have a choice of brands of medication but will have to take whatever equivalent generic pharmaceutical the pharmacy stocks. Some HMOs have expanded on this theme and limit coverage to certain medications belonging to a broadly defined class, not permitting their doctors even to prescribe others. (For a while, some insurers would not pay for SSRI antidepressants and would insist that tricyclic antidepressants be tried first. Although this is no longer true, many insurers will require a trial of a generic medication before a brand-named one.)

There was a time when medical treatment was controlled by doctors and patients. That time has passed. Managed care methods save millions upon millions of health care dollars. Some people argue that this means more people have access to better medical care because the system is more efficient and effective. Others argue that *managed care* is an oxymoron. But whichever is the case, managed care methods are common in all types of insurance coverage now. Your type of medical insurance will almost certainly determine which hospital your child can be admitted to and may determine which doctor your child can see. Your insurance company will probably supervise the length of any hospitalizations, and limit the number of office visits, and even control which medications can be prescribed. All this means that you should closely scrutinize all aspects of insurance coverage for psychiatric illness—your existing policy and any new policies that you may have to choose from because of job changes. Don't put yourself in the position of getting an emergency room surprise.

Be sure to keep all the information you have gathered in one easily accessible document or folder. Make a list of important phone numbers and other key information you will need at a glance during an emergency. Some of the items you should include are shown in figure 18-1.

MORE ON SAFETY

The most dangerous emergency situation for adolescents with mood disorders, and one that frequently leads to hospitalization, is the development of suicidal thoughts and behaviors. As the parent of a depressed child, *never* lose sight of the fact that mood disorders are potentially fatal diseases.

No firearms should be kept in the home of an individual who has been se-

Psychiatrist			
Name:	Business phone:	After–hours phone:	
Therapist			
Name:	Business phone:	After–hours phone:	
Pharmacy		**Approved Hospital(s)**	
Name:	Phone:	Name:	ER Phone:
Primary Care M.D.			
Name:	Business phone:	After–hours phone:	
Insurance Info.			
Policyholder:	Policy number:	Group number:	Pre–admission contact:

Figure 18-1 Medical information chart. Complete a chart or list with this information and keep it up to date.

riously depressed. For an illness whose symptoms can include suicidal depression and heightened irritability with loss of inhibitions, there is never, *ever* any justification whatsoever for having a gun of any type in the home.

Some parents disagree with this stance. Whether they are in the military or law enforcement, or are simply avid sportsmen who prefer hunting, they will argue that firearms are a perfectly reasonable tool when treated with care and safety (locked in a safe, with the ammunition stored separately, and so on). We are not taking a philosophical stance on the right to bear arms here, but a practical one that is based on many years of scientific research on cold, hard facts. Every study that has ever looked at firearms and suicide risk shows unequivocally that the presence of guns in the home increases the risk of completed suicide.[1] As we discussed in chapter 14, research shows that whether a firearm is a handgun or a long gun, loaded or unloaded, locked away or not is immaterial in the risk of completed suicide. As psychiatrists, and as parents, our job is to minimize that risk as much as possible, which means removing guns from the home.

The appearance of self-destructive thoughts and impulses is frightening both to the adolescent and to those around her. The tremendous stigma and disgrace that have been associated with suicide for centuries still make people reluctant to discuss these thoughts when they occur. This stigma along with notions like "only crazy people kill themselves" complicate what is really a straightforward clinical issue: suicidal thinking is a serious symptom of mood disorders; this symptom must be evaluated quickly by a professional and must be managed swiftly and effectively. Individuals can be intensely ashamed of suicidal thoughts and feel that the development of self-destructive impulses is a kind of failure. It is not a failing in any way, of course, but a symptom of an illness. It is important to see the development of suicidal feelings in a depressed adolescent as a very dangerous symptom of serious illness, just like the onset of chest pains in someone with heart disease. When these symptoms occur, it's not time to wonder what they mean, *it's time to call for help*. And just as with the development of chest pains in a heart patient, the development of suicidal feelings in a person with a mood disorder is often a reason for hospitalization.

Psychiatric hospitalization can be experienced as a terrible failure, but the clinical perspective tells us otherwise. Although we have gotten much, much better at treating mood disorders, our treatment methods are by no means perfect. Sometimes, despite everyone's best efforts, relapses occur: the patient has serious symptoms, such as suicidal feelings, and requires hospitalization. When this happens, it's not time for self-blame or questions like "What did I do wrong?" Rather, it's time for healing.

One more reminder: serious depression can raise many issues of personal safety. These issues need to be anticipated, discussed, planned for, and promptly addressed if and when they occur. Put together a safety plan, and don't be afraid to use it if the time comes.

Looking Ahead

We have made enormous progress in the last several decades in the field of psychiatry. The diagnosis of depression, bipolar disorder, and other psychiatric illnesses is much more accurate than it was even when this book was first written a decade ago, and the available treatments for these illnesses are far more effective than even a few years ago. But such advances have come about through trial and error, not because of a better scientific understanding of the causes of these diseases. We still do not understand what is "broken" in the nervous systems of individuals with psychiatric illness.

Thousands of scientists are now working on two great enterprises that will eventually lead to a fuller understanding of these illnesses and to new and more effective treatment approaches. The first of these is the field of neuroscience: the study of the biology and chemistry of the brain and nervous system. At the beginning of the twentieth century, physical and psychiatric examinations of patients with brain disorders followed by microscopic study of their brain tissue after death was the only available method to investigate diseases of the brain. Animal experiments conducted along similar lines complemented these studies, but this work resulted in only the vaguest outline of the organization of brain function. The locations of brain areas important for speech, movement, vision, and so forth, were discovered, but psychiatric illnesses remained so mysterious that ideas that had nothing to do with biology—theories such as psychoanalysis—were the only ones that seemed to offer any hope of understanding these problems.

Throughout the last century, however, breakthrough followed breakthrough, mostly in the field of the chemistry of brain functioning, as neurotransmitters were discovered, more powerful electron microscopes allowed the visualization of synapses and other cellular structures, and sophisticated chemical probes allowed scientists to work out the mechanisms by which neurons grow and communicate with each other. The discovery of G proteins inside the cells was another huge step forward, and new discoveries about the workings of the brain are being made every day.

Now, with new technologies for brain imaging such as PET scans (positron emission tomography) and SPECT (single photon emission computed tomography), scientists for the first time can see the brain at work in living persons. These imaging techniques can show changes in blood flow within the brain, locate areas that are hyperactive or abnormally low in activity, and detect abnormally high or abnormally low levels of brain chemicals such as serotonin and dopamine. Functional MRI imaging can show which areas of the brain are active when a person is performing particular tasks and has been helpful in determining how the brain's function changes, in a visible way, when someone is in the throes of a major depression or mania. A similar technique, diffusion tensor imaging, can show the tracts of the brain, how one neuron is connected to another to convey information. All this information is revealing the importance of the interplay of activity between different brain areas in the regulation of mood and is making it possible to identify the responsible circuitry. These techniques are allowing us to see how the brain of a person with a mood disorder functions differently from that of a person who does not have a mood disorder and, perhaps even more interesting, what changes occur when a person receives treatment and is beginning to feel well again.

We should be clear in our message, however. There are some practitioners who, as of the writing of this text, claim that neural imaging or certain EEG techniques can give a definitive diagnosis of ADHD or of mood disorders. They say that they, and they alone, are qualified to make a true diagnosis and recommend treatment. As of now, there is no evidence that any sort of imaging or objective testing of this type is in any way superior to a good old-fashioned diagnostic evaluation with a knowledgeable, experienced psychiatrist. In fact, almost all scientific studies still use the clinical evaluation as the gold standard against which all other tests (whether they be imaging or pencil-and-paper) are compared. Although we all hope for the day when a functional MRI or an EEG can give us the definitive diagnosis, we are simply not there yet, and we would caution any readers to be wary of practitioners who recommend expensive, out-of-pocket tests with little evidence behind the practice.

The second of these great scientific enterprises is the field of genetics. We've covered some of the developments in chapter 15, but if we left any doubt, the future of medicine and of psychiatry lies in understanding how our DNA influences our mood and our functioning, and using this knowledge to target any deficiencies. Here again, the development of new biochemical methods and molecular probes is what has made this research possible. The Human Genome Project, completed in 2003, gives us the full road map of the human genetic material. This analysis has led to other techniques, such as the ability to find very small mutations in an individual's genetic structure that may explain a particular physical or mental variation. The identification of the genes that are associated with mood disorders is only one of the goals of work in this field. Just as important will be understanding the mechanisms by which genes turn on and off and other mechanisms that regulate the expression and work of the instructions encoded in the DNA molecule.

As the genetic basis of the mood disorders is discovered, we may find that our classification system for these disorders is all wrong and that we need a whole new diagnostic system for psychiatric illnesses that is based on which genes are involved in individual patients. Instead of *major depressive disorder* or *bipolar disorder* II, we may be diagnosing patients with something like *21q22 mood disorder*, a name derived from the location of a gene.

A new field within the larger one of genetics is that of *pharmacogenomics*. Rather than looking for genes that are associated with specific illnesses, this search is for genes that are associated with therapeutic response to particular medications, an approach that promises to take the guesswork out of psychiatric therapeutics. A simple blood test may indicate which medication will work best for a particular patient, ending the lengthy and frustrating trial-and-error approach we now must use in finding the right medication for an individual. The field which has perhaps seen the greatest explosion in practical pharmacogenomics is oncology, the study of cancer. Treatment regimens are now custom tailored, not only to the general type of cancer a person has, but to the individual genetic makeup of the cancerous cells and the genetics of the person herself. In the future, the diagnosis and treatment of a particular patient will likely be determined by analyzing a single drop of blood. The phrase "Prozac is probably the best match for your particular type of depression given your serotonin receptor allele, and is the least likely to cause you side effects given your liver enzyme genetic makeup," will sound less like science fiction and more like the next step in reality.

Another promising approach to understanding genetics is *epigenetics*. Although the old adage that "You can't change your genes" still holds true, it turns out that environmental factors can affect how genes operate and can have important implications for health and disease. In 2014, a team of geneticists at Johns Hopkins University led by Dr. Zachary Kaminski published a research paper showing that stress hormones could flip epigenetic "switches" on a particular gene, resulting in a change of gene activity that predicted suicide and suicidal behaviors in persons with depression. This finding suggests that it may be possible to identify depressed individuals who are at highest risk for suicidal behaviors with a simple blood test. Like pharmacogenomics, the promise of epigenetics is just beginning to be realized in the practice of psychiatry.

The two fields of neuroscience and psychiatric genetics are closing in on the causes and mechanisms of mood disorders from different directions. As these two enterprises advance, they will begin to inform each other— that is, advances in one field will lead to advances in the other. Discovering that a gene for a particular protein is associated with a particular mood disorder will tell neuroscientists that the protein is important in the regulation of mood. The discovery of some new enzyme in neurons that is important in neuronal signaling will tell geneticists to focus on the gene for that enzyme in their linkage studies. Little by little, the whole picture will become clearer and clearer.

Advances in many seemingly unrelated fields hold promise for better understanding of mood disorders, too: advances in computer technology, for example. Just as architects now use computers to visualize buildings before they are built, pharmacologists are using computers to visualize the three-dimensional structures of neurotransmitters, receptors, and pharmaceutical agents to design new drugs. It is hoped that new pharmaceuticals that have a better "fit" with receptors or other targets will work faster, at lower doses, and with fewer side effects. In fact, many atypical antipsychotics (including clozapine) and some SSRIs (including fluoxetine, or Prozac) were developed using precisely these methods. Computers are also being used to model and study brain activity. Remember that the brain is much more than just a sophisticated computer: more like a network of millions and millions of individual computers. Advanced computers using *nonsequential neural architecture* to build *neural networks* (made up of many interconnected but independently computing units) show properties that would not be predicted from known principles of computing. These properties are probably highly relevant to the study of human brain activity and psychiatric illness.

Our understanding of the biology of mood disorders is getting better all the time. With each advance we get closer to better diagnostic methods and to safer and more effective treatments. The number of new medications continues to grow, and many more new pharmaceuticals are in the pipeline. With the more sophisticated use of nonpharmaceutical treatments such as transcranial magnetic stimulation, perhaps we'll be able to use lower doses of medications or help medications to work more quickly.

As we take the step from isolating genes to determining the function of those genes, we'll be able to design treatments more effectively and more rationally. This work also holds out the possibility of gene therapy: repairing the code in the DNA that causes mood disorders. The obstacles to be overcome before we can look for this type of cure can only be called daunting, even monumental. But scientists are closing in on these illnesses little by little, and with enough time and enough hard work, a cure might be possible.

As the mechanisms of illness development become known and the genetic vulnerabilities are identified, another exciting possibility emerges: prevention. Genetic data and a better understanding of what triggers the illness may allow the development of prevention programs aimed at averting illness development in individuals known to be at higher risk for a particular disorder. Some people see a darker side to this sort of prevention.

Imagine that a test is developed to determine the genetic risk of a patient, say, developing schizophrenia later in life. Many people who have schizophrenia require expensive medications for a long time, perhaps their entire lives. Now imagine that this test can be given to a newborn, or even in utero. Parents and patients worry that this information will be available to interested parties such as insurance companies or potential employers, cutting off their child's future. This sort of dystopian consequence to our increasing knowledge has been the topic of many science fiction works. Protection of genetic information is still being worked out by legislative bodies, but promising developments include the Genetic Information Nondiscrimination Act of 2008, which aims to eliminate exactly these sorts of discriminatory practices.

People frequently ask us whether they or their child will have to take medication for the rest of their lives. We always tell them that no one knows the answer to this question because no one knows exactly what the treatment of mood disorders might be in the future. Physicians practicing in the 1930s probably could not have imagined that vaccines would one day almost eliminate diphtheria, polio, measles, and other childhood diseases, common, often crippling, and sometimes fatal illnesses they saw so frequently in their patients but were completely helpless to treat. The astonishing developments in neuroscience and genetics hold just this much promise for those afflicted with mood disorders. There is every reason to be hopeful that a time is not too far off when treatments for depression and other mood disorders will be more effective than we can now imagine. But for now, the best way to manage a serious mood disorder is by using every resource available to you. The current evidence suggests that the longer a person can stay well, the lower the person's chance of relapsing into depression or mania. Continued treatment with your child's psychiatrist and therapist is a critical element to your child achieving his full potential.

RESOURCES

Suggested Reading

Samuel H. Barondes, *Mood Genes: Hunting for the Origins of Mania and Depression* (New York: Oxford University Press, 1999).

> *A clearly written and engrossing account of the tough science involved in the search for the genetic basis of mood disorders. An excellent introduction to the science of genetics.*

Robert Hedaya, *The Antidepressant Survival Guide: The Clinically Proven Program to Enhance the Benefits and Beat the Side Effects of Your Medication* (New York: Three Rivers Press, 2001).

> *An ambitious program for avoiding medication side effects that includes prescriptions for diet, exercise, and other lifestyle changes.*

Kay Redfield Jamison, *An Unquiet Mind: A Memoir of Moods and Madness* (New York: Vintage Books, 1996).

> *A powerful and moving narrative written with grace and wit by an international expert on bipolar disorder who suffers from it herself. A treasure of a book that contains some of the most engrossing and vivid descriptions of the experience of bipolar disorder ever written. A "must read" for anyone touched by bipolar disorder.*

George McGovern, *Terry: My Daughter's Life-and-Death Struggle with Alcoholism* (New York: Villard Books, 1996).

> *Senator McGovern's moving account of his daughter Terry's terrible and ultimately fatal addiction to alcohol cannot be too highly recommended for families dealing with an addicted relative. The senator vividly captures the dilemmas and struggles of a family trying to find the balance between helping their daughter without enabling her illness.*

Francis Mark Mondimore, *Bipolar Disorder: A Guide for Patients and Families,* 3rd ed. (Baltimore: Johns Hopkins University Press, 2014).

> *We admit to being more than a little biased about recommending this one but think it's a great resource for learning about bipolar disorder in all its variations. If you found the book you're holding in your hands helpful and want more information in the same style on bipolar disorder, this is your book.*

Francis Mark Mondimore and Patrick Kelly, *Borderline Personality Disorder: New Reasons for Hope* (Baltimore: Johns Hopkins University Press, 2011)

> *Yet another bit of shameless self-promotion, but a book we hope you will find useful. As we've discussed, adolescents are frequently lost, trying to redefine their identity, sometimes doing so in self-destructive ways. This is exactly how a patient with borderline personality disorder exists in the world. If this sounds familiar to you or your family, this book may help unravel some of the mysteries wrapped up in this complex and convoluted syndrome.*

Rolf Muuss, *Theories of Adolescence,* 6th ed. (New York: McGraw-Hill, 1996).

> *This college textbook provides an excellent overview of adolescent psychology by means of well-written chapters on all the major psychological theories from G. Stanley Hall and Sigmund Freud to Erik Erikson and beyond.*

William Styron, *Darkness Visible: A Memoir of Madness* (New York: Vintage Books, 1990).

> *We recommend this book to medical students as one of the best accounts of the symptoms of depression available. A good book for family members to read to better understand the experience of serious depression.*

Support and Advocacy Organizations

All the following organizations provide information, educational resources, and often referrals to support groups and to clinicians in your community who are skilled in treating mood disorders. Get in touch with them all and become a member! In addition to the direct services they provide to consumers, these groups are active in combating the stigmatization of psychiatric illnesses, in advocating for better medical insurance coverage of psychiatric disorders, and in supporting research.

Depression and Bipolar Support Alliance (DBSA)
  55 E. Jackson Blvd., Suite 490
  Chicago, IL 60604
  800-826-3632
  www.dbsalliance.org

International Foundation for Research and Education on Depression (iFred)
> P.O. Box 17598
> Baltimore, MD 21297-1598
> www.ifred.org

Mental Health America (MHA)
> 2000 N. Beauregard Street, 6th floor
> Alexandria, VA 22311
> 800-969-NMHA
> www.nmha.org

National Alliance on Mental Illness (NAMI)
> 3803 N. Fairfax Drive, Suite 100
> Arlington, VA 22203
> 800-950-NAMI
> www.nami.org

Internet Resources

All the support and advocacy groups listed above have websites with links to many, many other useful resources. The astonishing range of resources on the Internet continues to grow, but remember that you'll also find inaccurate information, bias, and just plain nonsense online, and it's important to consider information sources very carefully. Here are a few more excellent resources.

American Academy of Child and Adolescent Psychiatry
> www.aacap.org

> *Information on child and adolescent psychiatry, including fact sheets for parents and caregivers.*

Internet Mental Health
> www.mentalhealth.com

> *An excellent site, with information on many different disorders and their treatments, information on many psychiatric medications, and hundreds of reference articles from popular and professional publications.*

Medscape
> www.medscape.com

> *This is primarily a news site for medical professionals, but it has a "patient information" section with many useful articles and links to other resources.*

The Surgeon General of the United States
www.surgeongeneral.gov

Read the surgeon general's reports online, including comprehensive reports on child and adolescent mental health issues.

U.S. National Library of Medicine
www.nlm.nih.gov

This site provides free access to Medline, the most comprehensive medical database in the world. You can access more than eight million references in thirty-eight hundred journals. An incredibly valuable resource.

WebMD Health
www.webmd.com

A comprehensive and reliable source of health information. Thousands of pages on many different disorders, including depression, bipolar disorder, ADHD, eating disorders, and other illnesses. Includes an extensive online discussion group and regular chats on mental health issues.

NOTES

Preface

1. Ruth Perou et al., "Mental Health Surveillance among Children—United States, 2005–2011." *Centers for Disease Control and Prevention Supplements* 62, no. 2 (2013): 1–35.

2. Peter Lewinsohn, Paul Rohde, John Seeley, Daniel Klein, and Ian Gotlib, "Natural Course of Adolescent Major Depressive Disorder in a Community Sample: Predictors of Recurrence in Young Adults," *American Journal of Psychiatry* 157, no. 10 (2000): 1584–91.

Chapter 1   Depression: Some Definitions

1. William James, *The Varieties of Religious Experience* (New York: Penguin Books, 1982), 147.

2. William Styron, *Darkness Visible: A Memoir of Madness* (New York: Vintage Books, 1990), 58.

3. J. K. Rowling, *Harry Potter and the Prisoner of Azkaban* (New York: Arthur A. Levine Books, 1999), 203.

4. *J. K. Rowling: A Year in the Life*, directed by James Runcie (UK: IWC Media, 2007), film.

5. Johann Wolfgang von Goethe, *The Sorrows of Young Werther*, trans. Elizabeth Mayer and Louise Bogan (New York: Random House, 1971), 114.

6. Hugo Wolf quoted in Kay Redfield Jamison, *Touched with Fire: Manic-Depressive Illness and the Artistic Temperament* (New York: Free Press, 1993), 21.

7. Styron, *Darkness Visible*, 19.

Chapter 2   Normal Adolescence and Depression in Adolescence

1. Leo Kanner, *Child Psychiatry*, 3rd ed. (Springfield, Ill.: Thomas, 1957).

2. Joseph Brennemann, "The Menace of Psychiatry," *American Journal of Diseases of Children* 42, no. 2 (1931): 376–402.

3. As quoted in Sebastian Kraemer, "'The Menace of Psychiatry': Does It Still Ring a Bell?" *Archives of Disease in Childhood* 94, no. 8 (2009): 570–72.

4. N. Ryan et al., "The Clinical Picture of Major Depression in Children and Adolescents," *Archives of General Psychiatry* 44 (1987): 854–61.

5. Jerald G Bachman et al., "Adolescent Self-Esteem: Differences by Race/Ethnicity, Gender, and Age," *Self and Identity* 10, no. 4 (2011): 445–73.

6. Michael Rutter, *Changing Youth in a Changing Society: Patterns of Adolescent Development and Disorder* (Cambridge: Harvard University Press, 1980), 87.

7. Erik Erikson, *Childhood and Society*, 2d ed. (New York: Norton, 1963), 228.

8. Erik Erikson, *Identity, Youth, and Crisis* (New York: Norton, 1968), 131.

9. See James Marcia, "The Empirical Study of Ego Identity," in *Identity and Development: An Interdisciplinary Approach*, ed. Harke Bosma, Tobi Graafsma, and Harold Grotevant (Thousand Oaks, Calif.: Sage, 1994).

10. Rutter, *Changing Youth in a Changing Society*, 39.

11. Jerome D. Frank, *Persuasion and Healing: A Comparative Study of Psychotherapy*, rev. ed. (New York: Schocken Books, 1974), 316.

12. Ibid., 314.

13. Anna Freud quoted in Rolf E. Muuss, *Theories of Adolescence*, 6th ed. (New York: McGraw-Hill, 1996), 368.

14. Alfred Kinsey, Wardell Pomeroy, and Clyde Martin, *Sexual Behavior in the Human Male* (Philadelphia: W. B. Saunders, 1948), 639.

Chapter 3   The Mood Disorders of Adolescence

1. The APA Task Force on Laboratory Tests in Psychiatry, "The Dexamethasone Suppression Test: An Overview of Its Current Status in Psychiatry," *American Journal of Psychiatry* 144, no. 10 (1987): 1253–62.

2. P. Lewinsohn, H. Hops, R. Roberts, J. Seeley, and J. Andrews, "Adolescent Psychopathology I: Prevalence and Incidence of Depression and Other DSM-III-R Disorders in High School Students," *Journal of Abnormal Psychology* 102 (1993): 133–44.

3. Boris Birmaher et al., "Childhood and Adolescent Depression: A Review of the Past 10 Years, Part I," *Journal of the American Academy of Child and Adolescent Psychiatry* 35, no. 11 (1996): 1427–39.

4. Douglas Williamson, Boris Birmaher, Barbara Anderson, Mayadah Al-Shab-bout, and Ryan Neal, "Stressful Life Events in Depressed Adolescents: The Role of Dependant Events during the Depressive Episode," *Journal of the American Academy of Child and Adolescent Psychiatry* 34, no. 5 (1995): 591–98.

5. Kenneth S. Kendler and Charles O. Gardner, "Dependent Stressful Life Events and Prior Depressive Episodes in the Prediction of Major Depression—The Problem of Causal Inference in Psychiatric Epidemiology," *Archives of General Psychiatry* 67, no. 11 (2010): 1120–27.

6. Ian M. Goodyer, "The Influence of Recent Life Events on the Onset and Outcome of Major Depression in Young People," in *Depressive Disorders in Children and Adolescents: Epidemiology, Risk Factors, and Treatment*, ed. Cecilia Ahmoi Essau and Franz Petermann (Northvale, N.J.: Jason Aronson, 1999), 241.

7. Ruth Perou et al., "Mental Health Surveillance among Children—United States, 2005–2011," *Centers for Disease Control and Prevention Supplements* 62, no. 2 (2013): 1–35.

8. Ronald C. Kessler et al., "The Epidemiology of Major Depressive Disorder: Results from the National Comorbidity Survey Replication (NCS-R)," *JAMA* 289, no. 23 (2003): 3095–3105.

9. S. Seedat et al., "Cross-National Associations between Gender and Mental Disorders in the World Health Organization World Mental Health Surveys," *Archives of General Psychiatry* 66, no. 7 (2009): 785–95.

10. Birmaher et al., "Childhood and Adolescent Depression."

11. John Curry et al., "Recovery and Recurrence following Treatment for Adolescent Major Depression," *Archives of General Psychiatry* 68, no. 3 (2011): 263–69.

12. Birmaher et al., "Childhood and Adolescent Depression."

13. Maria Kovacs, Hagop Akiskal, Constantine Gatsonis, and Phoebe Parrone, "Childhood-Onset Dysthymic Disorder," *Archives of General Psychiatry* 51 (1994): 365–74.

14. Birmaher et al., "Childhood and Adolescent Depression."

15. S. Gehlert et al., "The Prevalence of Premenstrual Dysphoric Disorder in a Randomly Selected Group of Urban and Rural Women," *Psychological Medicine* 39, no. 1 (2009): 129–36.

16. C. Moreno et al., "National Trends in the Outpatient Diagnosis and Treatment of Bipolar Disorder in Youth," *Archives of General Psychiatry* 64, no. 9 (2007): 1032–39.

17. A. R. Van Meter, A. L. Moreira, and E. A. Youngstrom, "Meta-Analysis of Epidemiologic Studies of Pediatric Bipolar Disorder," *Journal of Clinical Psychiatry* 72, no. 9 (2011): 1250–56.

18. A. Pfuntner, L. M. Wier, and C. Stocks, *Most Frequent Conditions in U.S. Hospitals, 2011*, Statistical Brief 162, Healthcare Cost and Utilization Project (HCUP) Statistical Briefs (Rockville, Md.: Agency for Healthcare Research and Quality, 2013).

19. DSM-5 Committee, *Diagnostic and Statistical Manual of Mental Disorders*, 5th ed. (Washington, D.C.: American Psychiatric Association, 2013). Accessed online at http://dsm.psychiatryonline.org/doi/full/10.1176/appi.books.9780890425596.dsm04#BCFBGAGG.

20. Ibid.

21. Peter Lewinsohn, Daniel Klein, and John Seeley, "Bipolar Disorders in a Community of Older Adolescents: Prevalence, Phenomenology, Comorbidity and Course," *Journal of the American Academy of Child and Adolescent Psychiatry* 34, no. 4 (1995): 454–63.

22. William Coryell, Nancy Andreason, Jean Endicott, and Martin Keller, "The Significance of Past Mania or Hypomania in the Course and Outcome of Major Depression," *American Journal of Psychiatry* 144 (1987): 309–15.

23. G. Cassano, H. Akiskal, M. Savina, L. Musetti, and G. Perugi, "Proposed Subtypes of Bipolar II and Related Disorders: With Hypomanic Episodes (or Cyclothymia) and with Hyperthymic Temperament," *Journal of Affective Disorders* 26 (1992): 127–40.

24. See Sylvia Simpson et al., "Bipolar II: The Most Common Bipolar Pheno-type?" *American Journal of Psychiatry* 150 (1993): 901–3.

25. Frederick K. Goodwin and Kay Redfield Jamison, *Manic-Depressive Illness* (New York: Oxford University Press, 1990), 69.

26. Hagop Akiskal et al., "Switching from 'Unipolar' to Bipolar II: An Eleven-Year Prospective Study of Clinical and Temperamental Predictors in 559 Patients," *Archives of General Psychiatry* 52 (1995): 114–23.

27. Lewinsohn et al., "Bipolar Disorders in a Community of Older Adolescents."

28. Hagop Akiskal, "The Prevalent Clinical Spectrum of Bipolar Disorders: Beyond DSM-IV," *Journal of Clinical Psychopharmacology* 16, suppl. (1996): 4S–14S.

29. Lewinsohn et al., "Bipolar Disorders in a Community of Older Adolescents."

30. Hagop Akiskal and Gopinath Mallya, "Criteria for 'Soft' Bipolar Spectrum: Treatment Implications," *Psychopharmacology Bulletin* 23, no. 1 (1987): 68–73.

31. Emil Kraepelin, *Manic-Depressive Insanity and Paranoia*, trans. R. M. Barclay, ed. G. M. Robertson (Edinburgh: Livingstone, 1921; reprinted New York: Arno Press, 1976), 1 (in reprint edition).

32. Joachim Puig-Antich et al., "The Psychosocial Functioning and Family Environment of Depressed Adolescents," *Journal of the American Academy of Child and Adolescent Psychiatry* 32, no. 2 (1993): 244–53.

33. Paul Rohde, Peter Lewinsohn, and John Seeley, "Are Adolescents Changed by an Episode of Major Depression?" *Journal of the American Academy of Child and Adolescent Psychiatry* 33, no. 9 (1994): 1289–98.

34. Kiyuri Naicker et al., "Social, Demographic, and Health Outcomes in the 10 Years following Adolescent Depression," *Journal of Adolescent Health* 52, no. 5 (2013): 533–38.

35. Mark Sanford et al., "Predicting the One-Year Course of Adolescent Major Depression," *Journal of the American Academy of Child and Adolescent Psychiatry* 34, no. 12 (1995): 1618–28.

36. Maria Kovacs, Stana Paulaudkas, Constantine Gatsonis, and Cheryl Richards, "Depressive Disorders in Childhood III: A Longitudinal Study of Comorbidity and Risk for Conduct Disorders," *Journal of Affective Disorders* 15 (1988): 205–17.

37. Uma Rao, "Relationship between Depression and Substance Abuse Disorders in Adolescent Women during the Transition to Adulthood," *Journal of the American Academy of Child and Adolescent Psychiatry* 39, no. 2 (2000): 215–22.

38. Uma Rao et al., "Unipolar Depression in Adolescents: Clinical Outcome in Adulthood," *Journal of the American Academy of Child and Adolescent Psychiatry* 34, no. 5 (1995): 566–78.

Chapter 4   Mood Disorders: A Summary of Diagnostic Categories in the DSM

1. American Psychiatric Association, *Diagnostic and Statistical Manual of Mental Disorders*, 4th ed. (Washington, D.C.: American Psychiatric Association, 1994), xvii. Note that epilepsy was considered to be a mental illness at the time.

2. Alfred Kinsey, Wardell Pomeroy, and Clyde Martin, *Sexual Behavior in the Human Male* (Philadelphia: Saunders, 1948), 639.

Chapter 5   Medication Issues in Adolescence

1. Nancy C. Andreason, *The Broken Brain: The Biological Revolution in Psychiatry* (New York: Harper and Row, 1985).

2. Roland Kuhn, "The Treatment of Depressive States with G 22355 (Imipramine Hydrochloride)," *American Journal of Psychiatry* 115 (1958): 459–64. This is an English translation of Kuhn's 1957 article.

Chapter 6   Antidepressant Medications

1. Roland Kuhn, "The Treatment of Depressive States with G 22355 (Imipramine Hydrochloride)," *American Journal of Psychiatry* 115 (1958): 459–64.

2. C. K. Varley and J. McClellan, "Case Study: Two Additional Sudden Deaths with Tricyclic Antidepressants," *Journal of the American Academy of Child and Adolescent Psychiatry* 36, no. 3 (1997): 390–94.

3. J. Daly and T. Wilens, "The Use of Tricyclic Antidepressants in Children and Adolescents," *Pediatric Clinics of North America: Child and Adolescent Psychopharmacology* 45, no. 5 (1998): 1123–35.

4. Ibid.

5. C. K. Conners, "Methodology of Antidepressant Drug Trials for Treating Depression in Adolescents," *Journal of Child and Adolescent Psychopharmacology* 2 (1992): 11–22.

6. P. Hazell and M. Mirzaie, "Tricyclic Drugs for Depression in Children and Adolescents," *Cochrane Database of Systematic Reviews* 6 (2013): CD002317.pub2.

7. Rudolf Hoehn-Saric, John Lipsey, and Godfrey Pearlson, "A Fluoxetine-Induced Frontal Lobe Syndrome in an Obsessive-Compulsive Patient," *Journal of Clinical Psychiatry* 52 (1990): 343–45.

8. J. Price, V. Cole, and G. M. Goodwin, "Emotional Side-Effects of Selective Serotonin Reuptake Inhibitors: Qualitative Study," *British Journal of Psychiatry: Journal of Mental Science* 195, no. 3 (2009): 211–17.

9. D. Brent et al., "Switching to Another SSRI or to Venlafaxine with or without Cognitive Behavioral Therapy for Adolescents with SSRI-Resistant Depression: The TORDIA Randomized Controlled Trial," *JAMA* 299, no. 8 (2008): 901–13.

10. R. L. Findling et al., "Venlafaxine in the Treatment of Children and Adolescents with Attention-Deficit/Hyperactivity Disorder," *Journal of Child and Adolescent Psychopharmacology* 17, no. 4 (2007): 433–45.

11. R. L. Barkin and S. Barkin, "The Role of Venlafaxine and Duloxetine in the Treatment of Depression with Decremental Changes in Somatic Symptoms of Pain, Chronic Pain, and the Pharmacokinetics and Clinical Considerations of Duloxetine Pharmacotherapy," *American Journal of Therapeutics* 12, no. 5 (2005): 431–38.

12. S. E. Hetrick et al., "Newer Generation Antidepressants for Depressive Disorders in Children and Adolescents," *Cochrane Database of Systematic Reviews* 11 (2012): CD004851.

1. Anastase Georgotas and Samuel Gershon, "Historical Perspectives and Current Highlights on Lithium Treatment in Manic-Depressive Illness," *Journal of Clinical Psychopharmacology* 1, no. 1 (1981): 27–31.

2. John F. J. Cade, "Lithium Salts in the Treatment of Psychotic Excitement," *Medical Journal of Australia* 36 (1949): 349–52.

3. Ibid., 350.

4. Ibid., 350–51.

5. Ronald R. Fieve, *Moodswing: The Third Revolution in Psychiatry* (New York: Bantam Books, 1975), 3.

6. M. Schou, N. Juel-Nielsen, E. Strömgren, and H. Voldby, "The Treatment of Manic Psychoses by the Administration of Lithium Salts," *Journal of Neurology, Neurosurgery, and Psychiatry* 17 (1954): 250–60.

7. Paul Baalstrup and Morgans Schou, "Lithium as a Prophylactic Agent: Its Effect against Recurrent Depressions and Manic-Depressive Psychosis," *Archives of General Psychiatry* 16, no. 2 (1967): 162–72.

8. E. P. Worrall, J. P. Moody, and M. Peet, "Controlled Studies of the Acute Antidepressant Effects of Lithium," *British Journal of Psychiatry* 135 (1979): 255–62.

9. F. Rouillon and P. Gorwood, "The Use of Lithium to Augment Antidepressant Medication," *Journal of Clinical Psychiatry* 59, suppl. 5 (1998): 32–39.

10. Robert Kowatch and John Bucci, "Mood Stabilizers and Anticonvulsants," *Pediatric Clinics of North America* 45, no. 5 (1998): 1173–86.

11. Morgans Schou, "Forty Years of Lithium Treatment," *Archives of General Psychiatry* 54 (1997): 9–13.

12. Ibid., 11.

13. Neal Ryan, Vinod Bhatara, and James Perel, "Mood Stabilizers in Children and Adolescents," *Journal of the American Academy of Child and Adolescent Psychiatry* 38, no. 5 (1999): 529–36.

14. Ibid.

15. G. Walter, B. Lyndon, and R. Kubb, "Lithium Augmentation of Venlafaxine in Adolescent Major Depression," *Australian and New Zealand Journal of Psychiatry* 32, no. 3 (1998): 457–59.

16. A. Cipriani, K. Hawton, S. Stockton, and J. R. Geddes, "Lithium in the Prevention of Suicide in Mood Disorders: Updated Systematic Review and Meta-Analysis," *BMJ* 346 (2013): f3646.

17. American Psychiatric Association, "Practice Guidelines for the Treatment of Bipolar Disorder," *American Journal of Psychiatry* 151, suppl. (1994): 7.

18. Patricia Roy and Jennifer L. Payne, "Treatment of Bipolar Disorder during and after Pregnancy," in *Bipolar Depression: Molecular Neurobiology, Clinical Diagnosis, and Pharmacotherapy*, ed. Carlos A. Zarate and Husseini K. Manji (Boston: Birkhäuser, 2009), 253–69.

19. Frederick K. Goodwin and Kay Redfield Jamison, *Manic-Depressive Illness* (New York: Oxford University Press, 1990), 707.

20. Charles Bowden and Susan McElroy, "History of the Development of Val-

proate for the Treatment of Bipolar Disorder," *Journal of Clinical Psychiatry* 56, suppl. 3 (1995): 3–5.

21. A. Cipriani et al., "Valproic Acid, Valproate and Divalproex in the Maintenance Treatment of Bipolar Disorder," *Cochrane Database of Systematic Reviews* 10 (2013): CD003196.

22. Charles L. Bowden, "Predictors of Response to Divalproex and Lithium," *Journal of Clinical Psychiatry* 56, suppl. 3 (1995): 25–29.

23. Susan McElroy, Paul Keck, Harrison Pope, and James Hudson, "Valproate in Psychiatric Disorders: Literature Review and Clinical Guidelines," *Journal of Clinical Psychiatry* 50, suppl. 3 (1989): 23–29.

24. American Psychiatric Association, "Practice Guidelines for the Treatment of Bipolar Disorder," 21. See also Alan Swann et al., "Depression during Mania: Treatment Response to Lithium or Divalproex," *Archives of General Psychiatry* 54 (1997): 37–42.

25. American Psychiatric Association, "Practice Guidelines for the Treatment of Bipolar Disorder," 10.

26. Frederick Jacobson, "Low-Dose Valproate: A New Treatment for Cyclothymia, Mild Rapid-Cycling Disorders and Premenstrual Syndrome," *Journal of Clinical Psychiatry* 54, no. 6 (1993): 229–34. See also J. A. Delito, "The Effect of Valproate on Bipolar Spectrum Temperamental Disorders," *Journal of Clinical Psychiatry* 54, no. 8 (1993): 300–304.

27. N. Huband et al., "Antiepileptics for Aggression and Associated Impulsivity," *Cochrane Database of Systematic Reviews* 2 (2010): CD003499.

28. Gary Sachs, "Bipolar Mood Disorder: Practical Strategies for Acute and Maintenance Phase Treatment," *Journal of Clinical Psychopharmacology* 16, no. 2, suppl. 1 (1996): 32S–47S.

29. F. E. Dreifuss, D. H. Langer, K. A. Moline, and J. E. Maxwell, "Valproic Acid Hepatic Fatalities II: US Experience since 1984," *Neurology* 39, no. 2, pt. 1 (1989): 201–7.

30. H. J. Talib and E. M. Alderman, "Gynecologic and Reproductive Health Concerns of Adolescents Using Selected Psychotropic Medications," *Journal of Pediatric and Adolescent Gynecology* 26, no. 1 (2013): 7–15.

31. J. C. Ballenger and R. M. Post, "Carbamazepine in Manic-Depressive Illness: A New Treatment," *American Journal of Psychiatry* 37, no. 7 (1980): 782–90.

32. R. A. Kowatch et al., "Effect Size of Lithium, Divalproex Sodium, and Carbamazepine in Children and Adolescents with Bipolar Disorder," *Journal of the American Academy of Child and Adolescent Psychiatry* 39, no. 6 (2000): 713–20.

33. B. Lerer, M. Moore, E. Meyendorff, S. R. Cho, and S. Gershon, "Carbamazepine versus Lithium in Mania: A Double Blind Study," *Journal of Clinical Psychiatry* 48 (1987): 89–93.

34. Robert Post, Thomas Uhde, James Ballenger, and Kathleen Squillace, "Prophylactic Efficacy of Carbamazepine in Manic-Depressive Illness," *American Journal of Psychiatry* 140 (1983): 1602–4.

35. Joseph Woolston, "Case Study: Carbamazepine Treatment of Juvenile-

Onset Bipolar Disorder," *Journal of the American Academy of Child and Adolescent Psychiatry* 38, no. 3 (1999): 335–38.

36. Jonathan Sporn and Gary Sachs, "The Anticonvulsant Lamotrigine in Treatment Resistant Manic-Depressive Illness," *Journal of Clinical Psychopharmacology* 17 (1997): 185–89.

37. A. Trankner, C. Sander, and P. Schonknecht, "A Critical Review of the Recent Literature and Selected Therapy Guidelines since 2006 on the Use of Lamotrigine in Bipolar Disorder," *Neuropsychiatric Disease and Treatment* 9 (2013): 101–11.

38. Joseph Calabrese, S. Hossein Fatemi, and Mark Woyshville, "Antidepressant Effects of Lamotrigine in Rapid Cycling Bipolar Disorder," *American Journal of Psychiatry* 153, no. 9 (1996): 1236.

39. Thomas Maltese, "Adjunctive Lamotrigine Treatment for Major Depression," *American Journal of Psychiatry* 156, no. 11 (1999): 1833.

40. Sporn and Sachs, "Anticonvulsant Lamotrigine in Treatment Resistant Manic-Depressive Illness."

41. Cipriani et al., "Lithium in the Prevention of Suicide in Mood Disorders."

42. Sean Stanton, Paul Keck, and Susan McElroy, "Treatment of Acute Mania with Gabapentin," *American Journal of Psychiatry* 154, no. 2 (1997): 287.

43. Marshall Teitlebaum, "Oxycarbazepine in Bipolar Disorder," *Journal of the American Academy of Child and Adolescent Psychiatry* 40, no. 9 (2001): 993–94.

44. For a discussion of all these issues, see Magda Campbell and Jeanette Cueva, "Psychopharmacology in Child and Adolescent Psychiatry: A Review of the Past Seven Years, Part II," *Journal of the American Academy of Child and Adolescent Psychiatry* 34, no. 10 (1995): 1262–72; and Ryan, Bhatara, and Perel, "Mood Stabilizers in Children and Adolescents."

Chapter 8   Other Medications and Treatments

1. B. Geller et al., "A Randomized Controlled Trial of Risperidone, Lithium, or Divalproex Sodium for Initial Treatment of Bipolar I Disorder, Manic or Mixed Phase, in Children and Adolescents," *Archives of General Psychiatry* 69, no. 5 (2012): 515–28.

2. Robert L. Findling et al., "Prolactin Levels during Long-Term Risperidone Treatment in Children and Adolescents," *Journal of Clinical Psychiatry* 64, no. 11 (2003): 1362–69.

3. In a study of 11,555 patients treated with clozapine, 73 (or 0.63 percent) developed agranulocytosis (of whom 2 died of the infectious complications of the condition). See Jose Alvir, Jeffrey Lieberman, Allan Safferman, Jeffrey Schwimmer, and John Schaaf, "Clozapine-Induced Agranulocytosis: Incidence and Risk Factors in the United States," *New England Journal of Medicine* 329 (1993): 162–67.

4. Magda Campbell, Judith L. Rapoport, and George M. Simpson, "Antipsychotics in Children and Adolescents," *Journal of the American Academy of Child and Adolescent Psychiatry* 38, no. 5 (1999): 537–45.

5. Mark Olfson et al., "National Trends in the Outpatient Treatment of Children and Adolescents with Antipsychotic Drugs," *Archives of General Psychiatry* 63, no. 6 (2006): 679–85.

6. Ric M. Procyshyn et al., "Prevalence and Patterns of Antipsychotic Use in Youth at the Time of Admission and Discharge from an Inpatient Psychiatric Facility," *Journal of Clinical Psychopharmacology* 34, no. 1 (2014): 17–22.

7. Gregory Kutz, *Foster Children: HHS Guidance Could Help States Improve Oversight of Psychotropic Prescriptions*, Testimony before the Subcommittee on Federal Financial Management, Government Information, Federal Services, and International Security, Committee on Homeland Security and Governmental Affairs, U.S. Senate (Washington, D.C.: United States Government Accountability Office, 2011).

8. K. Linde, G. Ramirez, C. D. Mulrow, A. Pauls, and W. Weidenhammer, "St. John's Wort for Depression—An Overview and Meta-analysis of Randomized Clinical Trials," *British Medical Journal* 3, no. 313 (1996): 253–58.

9. Michael Dörks et al., "Antidepressant Drug Use and Off-Label Prescribing in Children and Adolescents in Germany: Results from a Large Population-Based Cohort Study," *European Child and Adolescent Psychiatry* 22, no. 8 (2013): 511–18.

10. E. U. Vorbach, W. D. Hubner, and K. H. Arnoldt, "Effectiveness and Tolerance of the Hypericum Extract LI 160 in Comparison with Imipramine: Randomized Double-Blind Study with 135 Outpatients," *Journal of Geriatric Psychiatry and Neurology* 7, suppl. 1 (1994): S19–S23.

11. R. Bergman, J. Nuessner, and J. Demling, "Treatment of Mild to Moderate Depression: A Comparison between *Hypericum perforatum* and Amitriptyline," *Neurologie/Psychiatrie* 7 (1993): 235–40, summarized in Peter McWilliams, Mikael Nordfors, and Harold H. Bloomfield, *Hypericum and Depression* (Los Angeles: Prelude Press, 1996).

12. Richard Shelton et al., "Effectiveness of St. John's Wort in Major Depression: A Randomized Controlled Trial," *Journal of the American Medical Association* 285 (2001): 1978–86.

13. For a discussion of the plant origins and potent toxicity of several poisons, see Joel Hardman, Alfred Goodman Gilman, and Lee Limbird, *Goodman and Gilman's The Pharmacological Basis of Medical Therapeutics*, 9th ed. (New York: McGraw-Hill, Health Professions Division, 1996), 178–90 (strychnine and related compounds), 146–49 (amatoxins), and 149–54 (belladonna alkaloids).

14. Andrew Stoll et al., "Omega 3 Fatty Acids in Bipolar Disorder: A Preliminary Double-Blind, Placebo-Controlled Trial," *Archives of General Psychiatry* 56, no. 5 (1999): 407–12.

15. Lauren B. Marangell et al., "A Double-Blind, Placebo-Controlled Study of the Omega-3 Fatty Acid Docosahexaenoic Acid in the Treatment of Major Depression," *American Journal of Psychiatry* 160, no. 5 (2003): 996–98.

16. Hanah Nemets et al., "Omega-3 Treatment of Childhood Depression: A Controlled, Double-Blind Pilot Study," *American Journal of Psychiatry* 163, no. 6 (2006): 1098–1100.

17. Shima Jazayeri et al., "Comparison of Therapeutic Effects of Omega-3 Fatty Acid Eicosapentaenoic Acid and Fluoxetine, Separately and in Combination, in Major Depressive Disorder," *Australian and New Zealand Journal of Psychiatry* 42, no. 3 (2008): 192–98.

18. Michael Alvear, "A True Fish Story," www.salon.com, Sept. 9, 1999.

19. Hiroyasu Iso et al., "Intake of Fish and Omega-3 Fatty Acids and Risk of Stroke in Women," *Journal of the American Medical Association* 285, no. 3 (2001): 304–12.

20. Jazayeri et al., "Comparison of Therapeutic Effects of Omega-3 Fatty Acid Eicosapentaenoic Acid and Fluoxetine, Separately and in Combination, in Major Depressive Disorder."

21. Boris Nemets, Ziva Stahl, and R. H. Belmaker, "Addition of Omega-3 Fatty Acid to Maintenance Medication Treatment for Recurrent Unipolar Depressive Disorder," *American Journal of Psychiatry* 159, no. 3 (2002): 477–79.

22. Catherine Rothon et al., "Physical Activity and Depressive Symptoms in Adolescents: A Prospective Study," *BMC Medicine* 8, no. 1 (2010): 32.

23. Carroll W. Hughes et al., "Depressed Adolescents Treated with Exercise (DATE): A Pilot Randomized Controlled Trial to Test Feasibility and Establish Preliminary Effect Sizes," *Mental Health and Physical Activity* 6, no. 2 (2013): 119–31.

24. Joseph Rey and Garry Walter, "Half a Century of ECT Use in Young People," *American Journal of Psychiatry* 154, no. 5 (1997): 595–602.

25. Garry Walter, Karryn Koster, and Joseph Rey, "Electroconvulsive Therapy in Adolescents: Experience, Knowledge, and Attitudes of Recipients," *Journal of the American Academy of Child and Adolescent Psychiatry* 38, no. 5 (1999): 594–99. For an excellent discussion of the history and current practice of ECT, see Max Fink, *Electroshock: Restoring the Mind* (New York: Oxford University Press, 1999).

26. N. Ghaziuddin, S. P. Kutcher, and P. Knapp, "Summary of the Practice Parameter for the Use of Electroconvulsive Therapy with Adolescents," *Journal of the American Academy of Child and Adolescent Psychiatry* 43, no. 1 (2004): 119–22.

27. Larry Squire, Pamela Slater, and Patricia Miller, "Retrograde Amnesia and Bilateral Electroconvulsive Therapy: Long Term Follow-Up," *Archives of General Psychiatry* 38 (1981): 89–95.

28. C. P. L. Freeman, D. Weeks, and R. E. Kendell, "ECT III: Patients Who Complain," *British Journal of Psychiatry* 137 (1980): 17–25.

29. Larry R. Squire and Pamela C. Slater, "Electroconvulsive Therapy and Complaints of Memory Dysfunction: A Prospective Three-Year Follow-Up Study," *British Journal of Psychiatry* 142 (1983): 1–8.

30. S. Kutcher and H. Robertson, "Electroconvulsive Therapy in Treatment-Resistant Bipolar Youth," *Journal of Child and Adolescent Psychopharmacology* 5 (1995): 167–75.

31. David Cohen et al., "Absence of Cognitive Impairment at Long-Term Follow-up in Adolescents Treated with ECT for Severe Mood Disorder," *American Journal of Psychiatry* 157, no. 3 (2000): 460–62.

32. I. Perkins and K. Tanaka, "The Controversy That Will Not Die Is the Treatment That Can and Does Save Lives: Electroconvulsive Therapy," *Adolescence* 14 (1979): 607–17.

33. Sukeb Mukherjee, Harold Sackeim, and David Schnur, "Electroconvulsive Therapy of Acute Manic Episodes: A Review of 50 Years' Experience," *American Journal of Psychiatry* 151 (1994): 169–76.

34. S. Mukherjee, H. Sackheim, and C. Lee, "Unilateral ECT in the Treatment of Manic Episodes," *Convulsive Therapy* 4 (1988): 74–80.

35. Frederick K. Goodwin and Kay Redfield Jamison, *Manic-Depressive Illness* (New York: Oxford University Press, 1990), 661.

36. Olivier Taieb, David Cohen, Philippe Mezet, and Martine Flament, "Adolescents' Experiences with ECT," *Journal of the American Academy of Child and Adolescent Psychiatry* 39, no. 8 (2000): 934–44.

37. Paul E. Croarkin, Christopher A. Wall, and Jon Lee, "Applications of Transcranial Magnetic Stimulation (TMS) in Child and Adolescent Psychiatry," *International Review of Psychiatry* 23, no. 5 (2011): 445–53.

38. See Mark S. George, Eric Wasserman, and Robert Post, "Transcranial Magnetic Stimulation: A Neuropsychiatric Tool for the 21st Century," *Journal of Neuropsychiatry and Clinical Neurosciences* 8 (1996): 373–82.

39. Mark George et al., "Mood Improvement Following Daily Left Prefrontal Repetitive Transcranial Magnetic Stimulation in Patients with Depression: A Placebo-Controlled Crossover Trial," *American Journal of Psychiatry* 154 (1997): 1752–56.

40. Mark George et al., "A Controlled Trial of Daily Left Prefrontal Cortex TMS for Treating Depression," *Biological Psychiatry* 48 (2000): 962–70.

41. A. Pascual-Leone, B. Rubio, F. Pallardo, and M. D. Catala, "Beneficial Effect of Rapid-Rate Transcranial Magnetic Stimulation of the Left Dorsolateral Pre-frontal Cortex in Drug-Resistant Depression," *Lancet* 348 (1996): 233–37; and Charles Epstein, Gary Figiel, William McDonald, Jody Amazon-Leece, and Linda Figiel, "Rapid Rate Transcranial Magnetic Stimulation in Young and Middle-Aged Refractory Depressed Patients," *Psychiatric Annals* 28 (1998): 36–39.

42. A. John Rush et al., "Vagus Nerve Stimulation (VNS) for Treatment-Resistant Depression: A Multi-Center Study," *Biological Psychiatry* 47, no. 4 (2000): 276–86.

Chapter 9 Counseling and Psychotherapy

1. A. Wood, R. Harrington, and A. Moore, "A Controlled Trial of Brief Cognitive-Behavioral Intervention in Adolescent Patients with Depressive Disorders," *Journal of Child Psychology and Psychiatry* 37 (1996): 737–46.

2. Boris Birmaher et al., "Clinical Outcome after Short-Term Psychotherapy for Adolescents with Major Depressive Disorder," *Archives of General Psychiatry* 57 (2000): 29–36.

3. Dinah Jayson, "Which Depressed Patients Respond to Cognitive-Behavioral Treatment?" *Journal of the American Academy of Child and Adolescent Psychiatry* 37, no. 1 (1998): 35–39.

4. John March et al., "Fluoxetine, Cognitive-Behavioral Therapy, and Their Combination for Adolescents with Depression: Treatment for Adolescents with Depression Study (TADS) Randomized Controlled Trial," *JAMA* 292, no. 7 (2004): 807–20.

5. Jerome Frank, *Persuasion and Healing: A Comparative Study of Psychotherapy*, rev. ed. (New York: Schocken Books, 1974), xvi.

6. The standard work on cognitive-behavioral therapy is Aaron Beck, A. John Rush, Brian Shaw, and Gary Emery, *Cognitive Therapy of Depression* (New York: Guilford Press, 1979).

7. The area of comparison studies of cognitive-behavioral psychotherapy and medication in the treatment of depression can be accurately described as a hornet's nest of controversy. It's not difficult to find a study to support any possible view: superiority of medication over psychotherapy, superiority of psychotherapy over medication, and equal efficacy for both. For a nicely designed and well-executed study that found cognitive therapy to be as helpful as imipramine for 107 patients with major depressive disorder, see Steven Hollon et al., "Cognitive Therapy and Pharmacotherapy for Depression, Singly and in Combination," *Archives of General Psychiatry* 49 (1992): 774–81. For readers who would like to jump into the hornet's nest, we suggest Jacqueline B. Persons, Michael E. Thase, and Paul Crits-Christoph, "The Role of Psychotherapy in the Treatment of Depression," and the four (yes, four) accompanying rebuttal/commentary articles in the same issue of *Archives of General Psychiatry*.

8. Beck et al., *Cognitive Therapy of Depression*, 11.

9. Jeannette Rosselló and Guillermo Bernal, "The Efficacy of Cognitive-Behavioral and Interpersonal Treatments for Depression in Puerto Rican Adolescents," *Journal of Consulting and Clinical Psychology* 67, no. 5 (1999): 734.

10. Laura Mufson, Myra Weissman, Donna Morceau, and Robin Garfinkle, "Efficacy of Interpersonal Psychotherapy for Depressed Adolescents," *Archives of General Psychiatry* 56 (1999): 573–79.

11. Marsha M. Linehan, "Dialectical Behavioral Therapy: A Cognitive Behavioral Approach to Parasuicide," *Journal of Personality Disorders* 1, no. 4 (1987): 328–33.

12. Steven C. Hayes et al., "Acceptance and Commitment Therapy: Model, Processes and Outcomes," *Behaviour Research and Therapy* 44, no. 1 (2006): 1–25.

13. Louise Hayes, Candice P. Boyd, and Jessica Sewell, "Acceptance and Commitment Therapy for the Treatment of Adolescent Depression: A Pilot Study in a Psychiatric Outpatient Setting," *Mindfulness* 2, no. 2 (2011): 86–94.

Chapter 10   Attention-Deficit/Hyperactivity Disorder

1. George Still, "Some Abnormal Psychical Conditions in Childhood," *Lancet* 1 (1902): 1008–12.

2. Laurence Greenhill, Jeffrey Halperin, and Howard Abikoff, "Stimulant Medications," *Journal of the American Academy of Child and Adolescent Psychiatry* 38, no. 5 (1999): 503–12.

3. Arthur Robin, "Attention-Deficit/Hyperactivity Disorder in Adolescents," *Journal of the American Academy of Child and Adolescent Psychiatry* 45, no. 5 (1999): 1027–38.

4. MTA Cooperative Group, "Moderators and Mediators of Treatment Response for Children with Attention-Deficit/Hyperactivity Disorder: The Multimodal Treatment Study of Children with Attention-Deficit/Hyperactivity Disorder," *Archives of General Psychiatry* 56, no. 12 (1999): 1088.

5. Thomas Spencer, Joseph Biederman, and Timothy Wilens, "Attention-Deficit/Hyperactivity Disorder and Co-morbidity," *Pediatric Clinics of North America* 46, no. 5 (1999): 915–27.

6. J. Biederman et al., "Attention-Deficit Hyperactivity Disorder and Juvenile Mania: An Overlooked Comorbidity?" *Journal of the American Academy of Child and Adolescent Psychiatry* 35, no. 8 (1996): 997–1008.

7. Stephen Faraone, Joseph Biederman, Douglas Mennin, Janet Wozniak, and Thomas Spencer, "Attention-Deficit/Hyperactivity Disorder with Bipolar Disorder: A Familial Subtype?" *Journal of the American Academy of Child and Adolescent Psychiatry* 36, no. 10 (1997): 1378–87.

8. M. Strober et al., "Early Childhood Attention-Deficit/Hyperactivity Disorder Predicts Poorer Response to Acute Lithium Therapy in Adolescent Mania," *Journal of Affective Disorders* 51, no. 11 (1998): 145–51.

Chapter 11   Autism, Asperger's, and Related Disorders

1. Hans Asperger, "Die 'Autistischen Psychopathen' im Kindesalter," *European Archives of Psychiatry and Clinical Neuroscience* 117, no. 1 (1944): 76–136.

2. Leo Kanner, "Autistic Disturbances of Affective Contact," *Nervous Child* 2, no. 3 (1943): 217–50.

3. Dennis K. Flaherty, "The Vaccine-Autism Connection: A Public Health Crisis Caused by Unethical Medical Practices and Fraudulent Science," *Annals of Pharmacotherapy* 45, no. 10 (2011): 1302–4.

4. Lindsey Sterling et al., "Validity of the Revised Children's Anxiety and Depression Scale for Youth with Autism Spectrum Disorders," *Autism* (Jan. 2014), doi:10.1177/1362361313510066.

5. Susan Dickerson Mayes et al., "Variables Associated with Anxiety and Depression in Children with Autism," *Journal of Developmental and Physical Disabilities* 23, no. 4 (2011): 325–37.

6. Alexander Kolevzon, Karen A. Mathewson, and Eric Hollander, "Selective Serotonin Reuptake Inhibitors in Autism: A Review of Efficacy and Tolerability," *Journal of Clinical Psychiatry* 67, no. 3 (2006): 407–14.

7. Elisabeth M. Dykens et al., "Reducing Distress in Mothers of Children with Autism and Other Disabilities: A Randomized Trial," *Pediatrics* 134, no. 2 (2014): e454–e463.

Chapter 12   Alcohol and Drug Abuse

1. L. Johnston, P. O'Malley, J. Bachman, *Monitoring the Future: National Results on Adolescent Drug Abuse: Overview of Key Findings* (Bethesda, Md.: National Institute on Drug Abuse, 2001), 6.

2. Markus Henriksson et al., "Mental Disorders and Comorbidity in Suicide," *American Journal of Psychiatry* 150 (1993): 935–40.

3. Marjorie Hogan, "Diagnosis and Treatment of Teen Drug Use," *Medical Clinics of North America* 84, no. 4 (2000): 927–66.

4. Sandra Morrison, Peter Rogers, and Mark Thomas, "Alcohol and Adolescents," *Pediatric Clinics of North America* 42, no. 2 (1995): 371–87.

5. Andrew Johns, "Psychiatric Effects of Cannabis," *British Journal of Psychiatry* 178 (2001): 116–22.

6. Thomas Crowley, Marilyn Macdonald, Elizabeth Whitmore, and Susan Mikulich, "Cannabis Dependence, Withdrawal and Reinforcing Effects among Adolescents with Conduct Symptoms and Substance Abuse Disorders," *Drug and Alcohol Dependence* 50 (1998): 27–37.

7. Asbjørg Chrisopherson, "Amphetamine Designer Drugs—An Overview and Epidemiology," *Toxicology Letters* 112 (2000): 127–31.

8. Matthew Klam, "Experiencing Ecstasy," *New York Times*, Jan. 21, 2001, available at www.nytimes.com/2001/01/21/magazine/experiencing-ecstasy.html.

9. Andrew C. Parrott, "MDMA, Serotonergic Neurotoxicity, and the Diverse Functional Deficits of Recreational 'Ecstasy' Users," *Neuroscience and Biobehavioral Reviews* 37, no. 8 (2013): 1466–84.

10. For an excellent summary of MDMA's short-term and long-term effects on the brain, see Michael John Morgan, "Ecstasy (MDMA): A Review of Its Possible Persistent Psychological Effects," *Psychopharmacology* 152 (2000): 230–48.

11. Valerie Kremer, "Navy Medicine Rolls Out New Campaign to Deter 'Bath Salts' Designer Drug Use," *Navy Medicine*, Dec. 20, 2012, available at www.navy.mil/submit/display.asp?story_id=71211.

12. L. D. Johnston, P. M. O'Malley, R. A. Miech, J. G. Bachman, and J. E. Schulenberg, *Monitoring the Future National Results on Drug Use, 1975–2013: Overview, Key Findings on Adolescent Drug Use* (Ann Arbor: Institute for Social Research, University of Michigan, 2014).

13. Timothy Wilens, Joseph Biederman, Ana Abrantes, and Thomas Spencer, "Clinical Characteristics of Psychiatrically Referred Adolescent Outpatients with Substance Abuse Disorder," *Journal of the American Academy of Child and Adolescent Psychiatry* 36, no. 7 (1997): 941–47.

14. Judith Brook, Patricia Cohen, and David Brook, "Longitudinal Study of Co-occurring Psychiatric Disorders and Substance Use," *Journal of the American Academy of Child and Adolescent Psychiatry* 37, no. 3 (1998): 322–30.

15. Michael Lyvers, "'Loss of Control' in Alcoholism and Drug Addiction: A Neuroscientific Interpretation," *Experimental and Clinical Psychopharmacology* 8, no. 2 (2000): 225–49.

16. Paul Bergman, Maurice Smith, and Norman Hoffman, "Adolescent Treatment, Implications for Assessment, Practice Guidelines and Outcome Management," *Pediatric Clinics of North America* 42, no. 2 (1995): 453–72.

Chapter 13   Eating Disorders

1. The complete texts of all three historical accounts can be found in Arnold Anderson, *Practical Comprehensive Treatment of Anorexia and Bulimia* (Baltimore: Johns Hopkins University Press, 1985), 10–29.

2. Richard Kreipe and Susan Birndorf, "Eating Disorders in Adolescents," *Medical Clinics of North America* 84, no. 4 (2000): 1027–49.

3. Peter Lewinsohn, Ruth Striegel-Moore, and John Seeley, "Epidemiology and Natural Course of Eating Disorders in Young Women from Adolescence to Young Adulthood," *Journal of the American Academy of Child and Adolescent Psychiatry* 39, no. 10 (2000): 1284–92.

4. T. Zaider, J. Johnson, and S. Cockell, "Psychiatric Comorbidity Associated with Eating Disorder Symptomatology among Adolescents in the Community," *International Journal of Eating Disorders* 28, no. 1 (2000): 58–67.

5. Tracey Wade, Cynthia Bulik, Michael Neale, and Kenneth Kendler, "Anorexia Nervosa and Major Depression: Shared Genetic and Environmental Risk Factors," *American Journal of Psychiatry* 157, no. 3 (2000): 469–71.

6. A. Raffi, M. Rondini, S. Grandi, and G. Fava, "Life Events and Prodromal Symptoms in Bulimia Nervosa," *Psychological Medicine* 30, no. 3 (2000): 727–31.

7. David Jimerson, Barbara Wolfe, Andrew Brotman, and Eran Metzger, "Medications in the Treatment of Eating Disorders," *Psychiatric Clinics of North America* 19, no. 4 (1996): 739–54.

8. Walter Kaye, Kelly Gendell, and Michael Strober, "Serotonin Neuronal Function and Selective Serotonin Reuptake Inhibitor Treatment in Anorexia and Bulimia Nervosa," *Biological Psychiatry* 44 (1998): 825–38.

Chapter 14   *"Cutting" and Other Self-Harming Behaviors*

1. Paul R. McHugh and Phillip R. Slavney, *The Perspectives of Psychiatry*, 2nd ed. (Baltimore: Johns Hopkins University Press, 1999), 151.

2. Jennifer Egan, "The Thin Red Line," *New York Times Magazine*, July 27, 1997.

3. Armando Favazza, "The Coming of Age of Self-Mutilation," *Journal of Nervous and Mental Disease* 186, no. 5 (1998): 259–68.

4. Caron Zlotnick, Jill Mattia, and Mark Zimmerman, "Clinical Correlates of Self-Mutilation in a Sample of General Psychiatric Patients," *Journal of Nervous and Mental Diseases* 187, no. 5 (1999): 296–301.

5. Favazza, "Coming of Age of Self-Mutilation."

6. See Egan, "Thin Red Line"; and Marilee Strong, *A Bright Red Scream: Self-Mutilation and the Language of Pain* (New York: Penguin Books, 1999).

7. Stephen P. Lewis, Nancy L. Heath, Jill M. St. Denis, and Rick Noble, "The Scope of Nonsuicidal Self-Injury on YouTube," *Pediatrics* 127, no. 3 (2011): e552–e557.

8. See Armando Favazza, *Bodies under Siege: Self-Mutilation and Body Modification in Culture and Psychiatry*, 2d ed. (Baltimore: Johns Hopkins University Press, 1996), 241.

9. Marsha Linehan, *Cognitive-Behavioral Therapy of the Borderline Personality Disorder* (New York: Guilford Press, 1993).

10. Benedict Carey, "Expert on Mental Illness Reveals Her Own Fight," *New York Times*, June 23, 2011.

11. Alan Frances, "Introduction to Section on Self-Mutilation," *Journal of Personality Disorders* 1 (1987): 316.

12. All information on youth suicide statistics was obtained from the CDC Injury Statistics Query and Reporting System (WISQARS) website. All data are freely available and accessible at www.cdc.gov/injury/wisqars.

13. Matthew K. Nock et al., "Prevalence, Correlates, and Treatment of Lifetime Suicidal Behavior among Adolescents: Results from the National Comorbidity Survey Replication Adolescent Supplement," *JAMA Psychiatry* 70, no. 3 (2013): 300–310.

14. Iris Borowski, Marjorie Ireland, and Michael Resnick, "Adolescent Suicide Attempts: Risks and Protectors," *Pediatrics* 107, no. 3 (2001): 485–93.

15. Centers for Disease Control, "Effectiveness in Disease and Injury Prevention: Adolescent Suicide and Suicide Attempts—Santa Fe County, New Mexico, January 1985–May 1990," *Morbidity and Mortality Weekly Report* 40, no. 20 (1990): 329–31.

16. Sonja A. Swanson and Ian Colman, "Association between Exposure to Suicide and Suicidality Outcomes in Youth," *Canadian Medical Association Journal* 185, no. 10 (2013): 870–77.

17. D. Brent, J. Perper, C. Allman, G. Moritz, M. Wartella, and J. Zelenak, "The Presence and Accessibility of Firearms in the Homes of Adolescent Suicides: A Case Control Study," *Journal of the American Medical Association* 266, no. 21 (1991): 2989–95.

18. Danice K. Eaton et al., "Youth Risk Behavior Surveillance—United States, 2011," *Morbidity and Mortality Weekly Report: Surveillance Summaries* (*Washington, DC:* 2002) 61, no. 4 (2012): 1–162.

Chapter 15   The Genetics of Mood Disorders

1. Emil Kraepelin, *Manic-Depressive Insanity and Paranoia,* trans. R. M. Barclay, ed. G. M. Robertson (Edinburgh: Livingstone, 1921; reprinted New York: Arno Press, 1976), 165 (in reprint edition).

2. For a more detailed account, which includes references to the original articles, see Eliot Marshall, "Manic Depression: Highs and Lows on the Research Roller Coaster," *Science* 264 (1994): 1693–95.

3. Jonathan Flint and Kenneth S. Kendler, "The Genetics of Major Depression," *Neuron* 81, no. 3 (2014): 484–503.

4. See Elliot S. Gershon, "Genetics," in *Manic-Depressive Illness,* Frederick K. Goodwin and Kay Redfield Jamison (New York: Oxford University Press, 1990), 373–401.

5. For a very readable overview of some of these issues, see Doris Teichler Zallen, *Does It Run in the Family? A Consumer's Guide to DNA Testing for Genetic Disorders* (New Brunswick, N.J.: Rutgers University Press, 1997).

Chapter 16   Strategies for Successful Treatment

1. Emil Kraepelin, *Manic-Depressive Insanity and Paranoia,* trans. R. M. Barclay, ed. G. M. Robertson (Edinburgh: Livingstone, 1921; reprinted New York: Arno Press, 1976), 179–81 (in reprint edition).

2. Ian M. Goodyer, "The Influence of Recent Life Events on the Onset and Outcome of Major Depression in Young People," in *Depressive Disorders in Children and Adolescents: Epidemiology, Risk Factors, and Treatment,* ed. Cecilia Ahmoi Essau and Franz Petermann (Northvale, N.J.: Jason Aronson, 1999), 241.

3. For a complete discussion of these animal models of the kindling phenomenon, see Robert Post, "Transduction of Psychosocial Stress into the Neurobiology of Recurrent Affective Disorder," *American Journal of Psychiatry* 149 (1992): 999–1010.

4. Constance Hammen and Michael Gitlin, "Stress Reactivity in Bipolar Patients and Its Relation to Prior History of Disorder," *American Journal of Psychiatry* 154 (1997): 856–57.

5. Depression Guideline Panel, *Depression in Primary Care*, vol. 1, *Treatment of Major Depression: Clinical Practice Guidelines* (Rockville, Md.: U.S. Department of Health and Human Services, Public Health Service, Agency for Health Care Policy and Research, 1993).

6. George McGovern, *Terry: My Daughter's Life-and-Death Struggle with Alcoholism* (New York: Villard Books, 1996), 187.

7. See Peter Lewinsohn, Paul Rohde, John Seeley, Daniel Klein, and Ian Gotlib, "Natural Course of Adolescent Major Depressive Disorder in a Community Sample: Predictors of Recurrence in Young Adults," *American Journal of Psychiatry* 157, no. 10 (2000): 1584–91; and Mark Sanford et al., "Predicting the One-Year Course of Adolescent Major Depression," *Journal of the American Academy of Child and Adolescent Psychiatry* 34, no. 12 (1994): 1618–28.

Chapter 17   The Role of the Family

1. Stephen Strakowski, Susan McElroy, Paul Keck, and Scott West, "Suicidality among Patients with Mixed and Manic Bipolar Disorder," *American Journal of Psychiatry* 153 (1996): 674–76.

Chapter 18   Planning for Emergencies

1. See, for example, J. E. Bailey et al., "Risk Factors for Violent Death of Women in the Home," *Archives of Internal Medicine* 157 (1997): 777–82.

INDEX

antidepressants (*cont.*)
structure of, 119, 120; dosing of, 127, 137, 138; duration of treatment with, 312–13; for eating disorders, 267; efficacy of, 106, 121, 122–25, 135–36; lag time for improvement with, 137; lithium augmentation of, 144–45, 161; mania precipitated by, 79, 224; mechanisms of action of, 112–17, 119–21, 224; monoamine oxidase inhibitors, 133–35; off-label prescribing of, 103, 127; overdose of, 122, 130; response to, 138–39; side effects of, 121–22, 136–38; SNRIs, 130–31; SSRIs, 125–30; suicidality and, 1, 5, 126; tricyclic, 118–25, 341

antipsychotics, 155–56, 164, 165–72; for aggression in autism, 238; for children in foster care, 171; controversies about use of, 170–72; mechanism of action of, 166; side effects of, 168–70; therapeutic profile of, 167–68

anxiety: bipolar disorder and, 94; depression and, 29, 36, 37, 38, 44, 45, 87, 89, 93; substance use and, 35; eating disorders and, 265, 266; marijuana use and, 179, 180, 245; psychotherapy for, 204, 205, 206; self-mutilation due to, 269, 270; suicidality and, 276, 277

anxiety disorders, 68, 69, 294

anxiety medications, 164, 295; antidepressants, 136; antipsychotics, 166; in autism, 237; benzodiazepines, 172; valproate, 153

appetite changes, 12, 13, 21–22, 23, 25, 29, 41, 45, 47, 48, 91; in anorexia nervosa, 260–61; in autism, 235; in bipolar depression, 75; in dysthymic disorder, 58, 59; in mania, 64

appetite effects of drugs, 136, 137, 317; amphetamines, 247, 248; antipsychotics, 169; bupropion, 132; marijuana, 245; SSRIs, 128; valproate, 154

aripiprazole (Abilify), 166, 167, 238
asenapine (Saphris), 167
Asendin (amoxapine), 119
Asperger's syndrome, 213, 228, 236; vs. autism, 233–35
assumptive world, 37
Ativan (lorazepam), 173
atomoxetine (Strattera), 224–25
attention-deficit/hyperactivity disorder (ADHD), 45, 213, 215–25; autism and, 232; bipolar disorder and, 222–23, 294–95; consequences of, 219–20; depression and, 222–23; depression misdiagnosed as, 22–23; diagnosis of, 87, 95, 216–19; executive dysfunction and, 216; "medical" marijuana in, 179–80; medications for, 217, 220–21, 223–25; psychotherapy for, 220, 221, 225; substance abuse and, 252
autism spectrum disorders (ASD), 213, 226–38; ADHD and, 232; vs. Asperger's syndrome, 233–35; history of, 227–30; mood disorders and, 235–36; prevalence of, 226–27; symptoms of, 230–33; treatment of, 236–38; vaccines and, 229–30

"bath salts," 247, 250–51
behavioral activation, 178
behavioral problems, 32, 82, 83, 162, 295, 296, 298; in ADHD, 216–17; antipsychotics for, 172; conduct disorder, 83, 91, 161–62, 295; *DSM* diagnoses and, 95–97; family therapy for, 203; mood stabilizers for, 153, 161–62; oppositional defiant disorder, 96–97, 161, 295; self-mutilation, 269–74; substance abuse and, 252
behavioral regulation, 216
benzodiazepines, 172, 173, 246
bereavement, 11, 13, 18–19
binge-eating disorder, 260, 263
biological markers, 96
biology-psychology split, 192–94

dangerousness, 327, 341
Daytrana (methylphenidate), 221
death: drug- and alcohol-related, 241,
244; from lithium poisoning, 141, 146;
from MDMA, 249; from tobacco, 241;
by suicide, 275, 279; thoughts of, 29,
41, 48; from tricyclic antidepressants, 121–22
defense mechanisms, 243
delusions, 30, 48, 52, 52n, 91, 165; antipsychotics for, 165, 167; definition of,
30; in mania, 64; self-mutilation due
to, 270
demoralization, 37–38, 39, 40, 41, 46,
123, 124
deoxyribonucleic acid (DNA), 282–84,
285, 286, 289, 347
Depakene; Depakote. See valproate
depression: ADHD and, 222–23; atypical, 91, 132; autism and, 235–36; behavioral problems and, 83, 91, 96–97,
161–62, 295; biological vs. psychological, 39–40; in bipolar I, 71–73; in
bipolar II, 73–75; in bipolar spectrum
disorders, 77; in cyclothymic disorder, 75; definition of, 9–10; vs. demoralization, 37–38, 39, 40; drug-
induced, 25; due to another medical
condition, 95; eating disorders and,
266–67; genetics of, 285, 287; long-
lasting effects of, 82; major depressive disorder, 47–55, 80; not otherwise specified, 60, 66, 90–91, 92;
recurrences of, 83; relapse prevention for, 312–13; serious, 39–41; substance abuse and, 83, 244, 252, 253;
substance/medication-induced, 95;
symptoms of, 12–23, 28–31, 47–48;
unipolar vs. bipolar, 80
depressive illness, 2, 9, 13, 23–24, 27
depressive syndrome, 13–23, 28, 47
desipramine (Norpramin), 119, 121–22
desvenlafaxine (Pristiq), 130
development, psychological, 31–36, 81;

effect of substance abuse on, 256,
315; theories of, 32–39
dexamethasone suppression test, 46
dextroamphetamine (Dexedrine), 221
diagnosis, 2–3, 43–47, 78–81; brain imaging, 346–47; "chart viruses" and, 295;
errors in, 45; evolutions over time,
44–45, 295; mental status examination, 46; psychological testing, 296–
98; purposes of, 43, 44; time required
for, 298; for treatment planning, 3, 6,
294–98; use of DSM for, 84–97
*Diagnostic and Statistical Manual of
Mental Disorders (DSM)*, 7–8, 16, 60,
84–97; autism spectrum disorders in,
232, 234–35; controversies in use of,
95–97; fifth edition (DSM-5), 7, 44, 45,
60, 68–70, 79, 84, 88, 93–94; history
of, 84–87; mood disorder categories
in, 90–95; multiaxial diagnostic system of, 87–90
dialectical behavioral therapy (DBT),
206–8; for self-injury, 273
diazepam (Valium), 173, 246
diet, 175, 317; autism and, 232; caffeine
in, 316–17; eating disorders and, 262,
265–66, 272; MAOIs and, 134–35;
omega-3 fatty acids in, 175, 177; for
weight management, 149, 169, 317
disclosure of patient information,
321–22
discouragement, 38, 40, 278
disinhibited behavior, 67
disruptive mood dysregulation disorder (DMDD), 67–70
divalproex sodium. See valproate
dopamine, 113, 132–33, 166, 168, 224
dopamine-norepinephrine reuptake
inhibitors, 131, 132–33, 224
doxepin (Sinequan), 119
driving, 51, 220, 245
duloxetine (Cymbalta), 130
dynamic psychotherapy, 193–94,
204–5, 320

dysphoria, 48, 52; premenstrual dysphoric disorder, 59–61

dysthymic disorder, 55–59, 80; compared with major depressive disorder, 58–59; in *DSM*, 90, 92–93; as precursor of depression, 58–59, 78

eating disorders, 214, 257–69; anorexia nervosa, 260–62; binge-eating disorder, 260, 263; bulimia nervosa, 260, 262–63; history of, 259–60; mood disorders and, 266–68; online groups promoting, 35; self-mutilation and, 271, 272; understanding, 264–66

echolalia, 231

ecstasy (MDMA), 241, 248–50, 253

Effexor (venlafaxine), 130–31, 138

Elavil (amitriptyline), 119, 120, 174, 174n

Eldepryl (selegiline), 134

electrocardiogram, 122

electroconvulsive therapy (ECT), 99, 180–87; history of, 180–82; mechanism of action of, 185–86; memory loss induced by, 184–85; modern procedure for, 182–84; prescribing of, 182, 186–87

electroencephalogram (EEG), 346, 347

emergencies, 51, 292, 332–43; calling 911 in, 325; insurance issues and, 335, 336, 337, 338–41; knowing who to call in, 336–38; medical information chart for, 341, 342; planning for, 332–35; safety issues / suicidality, 324–25, 341–43

Emsan (selegiline), 135

energy level, 317; in depression, 11, 13, 15, 22, 47; in mania, 64, 66–67

epigenetics, 348

Epitol. *See* carbamazepine

Erikson, Erik, 32–36, 299

escitalopram (Lexapro), 127

Eskalith; Eskalith CR. *See* lithium

euthymia, 319

executive function, 216, 250

exercise, 178–79

extrapyramidal side effects, 167

family. *See* parents/family

family therapy, 202–4, 221, 316, 331

fatigue, 13, 21, 22, 48, 59, 68; of amphetamine crash, 247; in anorexia nervosa, 261; bupropion for, 132

fight or flight response, 224

firearms, 279, 329, 341–43

fish oil, 175–78

fluoxetine (Prozac), 77, 113, 125–27, 128, 136, 139, 224, 267, 348, 349

fluvoxamine (Luvox), 127, 129

Freud, Anna, 38, 243

Freud, Sigmund, 193, 194, 198, 243, 299

future issues, 345–50; computer technology and drug development, 348–49; genetics research, 288–89, 347–48, 349–50; neuroscience research, 345–47; prevention programs, 349–50

gabapentin (Neurontin), 103, 159–60

Gabatril (tiagabine), 160

gamma-aminobutyric acid (GABA), 152

Genetic Information Nondiscrimination Act, 350

genetics, 46, 214, 280–89; of ADHD, 222–23; of anorexia nervosa, 266–67; epigenetics, 348; genes, chromosomes, and DNA, 280–84, 347; genetic diseases, 284–87; of mood disorders, 285–89; pharmacogenomics, 139, 289, 347–48; research in, 288–89, 347–48, 349–50; stress and, 311; twin studies, 287

genetic testing, 289, 350

Geodon (ziprasidone), 167

Global Assessment of Functioning (GAF) Scale, 90

G proteins, 114–16, 281

group psychotherapy, 205–6

guanfacine (Intuniv; Tenex), 224

guilt feelings, 11, 13, 19–20, 29, 48, 91, 203, 319; in bulimia nervosa, 266; in dysthymic disorder, 58, 59; of parents, 330; self-mutilation and, 270, 273

gynecomastia, 169–70

halfway houses, 256

hallucinations, 30, 48, 60, 91, 165; antipsychotics for, 165, 166, 167; diagnosis of, 30–31; in mania, 64; self-mutilation due to, 270; substance–induced, 25, 248, 251

hallucinogens, 248

happiness, 9, 10, 17

headache, 13, 22, 29, 48, 89, 158

health insurance issues: choice of psychiatrist, 304–5, 336; copayments, 338; genetic testing, 289, 350; hospitalization coverage, 335, 336, 337, 338–41; managed care, 304, 339–41; medication coverage, 341

Health Insurance Portability and Accountability Act (HIPAA), 321

health maintenance organization (HMO), 212, 304–5, 335, 339–40, 341

history of child psychiatry, 27–28

hopelessness, 19, 270, 276, 277, 320, 327

hospitalization, 66, 68, 70, 155–56, 293, 326–29, 332–43; antipsychotic use and, 171; benzodiazepine use and, 172; for bipolar II disorder, 75; consent and assent for, 326; for dangerousness, 327, 341; for eating disorders, 262, 263, 266, 267–68; for electroconvulsive therapy, 182–83; indicated by GAF Scale, 90; insurance coverage for, 335, 336, 337, 338–41; involuntary, 325, 326–29, 333; parent involvement during, 321; partial/day, 339; pre-admission review for, 340; questions/preparation for, 337–38; return to school after, 211; for substance abuse, 254, 255, 256; for

suicidality, 51, 327, 333, 335, 341, 343; for treatment noncompliance, 330

"huffing," 241

Human Genome Project, 288, 347

hypomania, 64, 66, 68, 71; in bipolar II, 73–75, 92, 94; in cyclothymic disorder, 75–77, 92, 94; electroconvulsive therapy–induced, 187; family reactions to, 319, 330; lithium for, 150; in seasonal affective disorder, 94

identity crisis, 32

identity development, 35–37

identity diffusion, 35

imipramine, 112, 113, 118, 119, 120, 121, 174, 174n, 193, 366n7

impulsivity: in ADHD, 216, 218, 219, 220, 222, 224, 294; in autism, 232; dialectical behavioral therapy for, 208; in eating disorders, 262, 263, 266, 267; in mania, 66, 162; medications for, 162, 220, 224; self-mutilation and, 271; suicidality and, 275

inhalant abuse, 241

insight-oriented psychotherapy, 193–94, 204–5, 320

interpersonal psychotherapy (IPT), 201–2

Intuniv (guanfacine), 224

involuntary commitment, 325, 326–29, 333

iproniazid, 25, 112, 133

irritability, 11, 12–13, 18, 19, 21, 29, 41, 45, 86; in ADHD, 222; antipsychotics for, 167, 168; in autism, 235, 236; behavioral problems and, 295; in bipolar disorder, 67, 69, 74, 75; dialectical behavior therapy for, 206, 207, 208; in disruptive mood dysregulation disorder, 67, 68, 69–70, 93; in dysthymic disorder, 58, 59; eating disorders and, 267; family effects of, 203, 210, 318, 319, 320, 329, 330–31; in major depressive disorder, 48–53; in mania,

63, 64; mood stabilizers for, 162; SSRI-induced, 128; substance withdrawal and, 245; suicide and, 324, 342

Kapvay (clonidine), 224
kindling phenomenon, 67, 310–11
Klonopin (clonazepam), 173
Kraepelin, Emil, 78, 80, 280, 310

laboratory tests, 44, 45–46
lamotrigine (Lamictal), 157–59, 161; mechanism of action of, 157–58; side effects of, 158–59; therapeutic profile of, 158
Latuda (lurasidone), 167
laxative misuse, 261, 262
Lexapro (escitalopram), 127
Librium (chlordiazepoxide), 173
lifestyle modifications, 316–17
lisdexamfetamine (Vyvanse), 221
lithium (Eskalith, Eskalith CR, Lithobid, Lithonate, Lithotabs), 73, 140–51, 161, 162; for antidepressant augmentation, 144–45, 161; electroconvulsive therapy and, 184, 186; history of, 140–44, 193; interaction with diuretics, 149; for mania with ADHD, 223; mechanism of action of, 114–16, 286–87; nonadherence to, 330; to reduce suicidality, 148; for relapse prevention, 144, 146–47; selection of, 163; side effects of, 148–51, 163, 171, 175; therapeutic profile of, 145–48, 146n; toxicity of, 141, 146, 175; use in pregnancy, 150
lorazepam (Ativan), 173
loss of interest or pleasure, 2, 13, 14–15, 16–18, 29, 41, 47, 48, 52, 53, 59, 91, 132; amphetamine-induced, 247; eating disorders and, 267
LSD, 248
Ludiomil (maprotiline), 119
lurasidone (Latuda), 167
Luvox (fluvoxamine), 127, 129

major depressive disorder, 47–55, 80; case examples of, 14–15, 48–51; compared with dysthymic disorder, 58–59; in *DSM*, 90, 92–93; duration of, 55; major depressive episodes in, 54–55; with mostly irritable mood, 48–53; onset of, 47; prevalence of, 54; recurrence of, 55; stress-precipitated, 53–54; symptoms of, 47–48
managed care, 304, 339–41
mania, 62–65; vs. agitation, 165; antidepressant-precipitated, 79, 224; in bipolar I, 71–73; electroconvulsive therapy for, 186–87; mood stabilizers for, 140–63; stimulant-precipitated, 223; symptoms of, 64, 66–67, 69. *See also* bipolar affective disorder
manic-depressive illness, 63, 71, 72, 73, 77, 78
maprotiline (Ludiomil), 119
marijuana use, 241, 242, 244–47, 256; addiction and withdrawal from, 244–46; depression treatment and, 314–15; "medical," 179–80, 246; prevalence of, 244; "synthetic" marijuana, 246–47
MDA, 248, 249
MDMA (ecstasy), 241, 248–50, 253
medical conditions, 89; depressive disorder due to, 95
medical information chart, 341, 342
medications, 6, 24, 41, 99, 101–72; for ADHD, 217, 220–21, 223–25; antidepressants, 118–39; antipsychotics, 165–72; for autism, 236–37; benzodiazepines, 172, 173; choice of, 293; computer technology and development of, 348–49; dosing of, 105–7; duration of treatment with, 312–13, 350; efficacy of, 106; FDA and, 102–5; individual responses to, 77–78; insurance coverage for, 341; labeling of, 102, 104–5; mechanisms of action of, 107–17; mood stabilizers, 140–63; for

school performance, 37, 62, 81–82, 179; ADHD and, 219, 220, 221; alcoholism and, 242, 243; falling grades, 22, 41, 49–50, 52, 54, 56–57

seasonal affective disorder, 94–95, 133

second messengers, 114–16

seizures: benzodiazepine-withdrawal, 172; bupropion-induced, 132; eating disorders and, 132, 263; electroconvulsive therapy–induced, 181–82, 183–84, 187, 190; medications for, 151–60; transcranial magnetic stimulation–induced, 190; vagal nerve stimulation for, 191

selective serotonin reuptake inhibitors (SSRIs), 5, 119, 125–30, 164, 224, 341; dosing of, 127, 137; drug interactions with, 129–30; efficacy of, 135–36; response to, 138–39; side effects of, 127–29; suicidality and, 5, 126, 279; use of, in autism, 237

selegiline (Eldepryl; Emsam), 134, 135

self-attitude, 41, 47, 205

self-control, 216, 255, 264, 319

self-doubt, 11, 35, 37

self-mutilation, 269–74, 333; eating disorders and, 271, 272; mood disorders and, 271; prevalence of, 270, 272; treatment of, 272–74

Seroquel (quetiapine), 166–67

serotonin, 113, 114, 119, 127, 130, 166, 167, 224

serotonin-norepinephrine reuptake inhibitors (SNRIs), 130–31, 224

sertraline (Zoloft), 77, 103, 127

sexuality, 34; ADHD and, 220; SSRI effects on, 128–29

shame, 19, 20, 323; bulimia nervosa and, 262, 266; of parents, 330; self-mutilation and, 270; suicidality and, 324, 343

Sinequan (doxepin), 119

sleep disturbances, 12, 13, 15, 20–21, 22, 25, 29, 41, 45, 47, 48, 52, 53; in atypical depression, 91; in autism, 235; in bipolar depression, 75; in disruptive mood dysregulation disorder, 67; in dysthymic disorder, 58, 59; hypersomnia, 13, 20, 21, 48; insomnia, 13, 20, 21, 41, 48; in mania, 64

sleep effects of drugs, 106, 136; amphetamines, 247, 248; antipsychotics, 165; benzodiazepines, 172; bupropion, 132; carbamazepine, 157; gabapentin, 160; lamotrigine, 158; lithium, 162; MAOIs, 134; marijuana, 245; SSRIs, 128; tricyclic antidepressants, 121; valproate, 154

sleep habits, 316–17

smoking/tobacco use, 82, 133, 241

social media, 4–5, 35

social withdrawal, 13, 48, 59, 82, 235

social workers, 302–3

spinal reflex, 107–8, 109–10

split treatment, 212

St. John's wort, 172–75, 174n

stigma, 5, 211, 343

stimulants: abuse of, 241, 242, 247–51; for ADHD, 217, 220–21, 248; mania precipitated by, 223

Strattera (atomoxetine), 224–25

stressful life events, 31–32, 53–54, 310–12; kindling and, 310–11; lifestyle modifications and, 316–17; relapse and, 311; suicide and, 275–76

substance/medication-induced depressive disorder, 95

substance use/abuse, 35, 52, 83, 213–14, 239–56; in adolescence, 239–42; of alcohol, 241, 242–44; of amphetamines, 241, 242, 247–51; brain functioning and, 252–53, 255; of designer drugs, 248; enabling of, 315, 331; of "gateway" drugs, 241; legal consequences of, 241; of marijuana, 241, 242, 244–47; mood disorders and, 251–53, 313–16; prevalence of, 251; progression of, 240–41; relapses of,